Fuzzy Logic ER

How to Think Like An Emergency Veterinarian

Printed in the United States of America

First Edition, 2026

ISBN 978-1-955639-23-1

Cover design: Patience Parks-Young (patience-creative.com). Front cover animal images: Aaron Gruben. (Other images public domain.)

The pictures and photos not drawn by the illustrator and not radiographs/ultrasounds are public domain.
Every effort has been made to attribute correctly all the material reproduced in this book.
Every jot and tittle of the text by Aaron Gruben (except where otherwise noted).

Post Tenebras Lux Books

www.jaarongruben.com

www.posttenebrasluxbooks.com

Fuzzy Logic ER

How to Think Like an Emergency Veterinarian

Written by J. Aaron Gruben, DVM

Illustrations by Geneva Gruben
(some additional by J. Aaron Gruben)

Also by J. Aaron Gruben

Veterinary Books

Fuzzy Logic: How to Think Like a Veterinarian
Fuzzy Logic 2: How to Keep Thinking Like a Veterinarian
Fuzzy Logic ER: How to Think Like an Emergency Veterinarian
A Theology of Beasts: Christians and Veterinary Medicine
Animal Anatomy Coloring and Activity Books (Canine & Feline)

School Studies

Chivalry: An Ancient Code for Our Time (high school to adults)
Chivalry: A Study for Little Knights (elementary school study)
Whatever Happened to the Vikings? (middle grade school study)

Nonfiction

Kristmenn: The Epic Saga of Viking Conversion
King: A Christian's Call to Imitate Christ's Kingship

The Tangled Eons Series

Crescent Tides
Fatal Fogs
The Stalwart Supinator: Servant of the Streets!

The Medieval Muddles

Juvament!: A Mythical Mess
The Mubblefubbles: A Toothy Tangle

Children's

Elye of Saint Gilles: A Chanson de Geste Retold (Middle Grade)
Logan the Wanderer: Adventures of a Boy out of Time (Middle Grade)
Mishaps in Miklagard: Brom Belcher's Journal #1 (Middle Grade)
Heaps of Hobs: A Fun-Filled Fable in Old English Verse (Picture Book)
Will to Start: The Extraordinary Adventures of William Moorcroft (Comic Book)

TABLE OF CONTENTS

WELCOME TO ANOTHER ADVENTURE IN VETERINARY MEDICINE!

You may fondly recall your experiences as you learned to think like a veterinarian through cases in *Fuzzy Logics 1 and 2.* Now it's time to move beyond the daytime clinic for a new challenge: the veterinary ER!

It's your first shift on the night crew who haunt the midnight hours at Owlhoot Veterinary Emergency Clinic in Santa Fe, NM!

The dark is now your element.

Moonbeams are now your medium.

You will become a creature of the night.

It's a couple of weeks before Christmas, and these shifts couldn't have come at a better time. You need more money for Christmas presents and medical bills, though neither of those is for you. You contemplate the eventful past few months as you dewrinkle your scrubs in the dryer. Attention to some suspicious details of a case led to the arrest of one of your clients. But the sad side effect was that a 9-year-old kid named Sam could no longer afford the expensive (and experimental) treatment he needed for a rare neurologic disease when his family was sent to prison.

You generally don't become a veterinarian without a soft heart and fluffy insides. And so it surprised nobody when you promised to help Sam. But despite a social media drive and Medicaid, you're left picking up a considerable amount of financial responsibility. A glance at the latest adorable sketch from little Sam, pinned on your fridge, helps remind you that this kid is well worth putting in a few extra shifts for.

You slip on your coat and hop in your car to drive to the clinic, feeling pumped and terrified. It's a confusing mix of emotions. There are no appointments at this clinic; only walk-ins. Nobody else is open, and you are the first line of defense for whatever emergencies strike Santa Fe's pet owners from the chilly midnight shadows. You picture a big hospital building, gleaming with a medical aura that flows with state-of-the-art equipment.

"I wonder what new diagnostic tools will have," you wonder as you direct your car to an unfamiliar part of Santa Fe. "Maybe they'll have a CT scan, and high-flow oxygen, and a dialysis machine and…"

It gradually dawns why you've never been to this part of Santa Fe.

It looks scary.

You pull up in front of a clinic and check your GPS. Yeah… This is it. Maybe it looks nicer inside?

It doesn't. But you bravely look past the 1980s countertops, peeling paint, and cracked tile floors as you introduce yourself to the staff in the lobby.

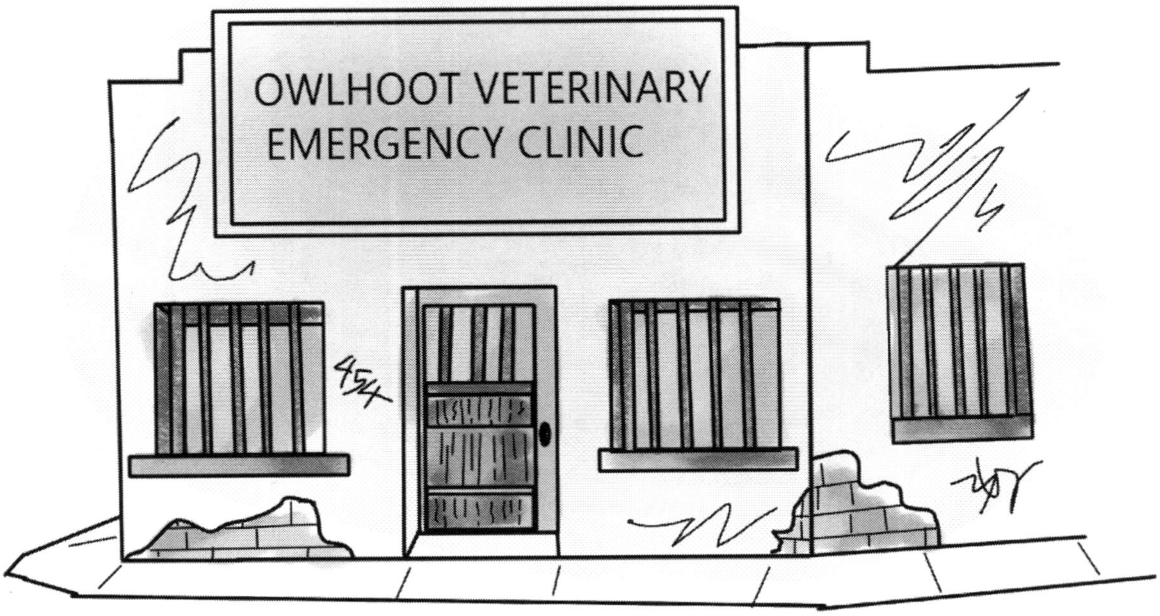

"Where's the first case?" you bravely ask Graham, the technician who let you in out of the frigid December air. He looks about 21. He seems friendly, sports a nose ring, and may have more tattoos than he has arm length. "I'm ready for action!"

You've practiced your basic ER vet phrases like, "Get me 0.2 mL epinephrine, STAT!" and "I need an ECG and a CBC and an AFAST on this HBC…STAT," and "Darn it Jim, I'm a doctor not a psychiatrist!"

You are eager, ready to take on the string of crazy emergencies with lab coat flapping heroically as you ride the waves of adrenaline that will get you through the night. Your new friends glance at each other, then at the empty lobby, with sheepish grins.

And then nothing happens.

Then more nothing happens.

Graham and your other technician for this shift, Lolita, show you around the clinic.

It's a small place, built many years ago. The lobby opens onto exam rooms. There's a pharmacy in a long hallway behind them. It's well-stocked for a little ER.

"Oh, I see you've even got fuzapladib for pancreatitis. That stuff's new and expensive!" You peruse the pharmacological tools that will make up your arsenal in the fight against emergency diseases. You make sure to say the drug names loudly to impress everyone with your knowledge. "Good selection for congestive heart disease here… Some pyrantel for deworming… Quite a few antibiotics, even some old ones! Is that tilmicosin? That's a cow antibiotic, isn't it?"

Graham laughs. "Sure, for respiratory infections, I think. Doctor Short will take on food animal cases if they're willing to come to the clinic. She started out as a livestock vet."

Dr. Celia Short manages this clinic and is the person who hired you.

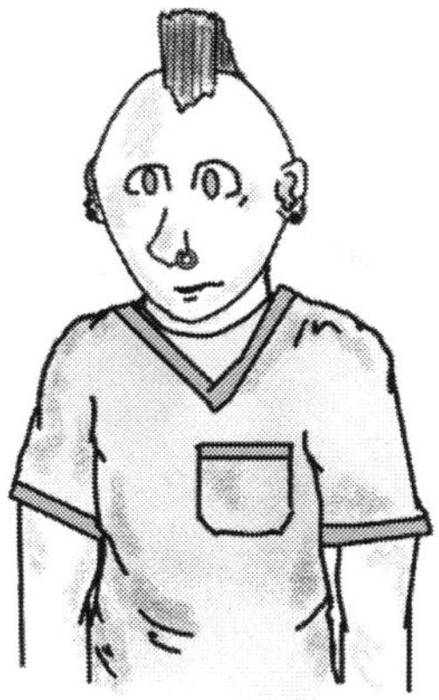

"What's with all the yellow labels on the vial?"

"That's because it's dangerous for people. Tilmicosin give you a heart attack if you poke yourself by accident..."

"Doesn't look like it's been used too often," you comment, noting the dust around the bottle. "But I'll stick to treating dogs and cats."

Sticking to what you know, and referring the critters you know little about (like cows and horses and snakes and wombats), is perfectly acceptable. There's a list of local clinics that will see large animals and exotics and you can send those emergencies their way.

Your techs walk you from the pharmacy, through a tiny surgery suite, into a treatment area with a wet table (that's like a big tub-sink with a grate on it). To the right is a hallway leading to a bunch of big dog runs and some creepy storage rooms. To the left is a big, open room with treatment tables, lined with smaller cages for little dogs and cats. An in-house lab (with a microscope and blood analyzers) sits on a counter along the other side of this room, along with a safe for controlled drugs. A closet-sized room for taking radiographs (X-rays) opens onto another side of this room. Next to that, a door leads to a small doctor's office. A door through the doctor's office opens to Dr. Short's private office: the dungeon where she suffers through the mental anguish of legal paperwork and taxes and budgets to keep the place open.

"And that's our clinic! It ain't much, but it does the job," Lolita grins.

You chat about life and get to know each other for a while. You spend an hour after that flipping through AVMA articles and sipping coffee in the doctor's office. Sometime around 11 pm your eyelids feel heavy with the crushing weight of boredom. You shut the door and lay down on the daybed in the doctor's office, wondering if it's truly legit and legal to get some shuteye on a shift, even though your boss assured you that getting some rest (as long as there are no current or hospitalized patients needing your attention) is a fine idea.

It is often legit to get rest on an ER shift. In many clinics it's encouraged (though in some it's against the rules). Long shifts, sometimes worked back-to-back, make doctors and staff prone to exhaustion, which leads to mistakes (some life threatening). This is a fact established by many controlled studies in the realm of occupational health, and more than one human hospital has come up with creative napping options too.

Lying around staring at the ceiling seems like the perfect time to review in your mind some of the diagnostic strategies you've learned are so helpful for solving the little mysteries you call "cases" in your job.

Contemplating differential lists and case logic is also a great way to fall asleep!

On the next page is a quick review of important information you'll want to remember from previous books in this series on how to THINK LIKE A VETERINARIAN…

You're ready to start! **Don't forget your helpful pals**, these gray boxes... They will explain terms and concepts, give you instructions and tips to help you through the cases, and mold your young gray cells into tiny but well-tuned detective think tanks! Read 'em!

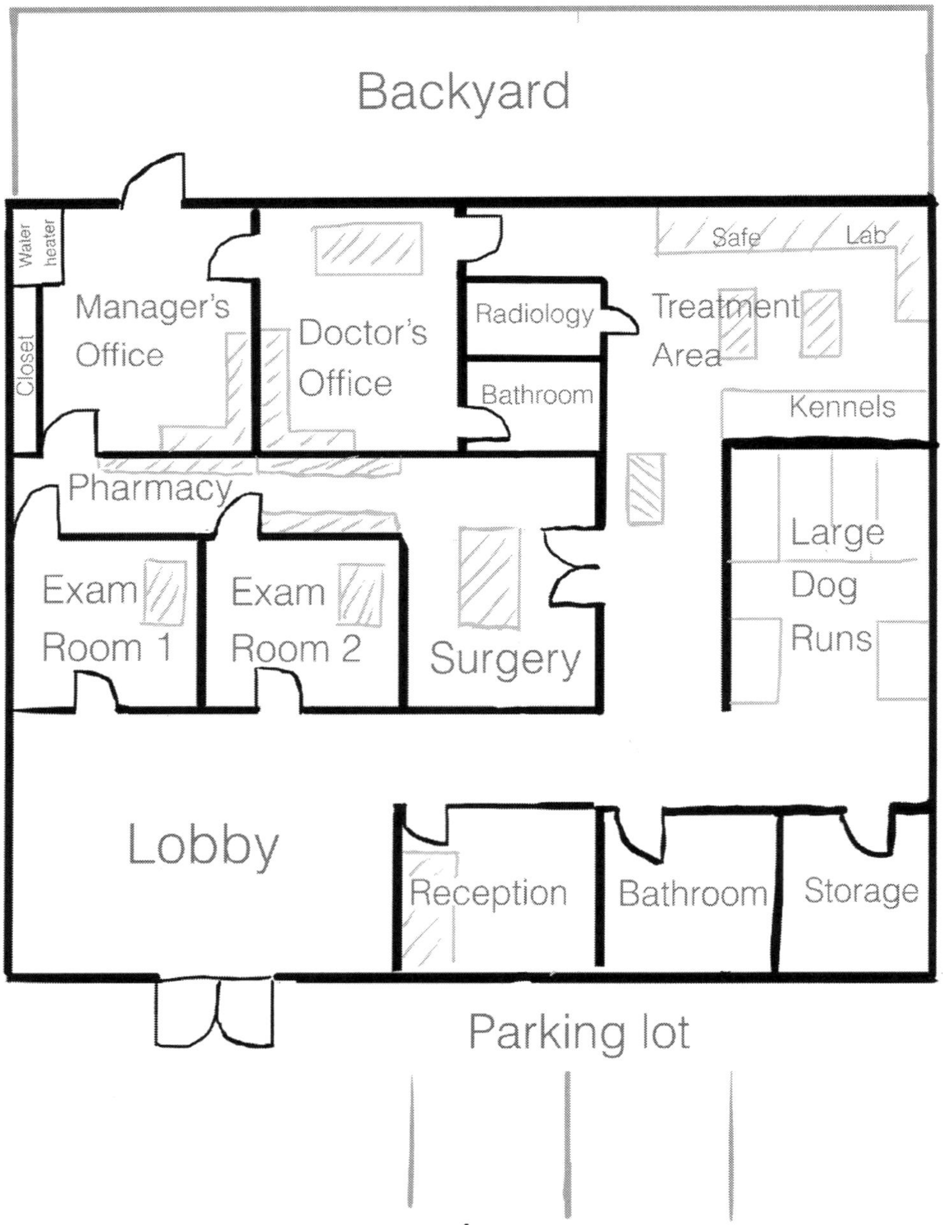

Whirlwind Reminder of the Logic of Medicine

Every case that comes into your clinic is a mystery! To be a good veterinarian, you need to think logically, like a detective *and* a doctor. Amazingly, laws of logic and philosophy can be quite practical in the trenches of medicine. Here's a quick overview of some important ideas you've been pondering.

Argument (sometimes called "inference"): working out a logical conclusion from a set of premises.

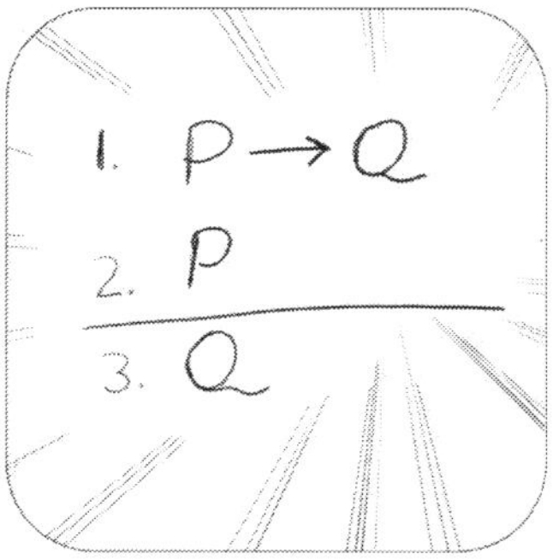

Deductive Reasoning

An argument from something general to something particular. Accepting the premise guarantees the truth of the conclusion. "Every baby is messy. This small person is messy. This small person must be a baby."

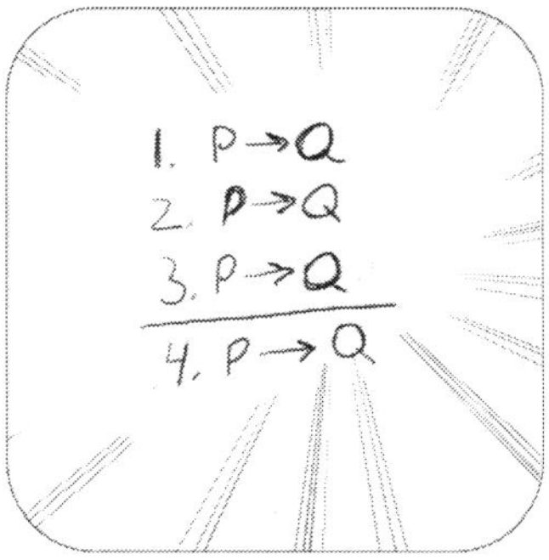

Inductive Reasoning

An argument from particular data points to make a generalization. The premise makes the conclusion more probable. "This baby's messy. Hey! This baby's messy too! Yowza! All babies must be messy."

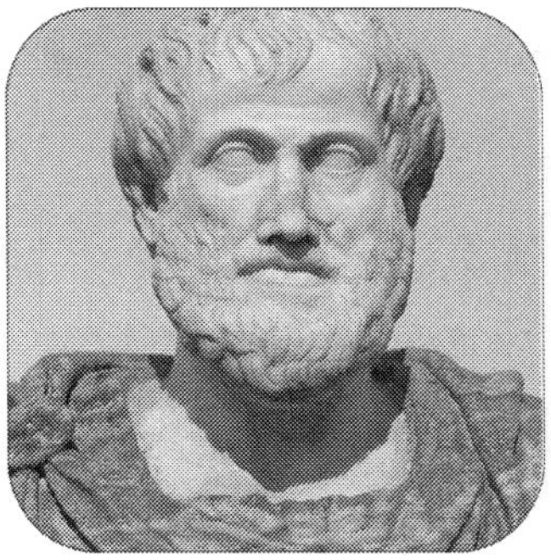

Syllogism

An old dead Greek guy with a beard named Aristotle discovered that the roots of a valid argument lie not in its particular claims so much as in the form of the argument. Thus, in more formal logic, we tend to say an argument is valid or invalid. In general, we know an argument is valid when it's impossible for its premise to be true and its conclusion false. The proper forms valid arguments can take are called syllogisms.

The best detective-doctors use a couple of important variations of classical deductive and inductive reasoning to get to the bottom of their cases.

Refutationism: essentially, the method of coming up with a theory based on your initial clues in the history and physical exam of a case, then using tests to refute the theory (i.e., prove it wrong). Rinse and repeat within the gilded bathtubs servicing the grand palace of your mind until you discover a theory you can't refute. This is a variety of deductive logic (arguing from an initial hypothesis downward).

Bayesian Induction: besides being super-fun to say (and making you sound oh-so-clever around your friends), this mental tool is a wonderful logical labradoodle crossbreed between inductive reasoning (arguing from observations upward) and statistical probability. It acknowledges that in the real world (you know, that nasty place where disease and injuries attack your patients), there aren't really any symptoms that fit a diagnosis with 100% ironclad accuracy. The real world gives us clues with a certain probability of occurring in a diagnosis. It uses scientific facts (based on studies), like "decreased vision occurs in 68% of visceral larval migrans (VLM) cases," to rank the likelihood that a symptom stems from a diagnosis. A doctor well-read in the latest medical studies should apply them (with at least vague probabilities like "this is more likely") in his mind while evaluating possibilities in cases. That's how we reason using "evidence-based medicine"—making our decisions based on published statistical evidence (instead of hearsay or experience).

> "In medicine, we make a list of the possibilities, and cross stuff off with tests until we get an answer."

In the simplest terms, a smart veterinarian-detective approaches a case using the clues in the history and physical exam to make a list of possible causes of the symptoms. This is called a differential list. Then you rank that list of possible diagnoses from the most likely to the least likely in your brain. Then you use tests (like bloodwork and X-rays) to cross things off the list that are least likely until you come to the most probable diagnosis. Thus, in medicine, we make a list of the logical possibilities for every problem affecting our critter patient, then cross stuff off with tests until we get an answer.

An' Bob's-yer-uncle, you've solved another case!

> "Once you eliminate the impossible, whatever remains, no matter how improbable, must be the truth."
>
> - Sherlock Holmes[i]

Differential list: the list of possible causes ("differentials") for a patient's problems. List of diseases that might make the patient sick.

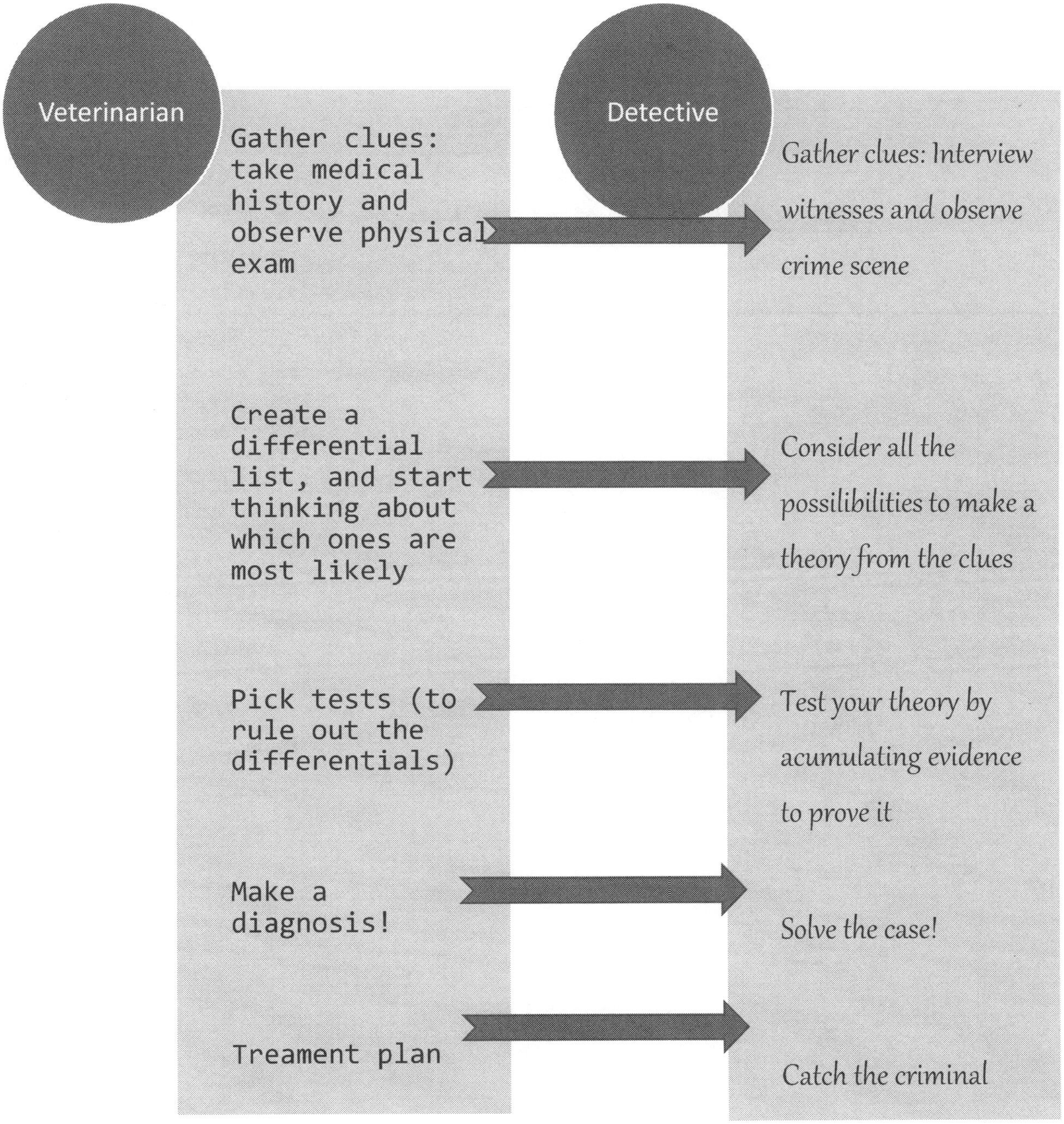

You may remember this diagram from Fuzzy Logic 1. It remains super-sweet, and you should peruse it again!

CASE APPROACH

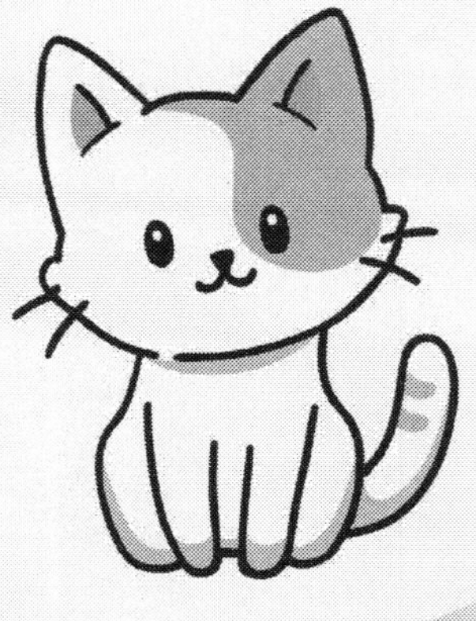

The basic outline we will use to work through cases...

1. ORGANIZE HISTORY

Take a detailed history of signalment and presenting complaints...

2. GATHER CLUES

Complete a physical examination of the patient...

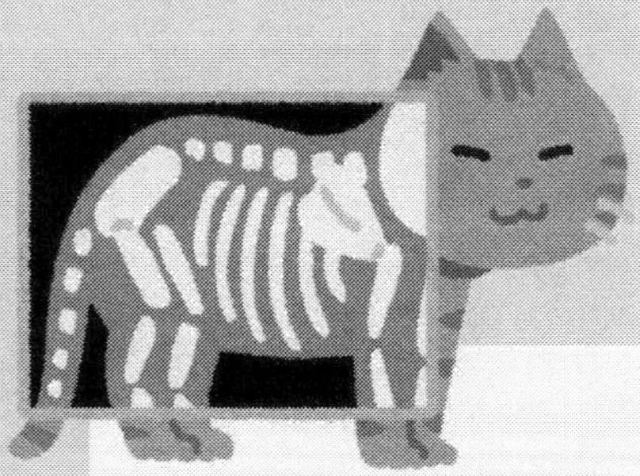

3. DIFFERENTIAL LIST

Create a list of the possible causes of the patient's symptoms...

4. PICK SOME TESTS

Pick tests logically to cross possibilities off your differential list...

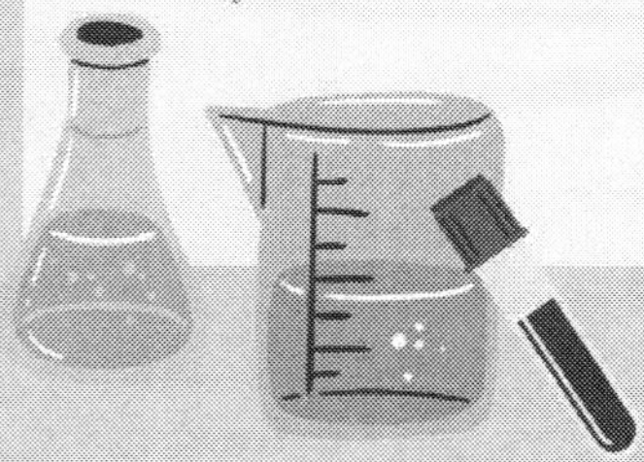

5. MAKE A DIAGNOSIS

Rule differentials out until you are left with the most likely possibility...

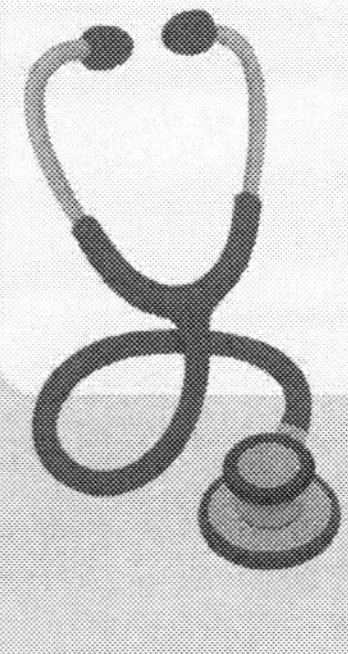

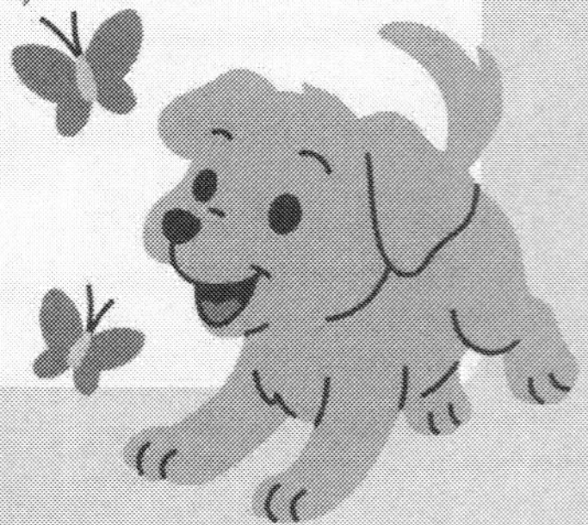

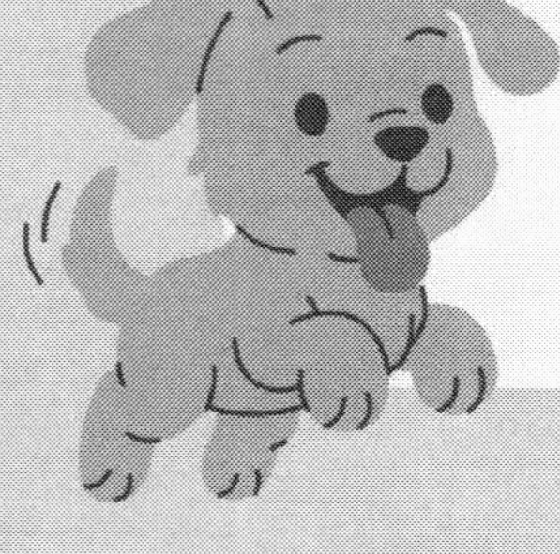

6. FORM A TREATMENT PLAN

Target your treatments to the diagnosis to make your sick patient well!

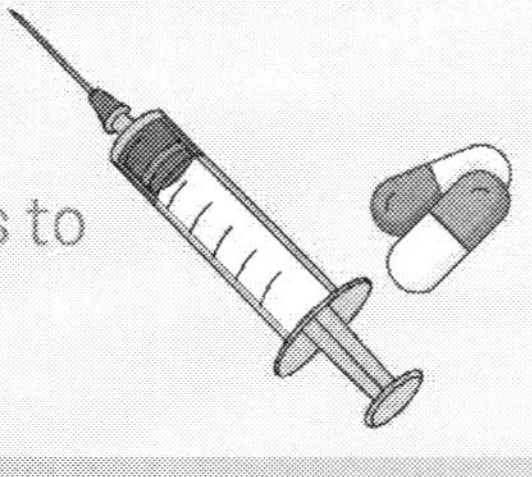

Differential List

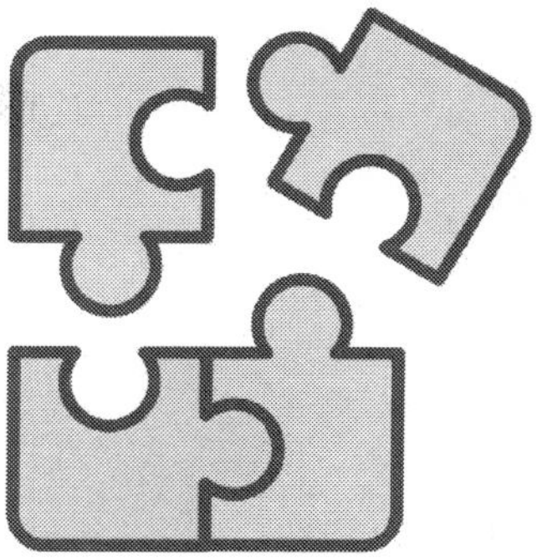

This is a special list of all the potential causes of a symptom ("differentials") we can think of, that we use in medicine as a roadmap to find our way to a diagnosis.

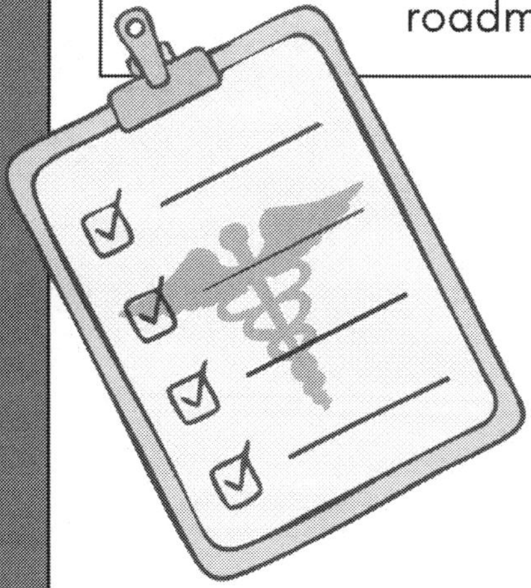

LIST THEM

List every possible cause you can think of for the symptoms your patient is presenting for. A good differential list can get quite long!

RANK THEM

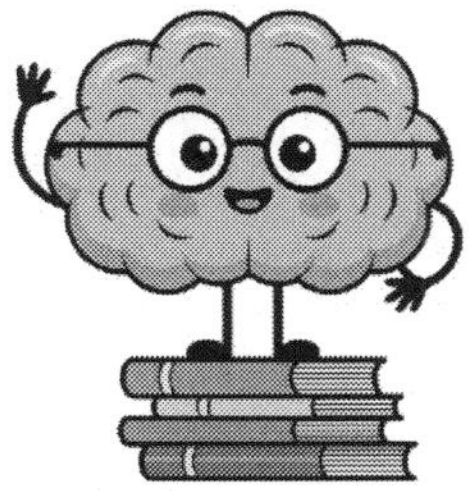

Organize your list from most likely to less likely. Knowing facts based on current studies (like disease incidence for your patient's population) helps.

CROSS THEM OFF

Now that you have a starting place, use tests to cross differentials off the list that are unlikely, until you reach a diagnosis.

As you become a more experienced doctor, much of this process will occur in your mind as you work your way through a case on the clinic floor!

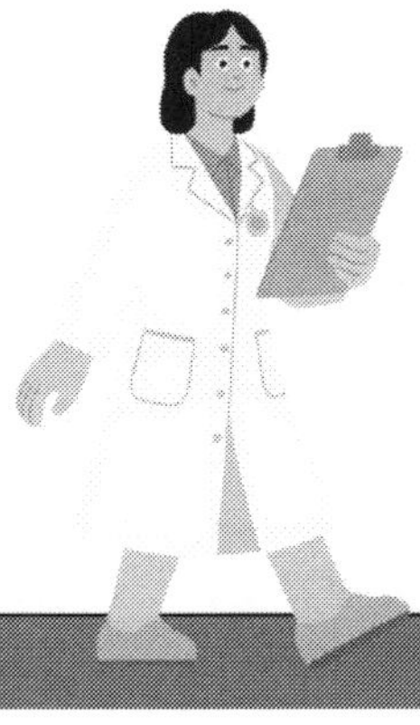

Case #1

An obnoxious knock upon the door of the office wakes you from a fitful doze. You rub your bleary eyes as the dulcet voice of technician Lolita cuts through your fuzzy brain cells like a midnight banshee. "Heads up, Doc! We've got a live one on the way…"

> If you get stumped by a big, scary medical term, do not fret! You can peruse the definitions of terms at the bottom of the pages when they first appear. You can also consult the handy, comprehensive glossary at the back of the book.

You wisely ask for more details.

A man called to say he's bringing in a Great Dane, which woke him up pacing and whining and trying to vomit. Those signs, in that breed, just might spell the "mother of all emergencies." You feel wide awake!

Ten minutes later, a beast that could be either a big dog or a small horse walks into the clinic with his human attached. Sigbert Farnsworth III is a purebred, merle-coated Great Dane supermodel that goes to dog shows. It's a stupid name, but nobody would listen to him when he tried to change it on his adoption papers. Now he is in serious distress and his owner, Greg Smith, is in distress right along with him.

"Something bad is going on! Siggy is in lots of pain and keeps trying to throw up. I think his belly looks big too. Could it be…"

It could.

It could indeed.

Step 1 – Organize the History

> In this book you'll learn to break down the logic of each case into a few simple steps. **Step 1** is to organize the information (history) so you don't miss anything important. This consists of A) the *signalment*: a fancy word for a description of the patient and B) *presenting complaints*: the problems the patient comes in for.

Signalment:

Great Dane

Male intact

5 years old

Presenting Complaints:

Acute pain

Pacing and restlessness

Retching (trying to vomit) without production

Abdominal distension

Signalment: the descriptive characteristics of the patient.

Gathering clues will be **Step 2** for each case. Remember that a veterinarian is like a detective and needs to gather clues early in a case to figure out what disease is making the patient sick. We do this by a *physical exam* (PE) first, then by running tests based on clues from the history and PE.

Step 2 – Gather Clues

Physical Examination (PE):

Abdominal palpation: Visibly distended (big belly!), marked splinting everywhere. Feels very tight on palpation. You suspect a ping on auscultation (listening with a stethoscope).

Attitude: BAR (bright, alert, responsive), distressed, restless, anxious.

Cardiac (heart): Tachycardia with a steady rhythm. No murmur noted. Weak, thready femoral pulses.

Ears: NSF (no significant findings).

Eyes: NSF.

Integument (skin): No wounds or sores noted, no rashes, no hair loss. Normal skin turgor.

Lymph Nodes: NSF.

Musculoskeletal: NSF, weight bearing on all four limbs.

Neurologic: BAR, normal menace response and palpebral reflexes noted OU (both eyes), normal conscious proprioception on all four paws.

Oronasal (mouth and nose): You decide against a full dental exam for the following reason: THIS DOG'S BELLY LOOKS LIKE IT'S GOING TO EXPLODE AND IT IS NOT A DENTAL

Ping: an "old-school" trick to listen for gas distention with your stethoscope. A "ping" is an airy high-pitched echo when thumping on the abdomen just behind the ribs, while listening with your stethoscope, *if* the stomach is filled with too much gas. In a normal stomach you won't hear a ping. Think of the sound a basketball makes when bounced off concrete…
BAR: Bright, alert, and responsive.
Distention: gastric distention means the stomach is dilated and bloated.
Integument: a fancy word for skin.
Lymph node: important structures for the immune system. "Hubs" of white blood cells and lymphatic drainage, to fight infection in specific places of the body. Small and bean-shaped, like the author of this book.
Menace response: a reflex that makes a patient close his eye when your hand is coming toward it.
Mucous membranes: the wet bits of a critter at the junction of skin and mucosa (like the gums in the mouth).
NSF: no significant findings (it's all normal looking)
OU: "oculus uterque," a fancy Latin phrase that means "both eyes."
Palpebral reflex: closing an eye when you touch the inside edge of the eyelid.
PE: Physical Examination.
Proprioception: a big neurology term (woo hoo!) for a reflex that causes an animal's paw to flip "right side up" when you turn it over. This is a postural reflex a related to the brain and the spinal cord useful to check in emergency cases.
Skin turgor: the tension or "stretchiness" of the skin, how well it falls back down when you tent (pull) it upward. This is a way we check the hydration status of a patient.
Splinting: tensing or tightening of the abdomen (often a specific region) because of pain or sometimes anxiety.
Tachycardia: a faster than normal heart rate.

PROBLEM!!!!!!!!! Sometimes even doctors have to be practical.

Respiratory: Tachypnea with no increase in respiratory effort. All lung fields sound clear with your stethoscope.

Urogenital (urinary and genital organs): Urinary bladder difficult to palpate due to patient splinting, no inflammation or abnormalities noted.

Vitals: Pale gums. Capillary Refill Time (CRT) over 3 seconds.

OK. Hopefully you've been thinking with that large brain of yours during your initial exam of this big guy. And you should think something like this: "What the bald monkey is going on!?!?!" Or in more correct medical terminology: "What might be on my differential list?"

Remember, a differential is a possible reason behind the patient's symptoms. And your differential list is your road map to diagnosis, your decoding list for the mystery, your first stop on this journey toward Sigmund Farnsworth III's recovery.

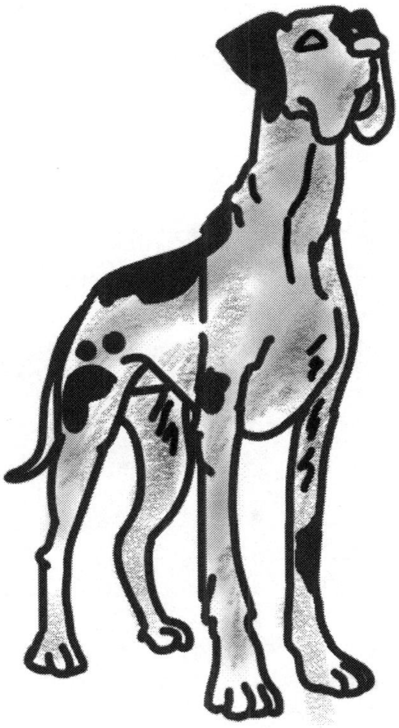

Capillary refill time (CRT): capillary refill time. A simple way to check blood flow (perfusion) by pushing down on the gums and counting how long it takes to pink up again in that spot. It should be less than 2 seconds in a healthy beast.

Oronasal: the mouth and nose.

Respiratory: all the bits for breathing; the body system that takes in oxygen and breathes out carbon dioxide.

Tachypnea: breathing fast.

Urogenital: urinary and genital organs.

Differential Diagnoses (some possible diseases):

Congestive heart failure

Gastric dilatation

Gastric dilatation-volvulus (GDV)

Gastric overdistension

Gastrointestinal foreign body/obstruction

Hemoabdomen

Neoplasia

Pancreatitis

Splenic torsion

Trauma

Differential Diagnoses: For every case you must have a running list of possible solutions (diagnoses) that you are working through, to reach a single, most likely diagnosis by process of elimination. In other words, it's a list of every possible cause you can think of for the problems. This essentially makes every case a really big multiple-choice question. This is the basic thought process in medicine. You use clues like tests and observations from PE and history to rule out the possibilities (*differentials*) until there's only one logical one left. And that is your diagnosis.

Alrighty. You have a pretty good list of possibilities (and may already have an idea of what's going on based on your physical exam, history, and signalment). Remember that each possibility comes with statistical probabilities. Here in the trenches, the probability of each disease condition being the real culprit is admittedly vague and complex. Basically, you can rank them as more or less likely in an "educated guess" based on studies you've read, the patient's signalment (age, sex, breed), presenting signs, physical exam findings and (eventually) your experience. All this is screaming through your head as you piece the puzzle together in real time.

But fortunately, you have another tool beyond logic and experience to help you narrow down that list of possibilities: you have clinical tests! It's time to use some tests to rule out the least likely possibilities and narrow those differentials down to a more exact diagnosis, so that you can know how to fix this beasty.

Congestive heart failure: right sided heart failure in particular can fill an abdomen up with fluid (which is called ascites)
Gastric dilatation: a stomach filled up and distended with gas.
Gastric dilatation-volvulus (GDV): a stomach filled up and distended with gas AND twisted out of its normal, happy position.
Gastric overdistension: This means a stomach "all swollen up" with food. It's often called "food bloat" and is exactly what it sounds like: a dog that ate way more than could fit in his stomach comfortably.
Hemoabdomen: This is a belly full of blood, from internal bleeding
Neoplasia: cancer.
Pancreatitis: inflammation in the pancreas, which is an organ that makes hormones and helps digestion.
Splenic torsion: a twisted spleen; rare but life-threatening, often occurs with a GDV. NOT morally twisted like an evil super-villain spleen, though a villainous spleen might be kinda cool.

Decision time!

What tests do you want to run first?

Here's what you can do in your clinic:

- ✓ Basic bloodwork (a chemistry panel and CBC)
- ✓ Benchtop Ethylene glycol test
- ✓ Blood gas analysis
- ✓ Clotting times
- ✓ Cytology
- ✓ Fecal flotation and direct saline exam
- ✓ FeLV/FIV test
- ✓ Giardia test
- ✓ Heartworm test (with rickettsial diseases)
- ✓ Leptospirosis test
- ✓ Pancreatic lipase
- ✓ Parvo test
- ✓ Pregnancy test
- ✓ Radiographs (X-rays)
- ✓ Skin scraping
- ✓ Thyroid hormone level (T4)
- ✓ Ultrasound
- ✓ Urinalysis

Here's where the rubber meets the road! Veterinarians have to make many choices for every case, each of which will have its own set of side effects and consequences (to the patient, the client, and the vet). If you're the sort of person who can never make a decision, then medicine may not be the career for you!

In this book you will choose two things for each case:
1) What tests to run.
2) What treatment to start.

Your choices should be based on what you read in the history and Physical Examination (PE), and what diagnoses you deduce from them. We'll walk you through the answers (and more importantly, the thought process algorithm) as you go.

Heartworms are real worms that live in the right side of an animal's heart and cause heart failure!

What tests do you want to run?

Pick one before you turn the page.

Blood gas analysis: a blood panel specifically designed to check chemistry related to respiration (like oxygen and bicarbonate levels) and blood pH.
Chemistry panel: blood panel with basic information on the function of the liver, kidneys, electrolyte levels, protein levels, blood glucose.
Clotting times: a test of the ability of blood to clot properly.
Cytology: looking at cells under a microscope. If you pick this, you have to pick where to get the cells from. Will it be scrapings from the skin? Or cells from a tumor with a needle (fine needle aspirate)? Or cells from a swab of ear gunk or snot?
FeLV/FIV: feline leukemia virus and feline immunodeficiency virus. These contagious diseases suppress the immune system in cats.
Giardia: a microscopic parasite that looks like a flying saucer with googly eyes. It causes a nasty infection in the intestines that produces diarrhea and vomiting.
Leptospirosis: a bacterial disease that causes kidney and liver failure, often contracted through contaminated water (much like giardia). This bug looks like a coiled, swimming pigtail.
Pancreatic Lipase: a test for pancreatitis. There's an fPL (feline pancreatic lipase) and a cPL (canine pancreatic lipase).
Parvo test: a test for canine parvovirus, which is a virus that attacks the GI tract in puppies.
Radiographs: X-rays. A way to use radiation to take pictures of an animal's insides.
Rickettsial diseases: some infectious diseases carried by ticks (Lyme is one of them).
Ultrasound: a way to use sound in ultrasonic frequencies to view pictures of an animal's insides.
Urinalysis: a test on urine, generally looking for infection or crystals from bladder stones.

There's one test you'll want to run ASAP: **radiographs**. In fact, you want to so badly that radiographs get taken even before we finish all the paperwork to check this patient in.

Why is that?

This patient is looking less than stable. That is a medical catchphrase to say that he could die soon…like any minute kinda soon. There's at least one item on your differential list that is very time sensitive: if this were a GDV (a twisted stomach) it could move beyond fixing if left too long. And so, to get the ball rolling in treating this unstable patient, you ask Graham to help you take a right lateral radiograph. It's a good thing you had some tech experience before going to vet school, and still remember how to use your hands. Night shifts are often understaffed, and you often need to play doctor *and* nurse to take care of patients.

You strain all your sad doctor muscles, which have atrophied after so many hours of studying in the ivory tower of vet school[1] and help get this monster of a dog onto the X-ray table. You stretch him out on his right side.

BEEP! says the machine as Graham steps on the foot switch.

Beep! says the veterinarian (to keep things G-rated).

This is not what you want to see, so you take another view hoping it will look better. It doesn't…

What do you think is going on with this dog?

Look over the radiographs on the next page and try to fill in the labels…

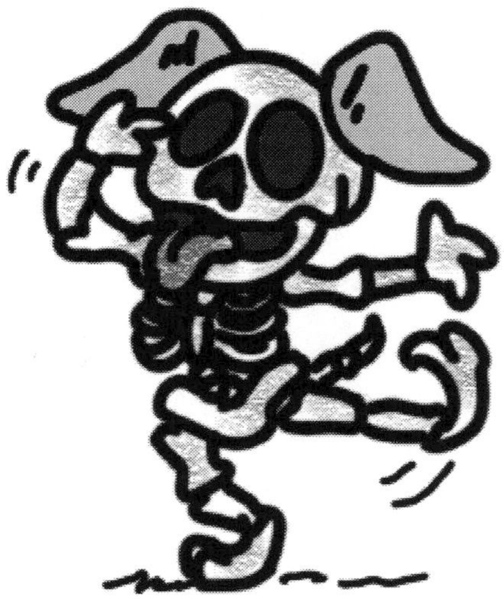

Lateral: on the side.

Right lateral: lying on the right side.

[1] Don't worry. After a few years of lifting big beasts like Sigbert you're probably going to be more buff and fit and jacked and stacked than you ever were before your years of inactivity in school.

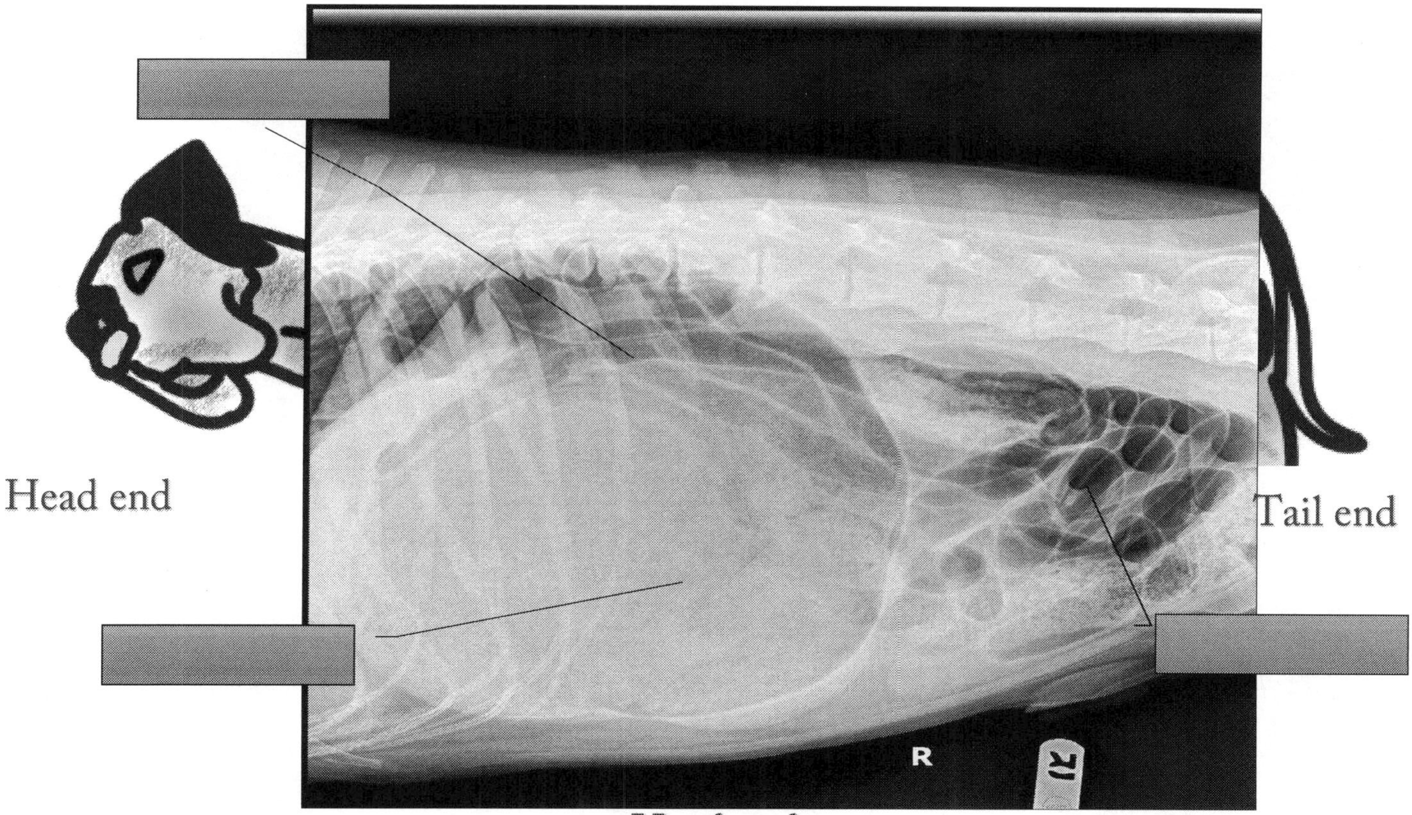
Head end
Tail end
R

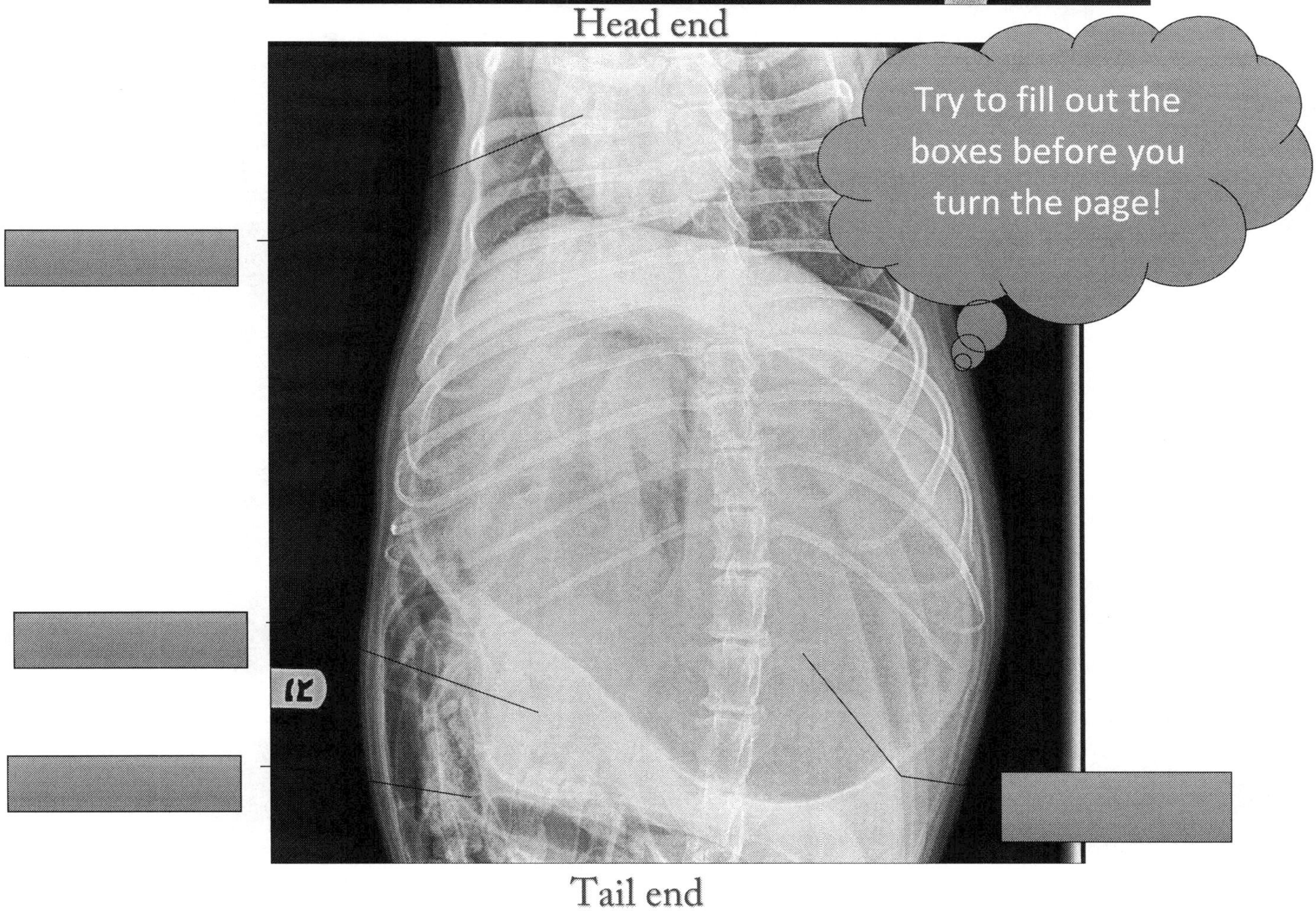
Head end
Try to fill out the boxes before you turn the page!
Tail end

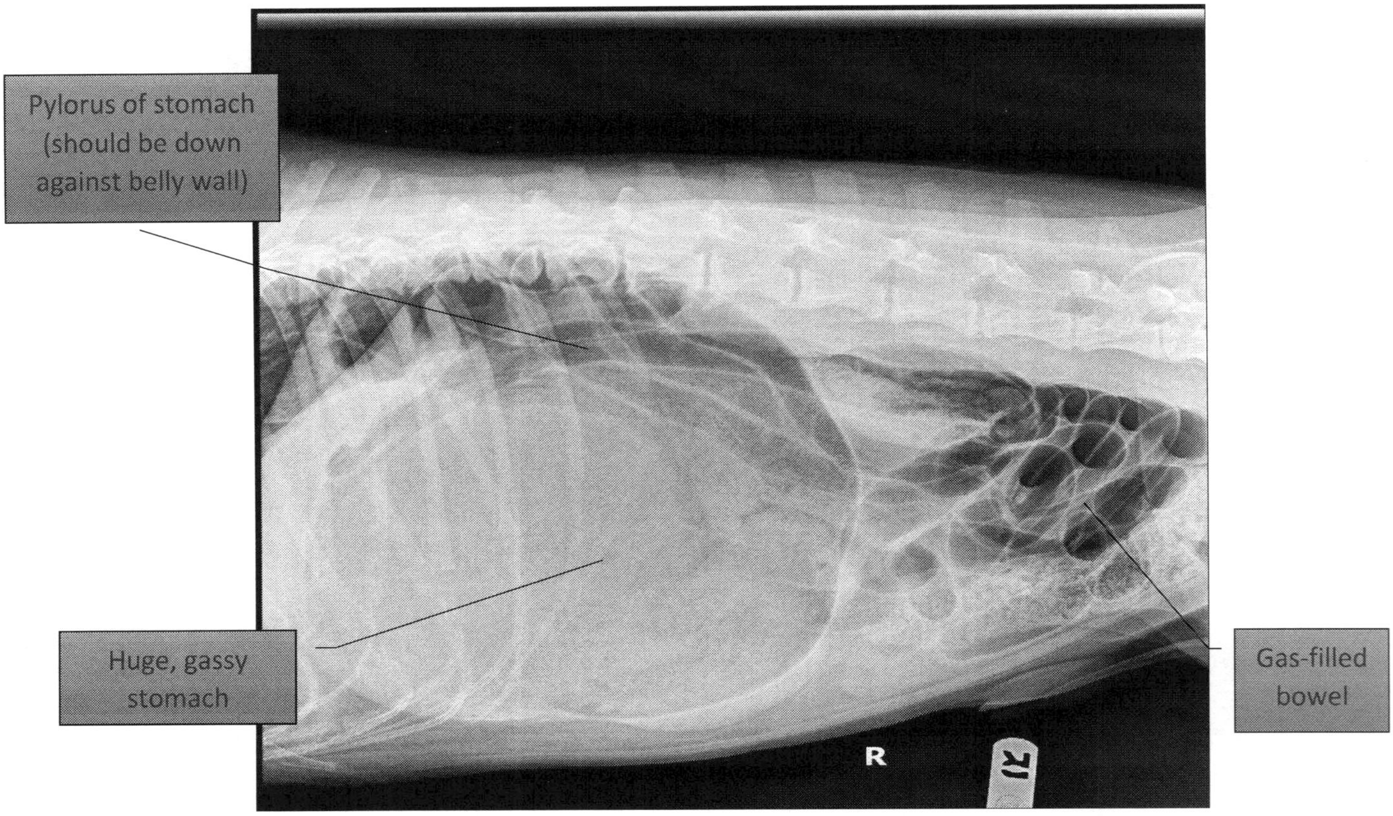
Pylorus of stomach (should be down against belly wall)
Huge, gassy stomach
Gas-filled bowel
R

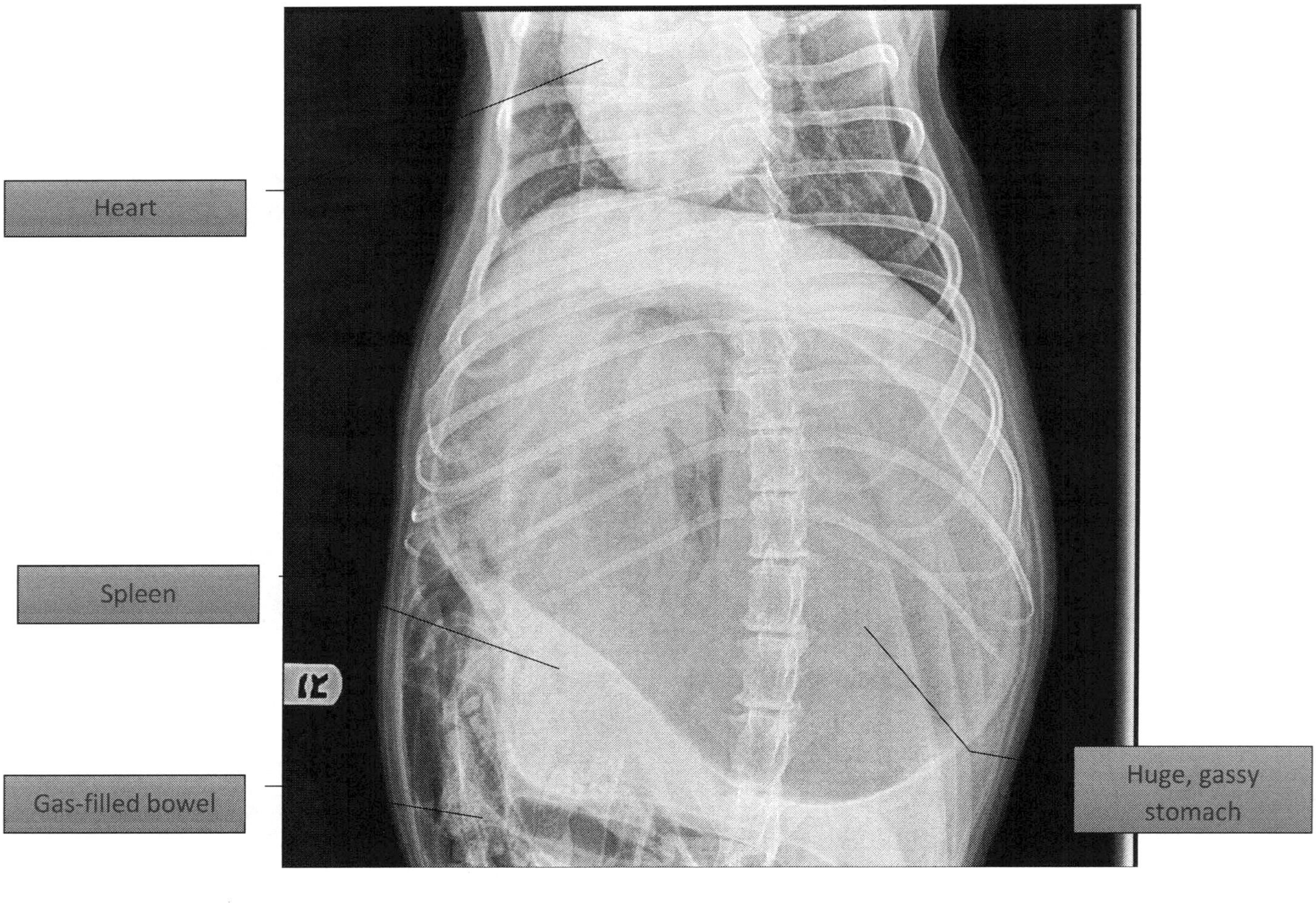
Heart
Spleen
Gas-filled bowel
Huge, gassy stomach

And your diagnosis is?

____

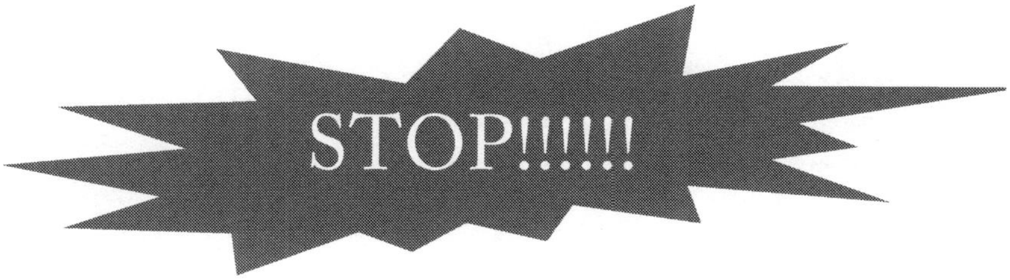

Before you turn the page,
try to ID the culprit...
What's the most likely cause of this patient's signs?
Go back a few pages to the disease differential list.

Notice: I said BEFORE you turn the page.

There's NO CHEATING in veterinary medicine.

I can't speak for those other types of doctors (like PhDs and those human doctors), but we veterinarians do not cheat. We do like workarounds and lifehacks, and we are better than average at shortcuts. But we do not cheat.

Remember!

You get down to the right answer by using clues to eliminate the improbable! That's why you'll find some detective (and other) quotes in this book.

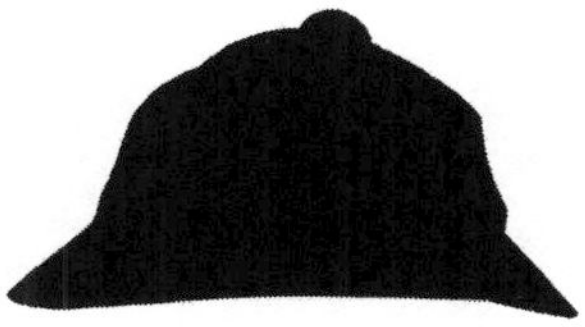

You are absolutely right. That is a big, distended, and flippéd stomach! This is the big one, the Mother of All Emergencies, that unspeakable three-letter word trotting in to anoint your very first ER shift with terror: **GDV**!

GDV stands for gastric dilatation-volvulus and involves the stomach distending with gas (dilatation), then flipping over on itself (volvulus). It is a major emergency because twisting of the stomach on its axis cuts off its circulation. This means the blood supply to the stomach gets twisted and kinked off, which leads to necrosis (tissue death) of the stomach walls quickly. Nobody likes their stomach rotting inside them.

Because the spleen is attached to the stomach, it tends to twist along with the stomach. This can result in splenic torsion (twisted spleen). To top off that little horror, since it's twisted up and cannot pass anything out into the intestines, the stomach continues to distend with air and fluid until it puts pressure on the chest. And to crown off this terrifying concatenation of disasters, the caudal vena cava and portal vein[2] can get stretched and twisted with the stomach. *That* can cause hypovolemic shock and contribute to dangerous heart arrhythmia. On the long list of things that are not good for you, GDV is pretty close to the top.

Nobody really knows what causes GDV. It is likely multifactorial (which is a fancy doctor word for "lots of things together cause this," and is a useful word to whip out when you want to avoid tedious explanations). It almost always occurs in big, deep-chested dogs because they have more space for their stomach to slither around inside their abdomen. That's never a good strategy: if you give that stomach an inch, it'll twist all over you.

The predisposition of big dog breeds toward GDV is so strong that many people get surgery done ahead of time to prevent GDV in these breeds. The surgery is called gastropexy, and it involves attaching the antrum part of the stomach to the body wall so that it can't flip. Other potential risk factors for GDV include GI foreign bodies (stuff stuck in the intestines), eating too fast, gasping air into the stomach (from things like over-excitement or eating from an elevated position), or eating too much at once.

So you've found the problem, and now everyone is running around panicking.

Caudal vena cava: big, important vein that drains blood back into the right side of the heart from organs in the abdomen.
Gastric antrum: lower, funnel-shaped portion of the stomach.
Gastropexy: a surgery to attach the stomach to the body wall so it can't flip and cause GDV.
Heart arrhythmia: irregular heartbeat, either too slow or too fast.
Hypovolemic shock: a whole-body drop in blood pressure in response to a problem, starving the tissues of oxygen.
Portal vein: a big vein that carries blood from the other organs in the abdomen to the liver, for filtering out bad juju.

[2] If you thought portal veins were vessels you could hop through to magically be transported to another dimension, I'm sorry to disappoint you.

What are you gonna do about this?

Choose several action items from this list of treatment options.

a) Antibiotics
b) Do more diagnostics before doing treatment
c) Euthanize the patient: we can't fix him
d) Flip the dog over 3-4 times to rotate his stomach back
e) IV fluids
f) Jab a hole into the stomach to let out the gas
g) Nausea drugs
h) Pain medications
i) Prescribe special food
j) Steroids
k) Surgery
l) Swear loudly, then go hide in a corner somewhere

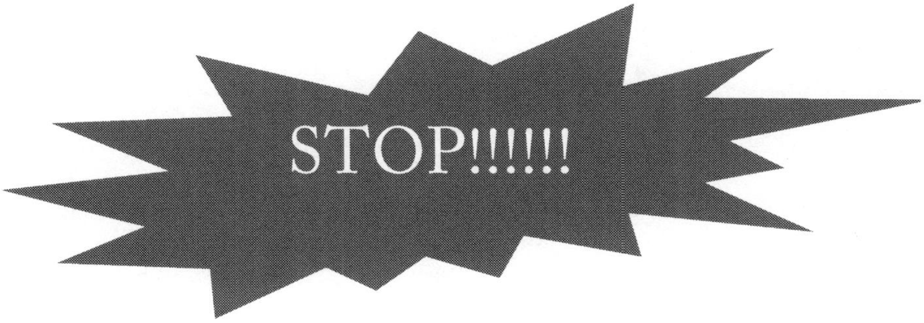

What main treatment plan are you going to go with?

What other things might you also need to do?

If you picked **k) surgery** as most important, then good on ya, champ!

Getting the gas out of the stomach and repositioning it surgically needs to happen ASAP. Time is limited. But if you are running right away to the surgical suite to scrub up, hold your horses, champ!

This is not a stable patient, and there are some things that need to be done first to give ol' Sigbert Farnsworth III a fighting chance at surviving the surgery.

There are two treatments to start right away before surgery: **h and e**.

You calculate a dose of **pain medications**. This is mainly because you're a nice human being, and don't like to let animals go through excruciating pain without some kind of pain relief. You also have your wonderful technician team place an IV catheter and give them directions for **IV fluids**.

IV fluids are needed to treat the signs of hypovolemic shock in this patient. This is not (as you know because you went to vet school) the "I'm really scared" kind of shock. It is a systemically low blood pressure from compromise of the circulatory system. Usually the mean arterial blood pressure (MAP) of a dog in shock is less than 60 mmHg. Low blood pressure to your patient's organs will cause hypoxia (not enough oxygen) because the blood carries the oxygen through its body. This then causes organ failure in multiple places and death… Game over. And on the long list of things not good for you, death is pretty close to the top.

So you give IV fluids at high rates quickly to build up pressure in those veins and arteries. Sometimes you have to give special fluids, either super concentrated (hypertonic saline) or with really big molecules (plasma or synthetic colloids) to treat shock that is not responding to normal IV fluids. The goal of those fluids is to pull water back into the veins and arteries through the mighty power of a force called osmosis (or oncotic pressure when we're talking about molecule size). In layman's terms[3] this means the fluid is pulled into places where there's a lot of big molecules to even concentrations out. The most important naturally occurring molecule in the body for this is albumen.

By the way, if you picked **swear loudly, then go hide in a corner somewhere**… You may want to consider another line of work. Emergency medicine may not be the right place for you. To be fair (and "real" and "legit," and all the other hip stuff kids say these days) sometimes even the best ER doctor occasionally needs to go cry in the corner. But you should try to avoid it on your first case on your first shift.

Circulatory system: the heart and blood vessels.
MAP: mean arterial blood pressure—average blood pressure.
Systemically: everywhere in the body.

[3] Something I generally picture myself wearing slippers and smoking a pipe in the sitting room while I say.

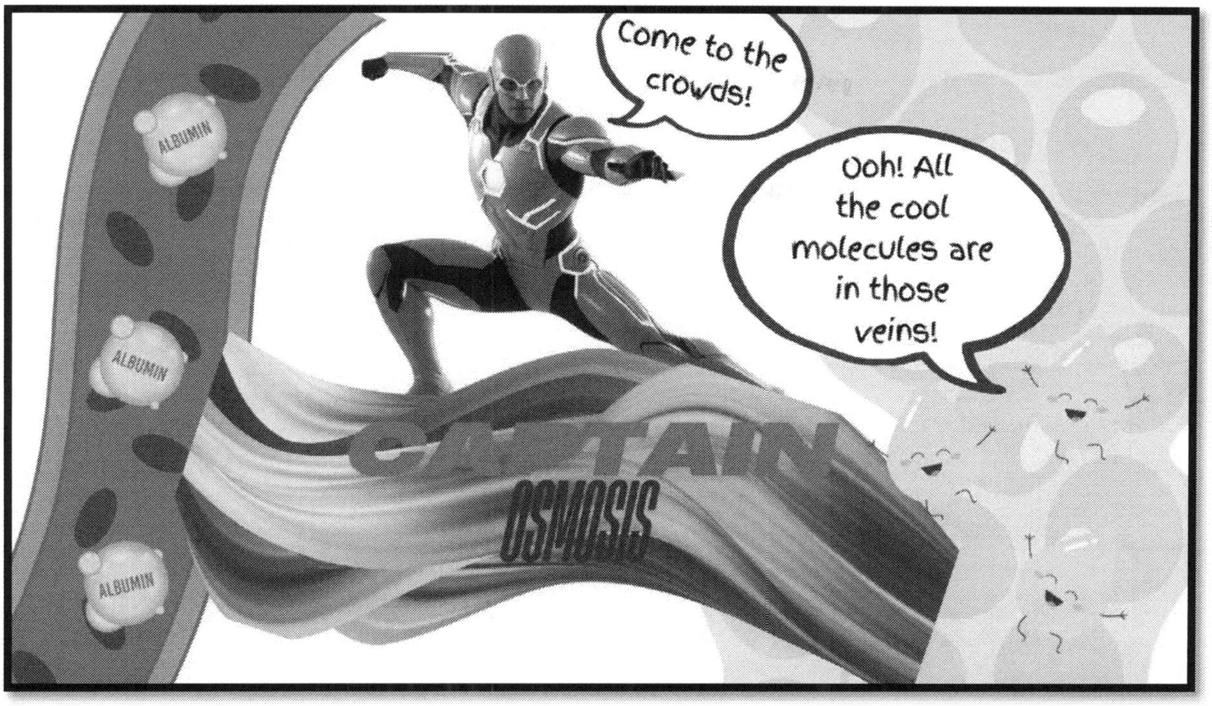

Things are happening quickly. And…before they happen so quickly they get out of control, you remember that this Great Dane came into the clinic with a human. You should talk to that human before you run up a huge bill and do a bunch of treatments they don't know about.

You find Greg Smith wringing his hands and pacing around the exam room. His designer sunglasses fall off as he almost runs into you in his eagerness to hear news of his hound.

"Hello, Mr. Smith…" you begin (feeling grateful that the long coat he wears is monogrammed to help you remember his name). But that's as far as you get before he interrupts you in choppy, staccato sentences.

"Yeah sure. Hi. What's happening with my dog?"

You are tempted to feel piqued but remember that this is a man panicked that his canine friend could be dying. So you refrain from the blunt words, "Well, you jerk, his stomach is about to explode, and he might not walk out of here." Instead, you tactfully and efficiently explain the situation.

"So he's gotta have surgery? Can you do it now? Let's get it done. This is my wife's favorite show dog, and he *cannot* die. We breed Great Danes, you know."

You tell him that you will do everything you can to hold off the fearsome, pale Specter of Death from wafting his sickle over Sigbert (well, you say something along those lines). And you tell him about the IV fluids and pain medications you've already started, and inform him you will work to get Sigbert ready while the technician goes over an estimate

"I don't need to see an estimate. Just go, man, go! Save our perfect paragon of a show dog…"

You go. But you are still going to make an estimate, having learned that many people "don't need to see an estimate" because they don't have money to pay their bill. You can generally tell how long someone has been a veterinarian by how emotionally traumatized and jaded they are…[4]

Greg Smith follows you to the lobby. "I'm gonna go check on my car. There was an…unsavory…character lounging around your parking lot when I drove up and I would not like him to scratch the paint job on my sportscar."

"That's probably Doug. He's homeless and hangs out sometimes. He's a few fries short of a happy meal, but not dangerous…" Graham offers, then shrugs as the client walks to the parking lot.

Things are happening fast and simultaneously now. You whip out an estimate for Graham to go over with Sigbert's wealthy and entitled owner while you work on more treatments.

There are a few other items on the list you should consider.

What are **three more things** you should probably do,

and what's a **fourth possibility** you should bring up with the owner?

"Logic takes care of itself; all we have to do is to look and see how it does it."
— Ludwig Wittgenstein[ii]

[4] Just kidding. There have been at least one or two veterinarians who stayed stable, optimistic, and happy throughout their entire career. At least, I've been told there are…

STOP!!!!!!

Formulate a more complete treatment plan…

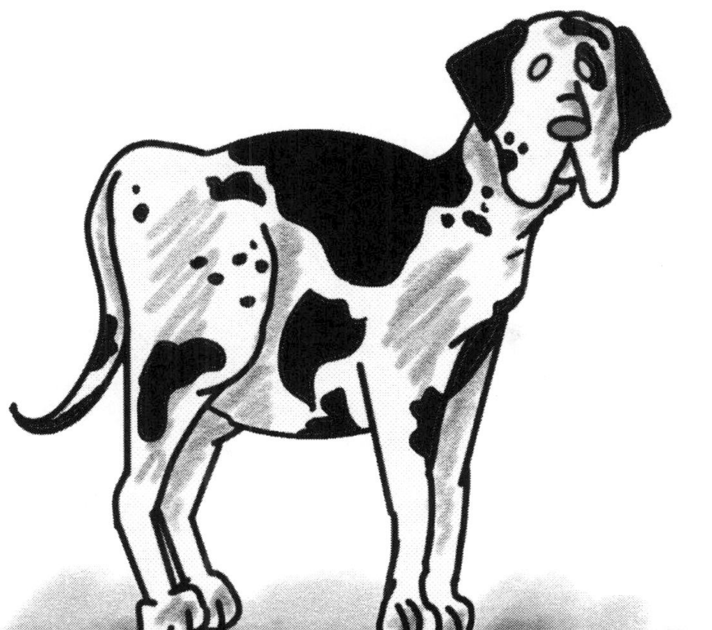

Let's think through options **a, b, c, and f**.

Giving some **antibiotics** as a treatment option would not be wrong. Some clinicians in GDV cases use antibiotics to preemptively treat infections you can get from bacteria slipping through damaged stomach wall, and from splenic blood supply compromise.

It's a good idea **do more diagnostics before doing treatment**. They should be quick, and you can move toward treatment while they're running. You help Lolita pull some blood to run a chemistry and CBC panel with blood gases when you get the green light from good ol' Greg. Then you put an ECG on the patient. The ECG looks OK other than a fast heart rate.

You move on to another important part of treatment (one you warned the owner you would do): **jab a hole into the stomach to let out the gas**. (I bet some of you didn't pick this one!)

There is a fancy word for this barbaric sounding procedure. Well, two fancy words, depending on which method you use. Trocharization is the common term to use, but technically this means you are using a special stabby tool called a trochar, which is more common in livestock medicine. Gastrocentesis is the word for when we use a large sized IV catheter, a more common method in dogs.

What you do is take this stabby tool, and stab the dog in the belly with it to release gas from the stomach before it kills him. OK, so it's a little more finessed and less horrible… First you shave and aesthetically prep a patch of the dog behind his ribs on the right side (where you will be less likely to hit important things internally). You ca percuss the spot first (listen for that "ping" sound with a stethoscope while you thump the body wall) to avoid the spleen. Usually we have given a pain injection that sedates the patient a bit, as well as local anesthetic to numb the skin where you are gonna poke. Then you carefully poke your tool into the abdomen behind the ribs.

You follow the steps and are gratified and disgusted at the same time to hear a hiss of gas from the catheter. You smell a rank, fermented, bog-of-death kind of smell as the evil vapors are released from that angry stomach. You wait until there's no more gas, then you do it one more time to get out as much as you can. Now you hopefully have a little more time to stabilize this patient and get him to surgery. The stomach is still flipped, even if you deflated some of it.

An alternative to trocharization and gastrocentesis that many vets try is to slide a stomach tube down the esophagus into the stomach. Usually, the stomach is so twisted that a stomach tube won't get past the esophageal sphincter (the place where the esophagus goes into the stomach), and you still must trocharize.

One more possibility I would not chide you for choosing: **euthanize this patient**.

This is undeniably sad. BUT we have a patient in extreme amounts of pain, whose stomach is rolled up and rotting inside of him. Prognosis for GDV is highly variable (with studies reporting a mortality rate anywhere between 10-45%). Factors like the degree of stomach necrosis, splenic involvement, and complications like sepsis and arrhythmias can all worsen the prognosis considerably. Especially in those cases where prompt treatment and surgery are not realistic, the next best thing you can advise is ending the patient's suffering.

What you absolutely don't want to do is say the dog will be fine, and let him go without surgery. That will invariably result in a dead patient who has suffered excruciating pain in their last moments.

You get up off the floor after performing gastrocentesis and find Graham looking flustered.

"Well, Doc... Mr. Smith says he can't pay eight grand for surgery and post-op care. He says that's almost as much as Sigbert cost as a puppy."

Oh boy. This may be your least favorite part of veterinary medicine. The high cost of human medicine is usually "hidden" within insurance company payments and government assistance that patients often don't see. In animal medicine, a client sees all the cost up front. And even if they have pet insurance, it is almost universally retroactive: meaning you still must get a full payment from the owner, then later they might be paid back by insurance.

And thus it cometh about that our hero is oft trapped in betwixt the moral conundrum of working for a service-based business they must not steal from (by doing stuff for free) and the noble desire to do all they can for the patient suffering before them.

In this case you suspect your monogrammed, Dane-breeding client cannot pay the bill because he's maxed his credit card limit. You march into the exam room to do some slick negotiations.

You march back out of the exam room to call your boss who owns the clinic. It turns out Greg really can't afford surgery because of the payments for the Lamborghini he drove to the clinic, and his monthly golf club fees. He applied for medical credit cards and was declined. Greg, it seems, is the captain of a sinking ship, keeping up a rich man's lifestyle he's having trouble affording.

Annnnnnd, you can't get ahold of the clinic owner. In her defense, it is 2 am.

"I mean, I totally understand," Graham tries to ease a growing tension. "I'm broke all the time, trying to pay for school. That's why I work so many shifts..."

You nod nervously. Understanding financial difficulty is one thing, giving away thousands of dollars of free services is another. You're going to have to make a tough choice. It would seem that (even though nobody said you have financial authority) the buck stops with you for now.

What are you going to do?

a) Just do surgery and take whatever deposit the client can come up with.
b) Tell Mr. Smith you can't help him and give him the phone numbers of vets you don't get along with much, so he can call and bug them next.
c) Discuss options like euthanasia.
d) Tell your technician they have to make the decisions now cuz it's too hard for you.
e) Pull out your bank card and pay his bill yourself.
f) Contact local dog rescues and charity groups.

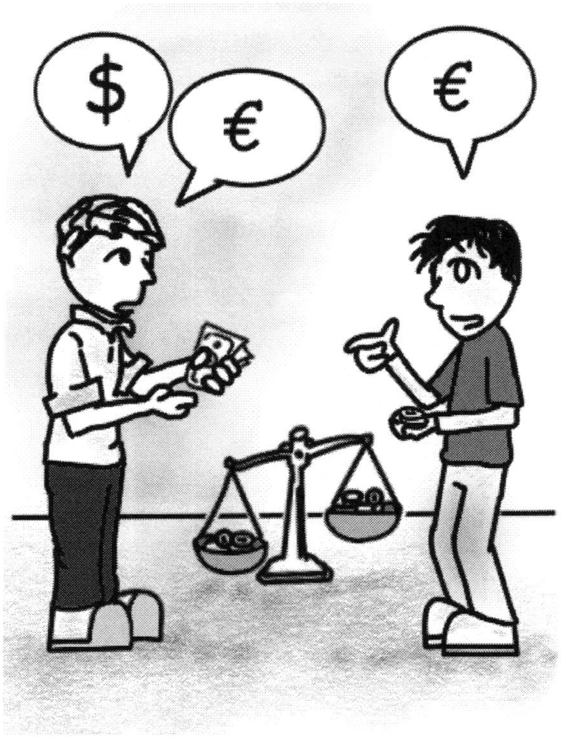

STOP!!!!!!

Don't turn the page until you've picked some options…

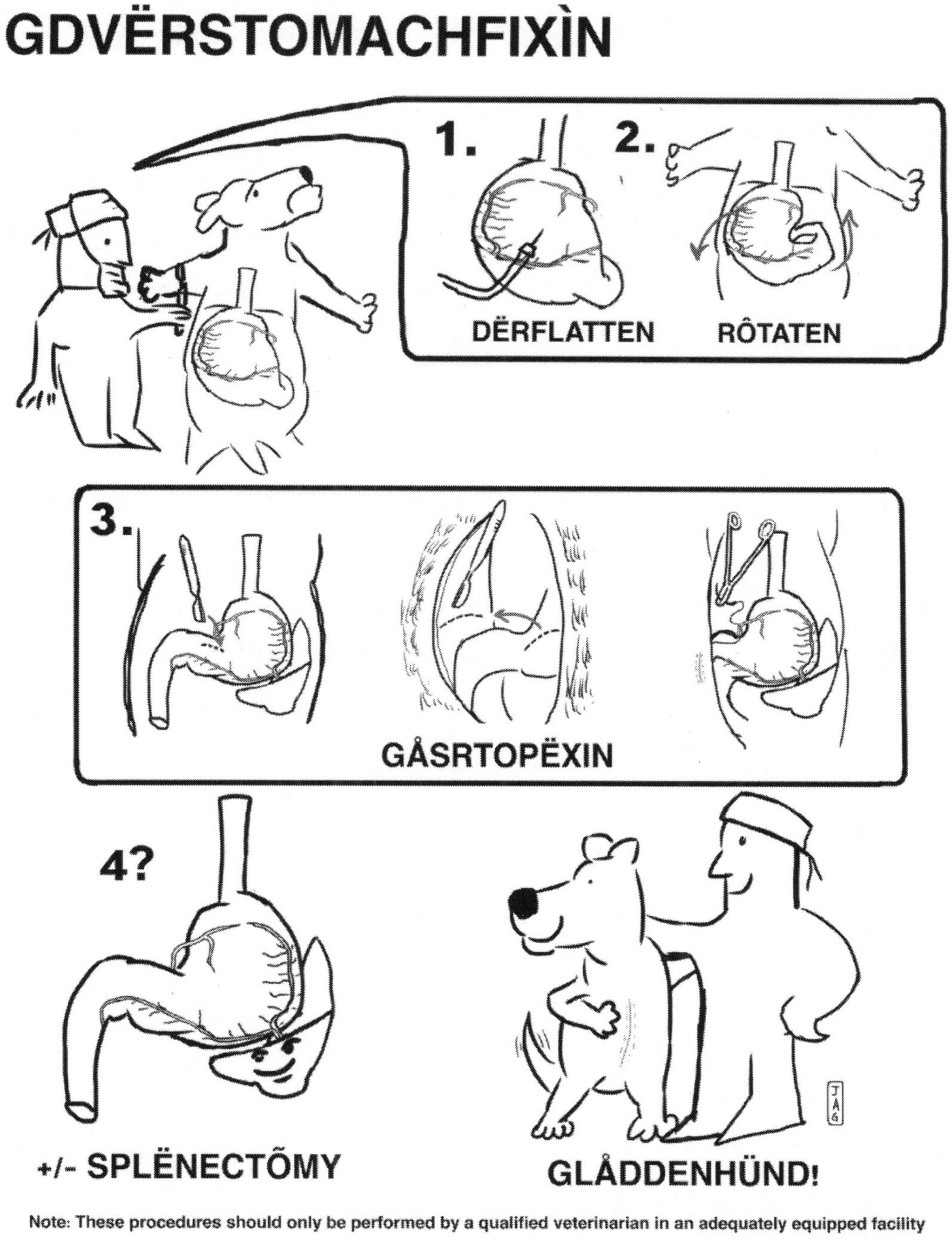

What I would do is a bit of a combination of the options: **a, c, f**.

This is a hard one, and a situation I often encounter in the grimy real-world trenches of clinical practice. What we have here is a less-than-perfect situation with no great solution.

Start by explaining the options other than surgery (i.e. humane euthanasia) and why they might be considered. Any information you can gather about the patient's predicted chances of getting through this alive will be very important, of course. If this is a really old dog already on medications for heart failure, and has really bad bloodwork, for example, you should probably be clear with the owner about a really bad prognosis regardless of money.

I would have some staff work through any creative financial options available (applying for assistance programs and charities if you have that option, other medical credit card applications, etc). I'd still want to hurry things along, and move Sigbert toward surgery, if surgery is still a possibility. The longer we put off untwisting the stomach, the bigger the chances are that his stomach lining necroses and he can't be saved. And in some cases, if all the options have been exhausted, I might go ahead with things, trying to keep cost as low as possible and hoping my boss will forgive me later.

By the way, if you picked **pay his bill yourself** then I'd very much like to be your friend, and maybe have whatever job gives you that much cash. I'd pick that option more often, only I have six kids to support. That's why I'm so happy you bought this book in the first place.

The conversation takes some tact in the case of Mr. Smith, but he does take the discussion better than you expected. He tells you he needs Sigbert to get through this. His wife is already angry at him for mismanaging their finances, and she will murder him gruesomely in the night if he lets Siggy die without trying everything. He can pay about a quarter of the bill tonight and will get the rest paid as soon as he can. Good enough, you say. You'll stick your neck out and do the surgery without being sure it can be paid for.

Here goes! IV fluids are running, your patient has some strong pain medication, and is not in hypovolemic shock. You give him some magic sleepy drugs, and have your techs prep him for surgery. Because you have learned already in your brief time as a veterinarian to second guess everything you think you know, you breeze through an entry in a textbook to remind yourself of the procedure you are about to perform.

Whilst your technicians scrub the dog's belly, you scrub your hands. You'll never feel quite so clean as when prepping for surgery! When I went to school (back in the dark ages when cavemen ran around with clubs and stuff) they taught me to scrub each plane of my hand and forearm, and each finger 10x with a special surgical brush packed with surgical scrub. It's nice for cleaning out your pores. But what's also nice, and is the real goal, is that it helps you be sterile (free from bacteria). You use a special technique known

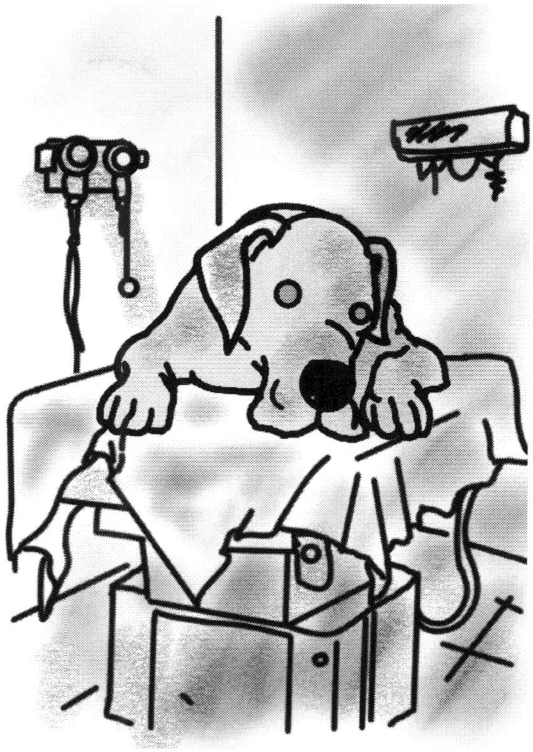

only to the wise and initiated to don your sterile gloves and gown. You've hopefully already remembered to put on your cap and booties and mask (otherwise you must start the whole process all over). Great! You're ready to rock and roll.

You feel just a little worn out from all that scrubbing and glove and gown donning. But brace yourself, 'cuz now's the hard part! Your patient is now on the table on his back, bloated tummy staring up at you, and it's your show.

Here's what you do...

Taking your scalpel blade, you make an incision in the ventral abdomen and get inside there. You do an initial explore (which is usually a bit limited due to the massive stomach pushing everything away from where it should be). The good news is that the stomach is mostly pinkish, other than a broad patch of red irritation. What you don't want to see is a purple or black color to the stomach, which would be signs that its wall is dead. You discover the pylorus (the narrowed part of the stomach that flows out to the intestines) way up near this guy's spine, a bit right of his midline. That's not where it should be. You have an approximately 270 degree torsion. Your mission, should you choose to accept it, is to grab that sucker and untwist him. Your immediate problem is that the stomach is so massive and tight with gas against the body wall that there's no way you can turn it anywhere.

What should you do? Well, remember that whole gastroecentesis thing? That works great here too! You have Lolita hand you a needle (using a super-secret sterile technique only known to the wise and initiated). This you jab into the stomach (at the pinkest part you can find) and connect to surgical suction. FWOOOOOP! SLOOORP!

Hohohohoho!

That was fun. The stomach deflates like paper bag being sucked on by a kid. Now you've got plenty of room to move it back into position. Because you looked earlier at your textbook you remember that most GDV stomachs turn in a clockwise direction. This is from where the surgeon stands, viewed from a dog's

Greater curvature: the big part of the stomach.
Pylorus: the narrowed part of the stomach that flows out to the intestines.
Ventral: lower body surface; toward the belly.

right side facing his head, with the dog on its back. So you do this heroic move: you reach down and grab the pylorus with your right hand (plunging it into a cavern of squishy organs that shplorp juicily, of course). You put your other hand on the greater curvature (the big part of the stomach). Then you push with your left toward the table, and pull up with your right hand away from the table. SHHHHHPLORP! Good work! That twisted stomach moved right back into place!

You spend a little time looking around and making sure things are back where they should be. The pylorus is back on the dog's right ventral side. You can reach down and feel normal tension on the esophagus, where it comes into the stomach just past the liver. You still don't see any purple or black stomach walls. The gastrosplenic ligament (a band that connects the spleen to the stomach) is not too tight. You also feel all the guts to make sure there's not a blockage that started this GDV. Good so far.

Graham snags a big rubber tube, pre-measured from mouth down to the xiphoid (that pokey bit at the end of the breastbone) and pushes it from the patient's mouth down into the stomach. In a fully twisted stomach, the tube won't go in. Now that you've untwisted the stomach, the tube goes in fine. You reach down there and feel the end of the esophagus while he passes the tube, so you can be sure it doesn't have unusual resistance. It helps calm that angry stomach to lavage it with warm water. Graham takes a special pump and a bucket of warm water, and pumps water into the stomach, creating a siphon that flows disgusting gastric fluid and fermented, foul-smelling dog food back out into the bucket when he disconnects it. Doing that a few times helps make the poor traumatized stomach lining a bit less angry, and gives you a chance to laugh at your poor grossed-out tech.

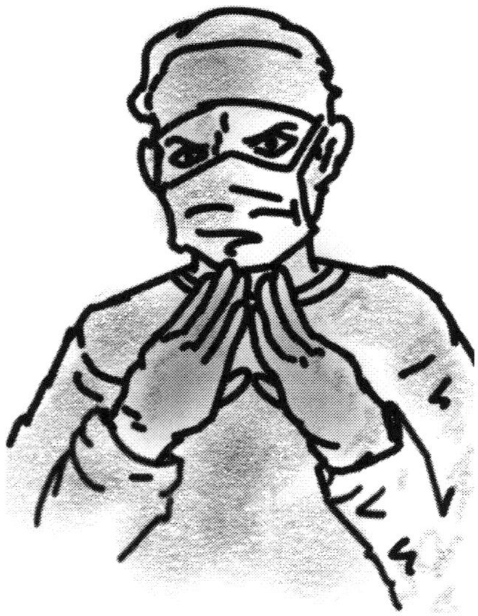

Because you don't want Sigbert to go through all this again, you do a gastropexy next. This surgical procedure attaches the stomach to the body wall to prevent it from flipping again. There are a few different techniques surgeons use, but you pick one called incisional gastropexy (probably the most common one, and my own personal favorite).

First, you make an incision in the stomach's antrum (the bit between its narrow pylorus and its big, fat body), then you "kiss it" (not with your lips!) up against the right abdominal wall to make a little line of blood impressed along the wall. That blood smear helps guide you to make a matching incision in the

gastrosplenic ligament: a band that connects the spleen to the stomach.
xiphoid: pokey bit at the front of the breastbone.

abdomen lining. Then you suture the stomach to the body wall by matching the two incisions, using a separate line of suture along each side of the incision.

What does that get you? Good question! You're a smart reader. It sticks together the muscle layers of the stomach and the abdominal wall, and lets these scar and fuse together over time to help hold the stomach in place. By the time you're all done, you are sweating and feeling a bit dizzy from nearly standing on your head looking down into the deep Great Dane cavern to suture things backward.

But you did it!

Time to get out of here and go sip some coffee…

Wait. Why is the spleen about as big as a salmon, and extra dark with purple, with black blotches? That's one angry spleen!

Hmm… What should you do?

Do you…

a) Inject antibiotics into the spleen
b) Get out of surgery and consult a textbook
c) Let it ride
d) Perform a total splenectomy
e) Take a biopsy of those yucky colored bits of spleen
f) Throw up your hands and weep, because this is all just too much

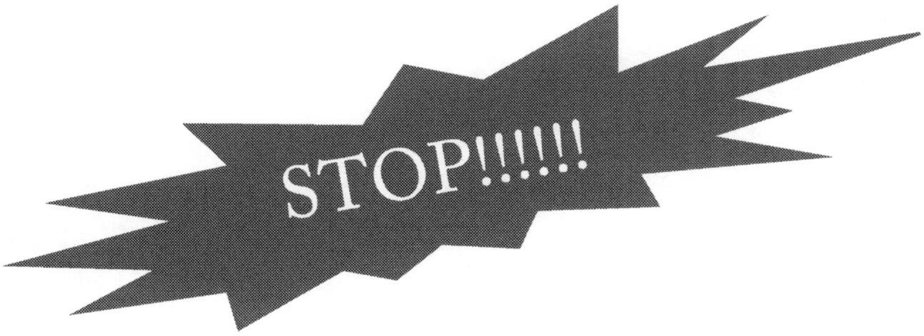

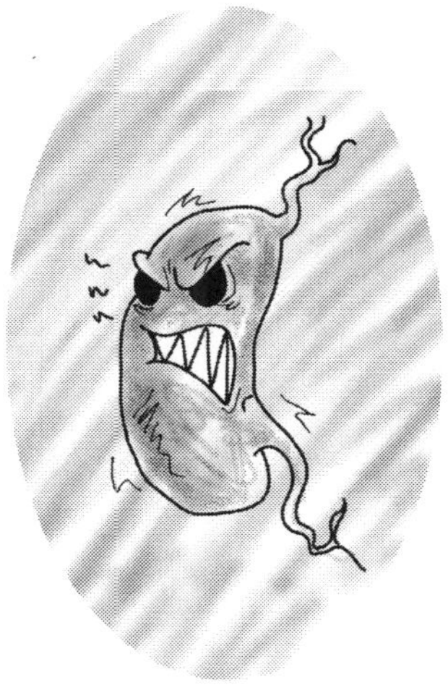
[5]

[5] Artistic rendition of an angry spleen: any resemblance to an actual spleen is purely coincidental (and highly frightening).

The correct answer is **d) perform a total splenectomy**.

Get that fella out! Remember that the spleen is attached to the stomach and can get twisted up with it, cutting off its blood supply. Signs of splenic necrosis mean the spleen is shot, and is going to become a rotting source of inflammation.

Note that important decisions need to be made in the middle of surgery. This is one of the big challenges of surgery. You generally don't have the luxury of consulting a textbook or phoning a friend in the middle of an operation, so you want to prepare mentally and logistically. You probably don't want to take biopsies of the spleen, as splenic tissue bleeds a lot, *and* because the whole spleen is yucky.

You sigh and dive back in. You double ligate all the little blood vessels going into the underside of the spleen, and it takes FOREVER. Then you transect the vessels, remove that big ol' nasty spleen (holding it up for your technician to see, like some kind of proud fisherman), and check for any bleeding. If your clinic was fancier you might have a cool tool that cauterizes and cuts blood vessels with electricity that would make this go faster. But you work with what you have.

There are several good surgical methods to choose from for this procedure (as is the case with many surgeries). The important part is that the spleen is out, and your ligated vessels are not bleeding when you double check, and the other important organs near the spleen still look fine.

You close up your patient and get out of there. That was a lot of time bending over a surgery table, and your back hurts! You're about tired of this case, but you're not done yet.

Now you need to decide what to do for Sigbert post operatively. You've already let Mr. Smith know Siggy will be staying the night, and needs to be transferred to his primary care vet in the morning for at least 24 hours monitoring in a hospital post op.

Ligate: to bind/tie off, usually using a suture.

Transect: cutting, often after ligation.

What medications and treatments does Siggy need tonight?

a) Acupuncture

b) Antacids — Provides relief from indigestion, acid reflux, ulcers, gastritis, etc.

c) Antibiotics

d) Eggnog and hot cocoa… Lots and lots of eggnog, with nutmeg sprinkled on top…

e) Heart medications

f) IV fluids

g) Nausea medications

h) Pain medications

i) Plasma transfusion

j) Vitamin E

STOP!!!!!!

"I find it hard enough to tackle facts, Holmes, without flying away after theories and fancies."

—Arthur Conan Doyle,
The Boscombe Valley Mystery[iii]

Here's what I would pick: **b, c, e, f, g, h**.

IV fluids are very important after surgery to help keep up the blood pressure and provide hydration and electrolytes to a patient who is not ready to eat and drink on his own. If you answered **pain medications**, great work! This guy needs lots of those. Generally, we use pain medications called opioids for the first day post op, and often we use really strong continuous rate infusions (i.e. pain medications continually through an IV pump). **Antibiotics** are given just before surgery and during surgery, and if there are signs of damaged stomach lining (and/or leakage of bacteria contaminating the abdomen) they are sometimes continued post-op. The stomach has taken a big hit in this patient so **antacids** and **nausea drugs** help. The **heart medication** to consider in this case is called lidocaine. It is generally used to numb a patient, but also slows the heart rate when given IV. A major concern post op in GDV cases is a heart arrhythmia that causes fast heart rate and irregular contractions. We usually monitor ECGs for the first 12-24 hours post-op, and start lidocaine if needed. Many veterinarians will start a low-rate lidocaine CRI regardless, even during surgery on GDV cases. It also helps with painful abdominal organs.

Your reward for powering through a physically demanding surgery in the wee hours of the morning is the chance to make your tired brain calculate a bunch of drug doses for this patient. Good work! You get everything set up for this guy, waiting around the ICU while the technicians monitor his ECG and vitals. Everything looks fine. You become conscious that Lolita and Graham are staring at you in embarrassing silence while the early morning hours tick by, and you decide to head back to your office. They are good at their job and will get you if something changes.

You pull out the latest medical journal and read through a couple of studies. That was a mistake. Halfway through a riveting article entitled *Evaluation of Current Anthemintics for Treatment of c. Toxascara in A Population of Greyhounds* your head slumps down and you start drooling on the pages as slumber overtakes you.

Case #2

A loud knock bursts through the silence about half an hour later, and you jump up with a start, and fall off your chair. "Who? Wha?? How?!?" You mutter eloquently before opening the door to find Lolita standing there with a tablet and a history for a new patient. You glance at the clock, hoping you get to go home soon. It's 4 am. You've got four more hours of this…

"Got another patient for you, Doc," your technician yawns. "Another distended abdomen…"

Wait a second! That's not fair. I already saw one of those!

You'll soon learn that, for some unknown cosmic reason, ER shifts often have a "theme of the night." Distended bellies is not a good theme. This time you find that your new patient is a little corgi called Monkfruit with a fat, fat tummy.

Monkfruit's owner is a blond college girl who looks like she jumped out of bed and threw on whatever clothes were handy… Her old flannel shirt has dried soup of some kind and coffee stains, and more than one string hanging off the frayed sleeves. Her bright yellow pants clash horribly, and have so many wrinkles they could pass as Shar Pei skin. To be fair, it is 4 am and most of us don't look our best at that hour. It seems Ms. Piper Larsen got up in the middle of the night to get some water and noticed that her beloved dog-beast looked different. He was breathing heavy, and when she woke him up, he acted listless and vomited all over her bed. That's when she noticed that his belly seemed big.

"What's wrong with him?" she asks.

"Well, Miss Larsen, let me take a look…"

Step 1 – Organize the History

Signalment:

Male neutered (MN)

11 years old

Welsh Corgi

Presenting Complaints:

Vomiting and inappetence

Lethargy

Abdominal distention

Step 2 – Gather Clues

Physical Exam:

Abdominal palpation: Suspect a distended abdomen (big belly!), only mild splinting noted in the cranial abdomen. Possible fluid wave on palpation.

> This is a soggy bounce to the belly, which feels a bit like a water balloon, and can be a sign of fluid building up in the abdomen.

Attitude: Quiet, alert, and responsive.

Cardiac: No murmur or arrhythmia noted. Weak but synchronous femoral pulses.

Ears: NSF.

> Remember, NSF means "No Significant Findings."

Eyes: NSF.

Integument: No wounds or sores noted, no rashes, no hair loss. Normal skin turgor.

Lymph Nodes: NSF.

Musculoskeletal: NSF, weight bearing on all four limbs.

Neurologic: BAR, normal menace response and palpebral reflexes noted OU (both eyes), normal conscious proprioception on all four paws.

> Remember, BAR means "Bright, Alert, Responsive."

Oronasal: Gunky gums and dirty teeth.

Oronasal: WNL.

Respiratory: Normal respiratory rate and mild increase in respiratory effort. All lung fields sound clear with your stethoscope.

Urogenital: Urinary bladder difficult to palpate due to patient splinting and fat belly, no other inflammation or abnormalities noted.

Vitals: Pale gums, CRT over 3 seconds

Piper stares at you through glasses covered in grime and asks what should be done next. You're a little distracted wondering if she can see you through that dust-storm over her eyes.

"W…we should probably do some tests?" you stammer.

Heeeeeey! That's a good idea….

Synchronous: coordinated with the heartbeat.

WNL: Within Normal Limits.

But first, you need to make a differential list to guide what tests might be helpful.

Remember, you are making a list of all the possibilities you can think of "off the cuff" as a starting point you can rule unlikely diagnoses from.

See what you can come up with before you turn the page.

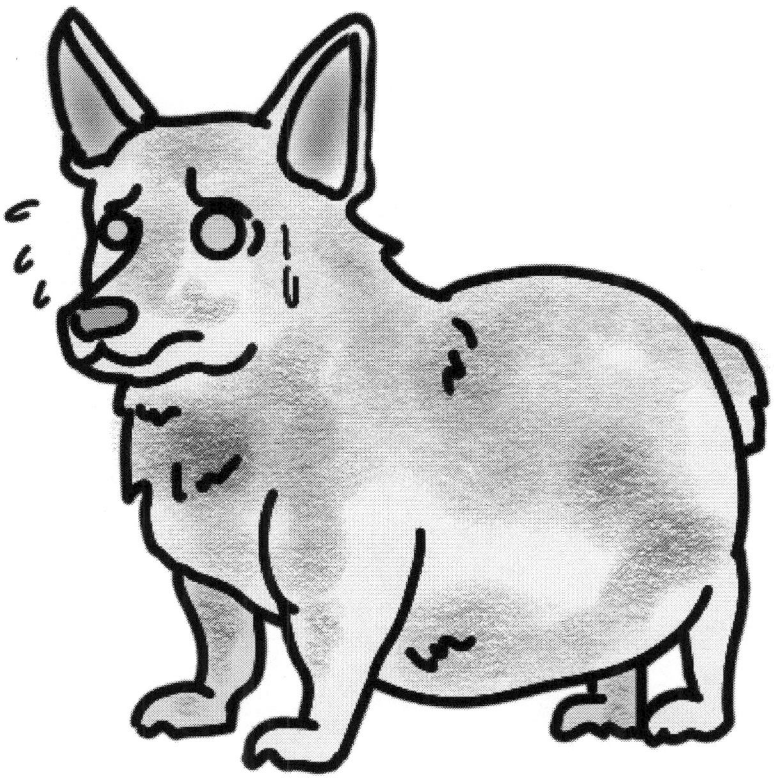

Differential Diagnoses (the possible diseases for a distended abdomen):

- Ascites — Clear fluid filling up the abdomen.
- Cushing's disease — A disease of the adrenal glands that makes the abdominal muscles weak (and other stuff).
- GD (gastric dilitation) — No volvulus here: i.e. stomach not twisted
- GDV (gastric dilitation and volvulus) — A problem you know a lot about now!
- Food bloat — A distended stomach from good old-fashioned gluttony.
- Hemoabdomen — Blood filling up the abdomen.
- Infection/peritonitis — An infection in the lining of the abdomen itself can cause it to fill up with fluid.
- Pain — Can make a patient tense his abdomen up to seem distended.
- Uroabdomen — Urine filling up the abdomen.

If you got some of those on your list, great job! You may have noticed something tricky. Some of these differentials are more like categories or side effects from other disease processes. That means they have differential lists of their own! Ascites, hemoabdomen, and uroabdomen are good examples. They are differentials for a distended abdomen, but they're also signs of whole other lists of causes.

Following are a few potential differentials for them…

Ascites

- Extremely low protein — if enough protein is lost through the kidneys or intestines too fast fluid leaks out into the abdomen and other places because of Captain Osmosis.
- Heart failure (right heart failure in particular)
- Liver failure
- GI parasites — Really large amounts of them.
- Neoplasia

Hemoabdomen

- Anaphylaxis — A serious allergic reaction that can affect the whole body, and sometimes causes internal bleeding)
- Neoplasia
- Trauma

Uroabdomen

- Ruptured urinary bladder
- Ruptured ureter — One of the tubes going from the kidneys to the bladder.
- Ruptured urethra — The tube going from the bladder to exit the dog.

Hint: It's sounding like we need to decide if there is fluid in the abdomen of this dog. That would automatically rule in or out several of these possibilities. So what tests should we run?

Decision time!

Here's what you can do in your clinic:

- ✓ Basic bloodwork (a chemistry panel and CBC)
- ✓ Benchtop Ethylene glycol test
- ✓ Blood gas analysis
- ✓ Clotting times
- ✓ Cytology
- ✓ Fecal floatation and direct saline exam
- ✓ Fluid analysis
- ✓ FeLV/FIV test
- ✓ Giardia test
- ✓ Heartworm test (with rickettsial diseases)
- ✓ Leptospirosis test
- ✓ Pancreatic lipase
- ✓ Parvo test
- ✓ Pregnancy test
- ✓ Radiographs (X-rays)
- ✓ Skin scraping
- ✓ Thyroid hormone level (T4)
- ✓ Ultrasound
- ✓ Urinalysis

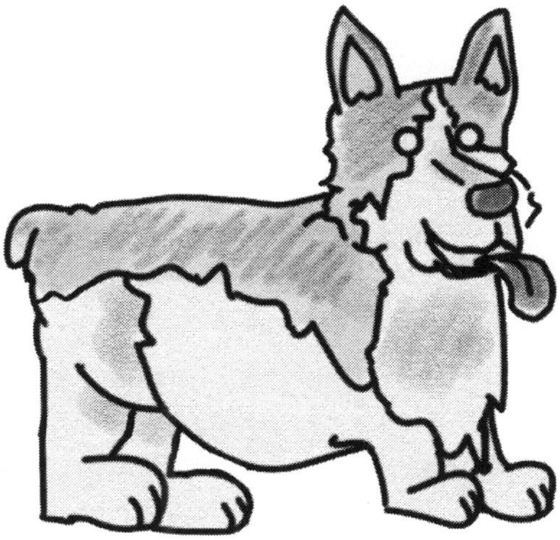

What tests do you want to run?

STOP!!!!!

This is a case where I would probably do an **ultrasound** first.

Other tests that might make sense include abdominal radiographs, general bloodwork, and clotting times. But with a distended belly *and* a suspected fluid wave, there is a good chance an ultrasound will show what you need to know: because ultrasounds are good at looking for fluid and through fluid.

An AFAST ultrasound would make sense in particular. AFAST stands for Abdominal Focused Assessment with Sonography for Trauma. That's a mouthful of words! It is essentially a quick peek at four very specific spots on a patient's abdomen to look for fluid. There's a lot of other helpful stuff you may see on an AFAST, but finding fluid is the main goal of this type of ultrasound.

On an ultrasound, fluid looks like black patches (or "anechoic"). You're looking specifically for "free fluid," meaning fluid just floating in the abdominal cavity around internal organs. Look especially for patches of black with square-ish or triangular shapes. You calculate an abdominal fluid score (AFS) then by adding 1 for every view you see fluid in, to get a score of 1-4 out of 4 (some doctors use 0.5 for ultrasound views with tiny bits of free fluid).

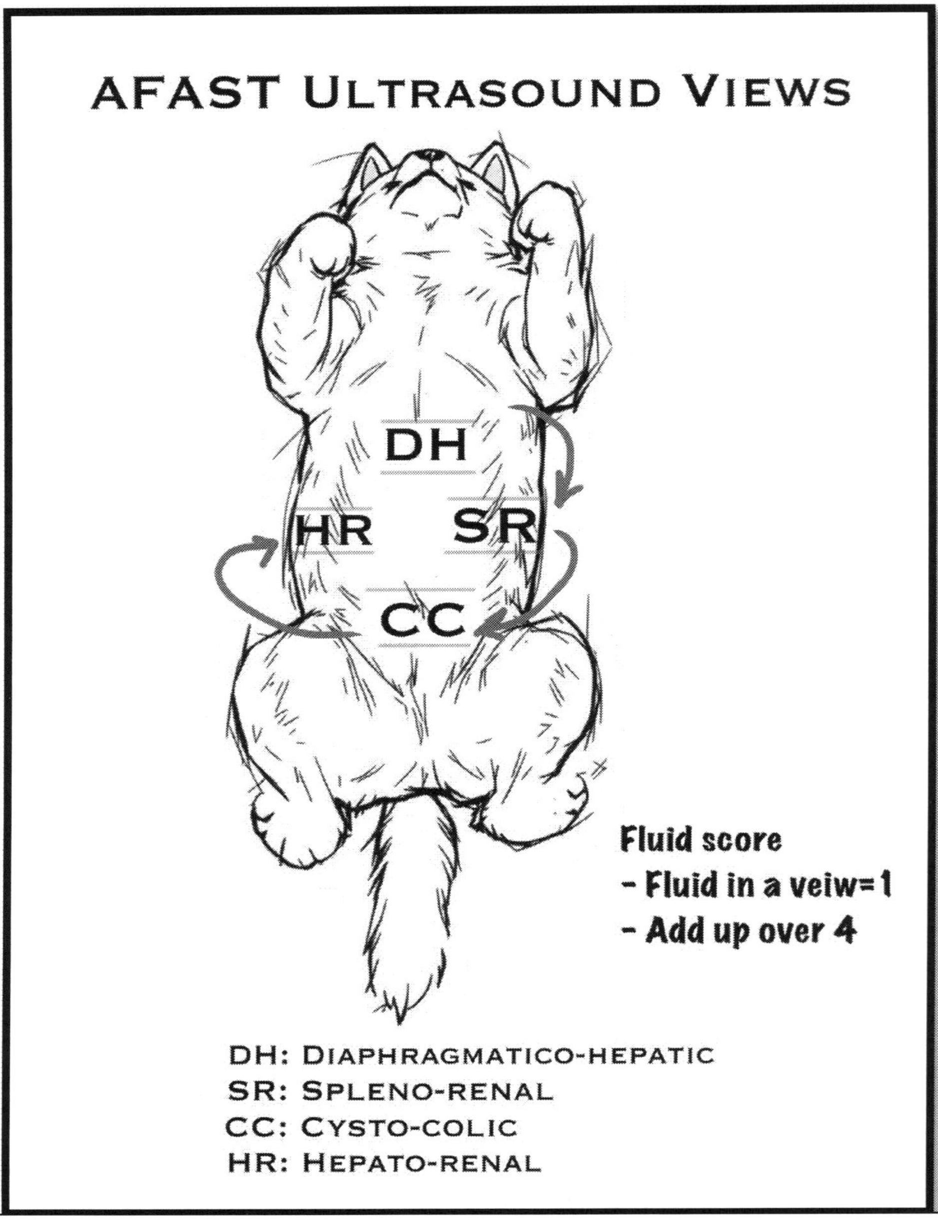

On the next page is what you find in Monkfruit. **Can you fill in any of the blanks?**

AFS: abdominal fluid score

Da Ultrasound!

You can see the location of the images in their top left corners. Try to think of what organs might be in those locations (refer to the diagram on the previous page).

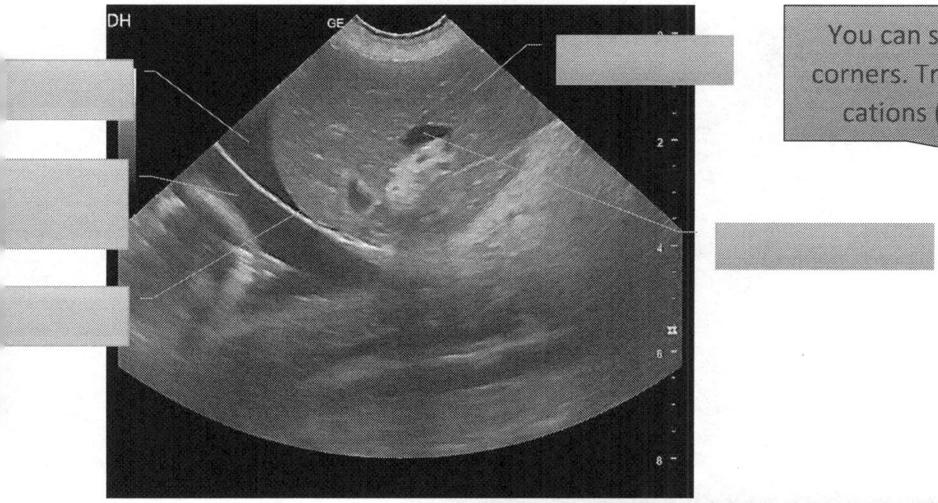

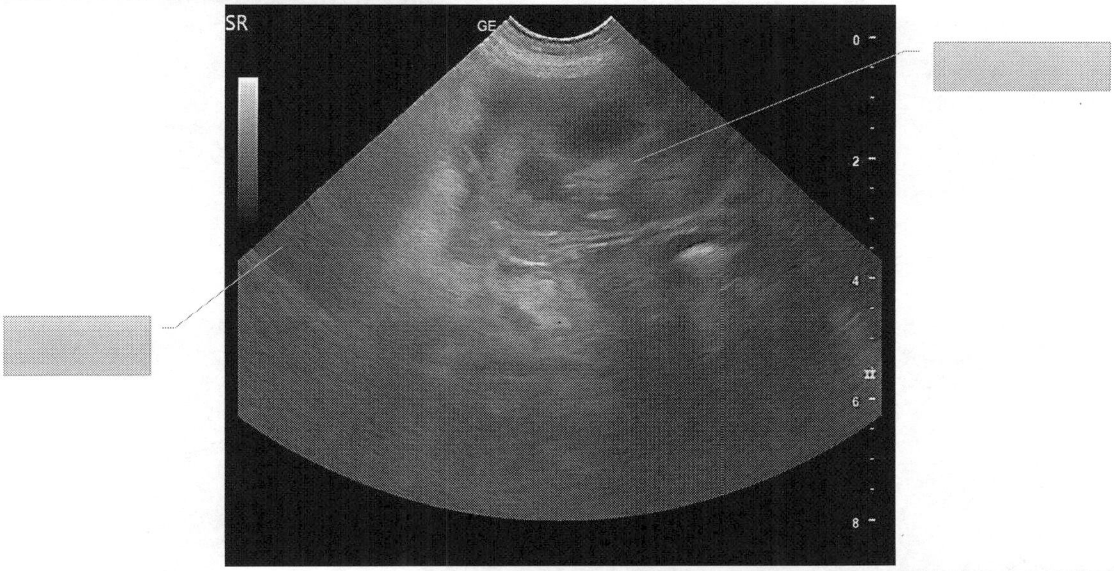

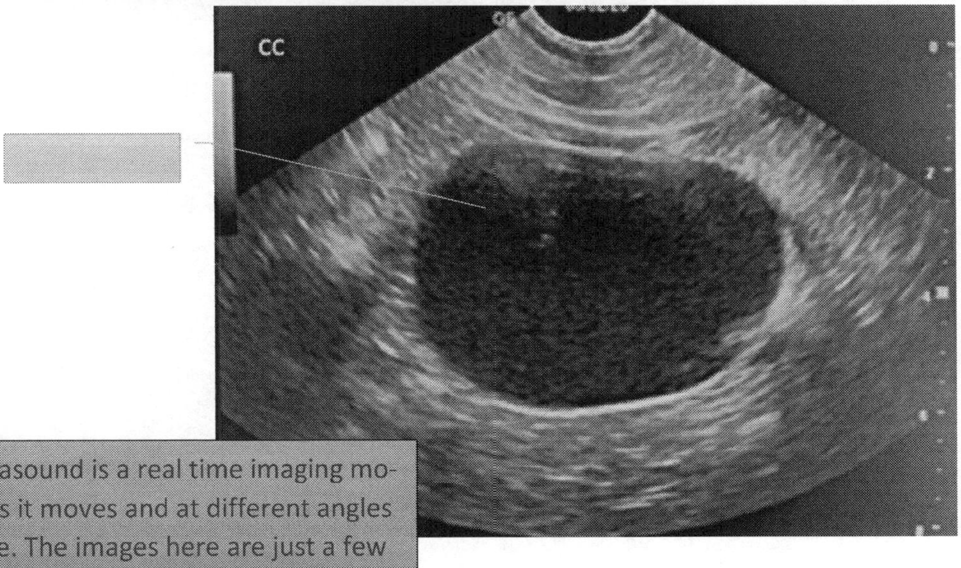

Remember that an ultrasound is a real time imaging modality: you see tissue as it moves and at different angles as you move the probe. The images here are just a few snapshots of your entire exam of this patient's innards.

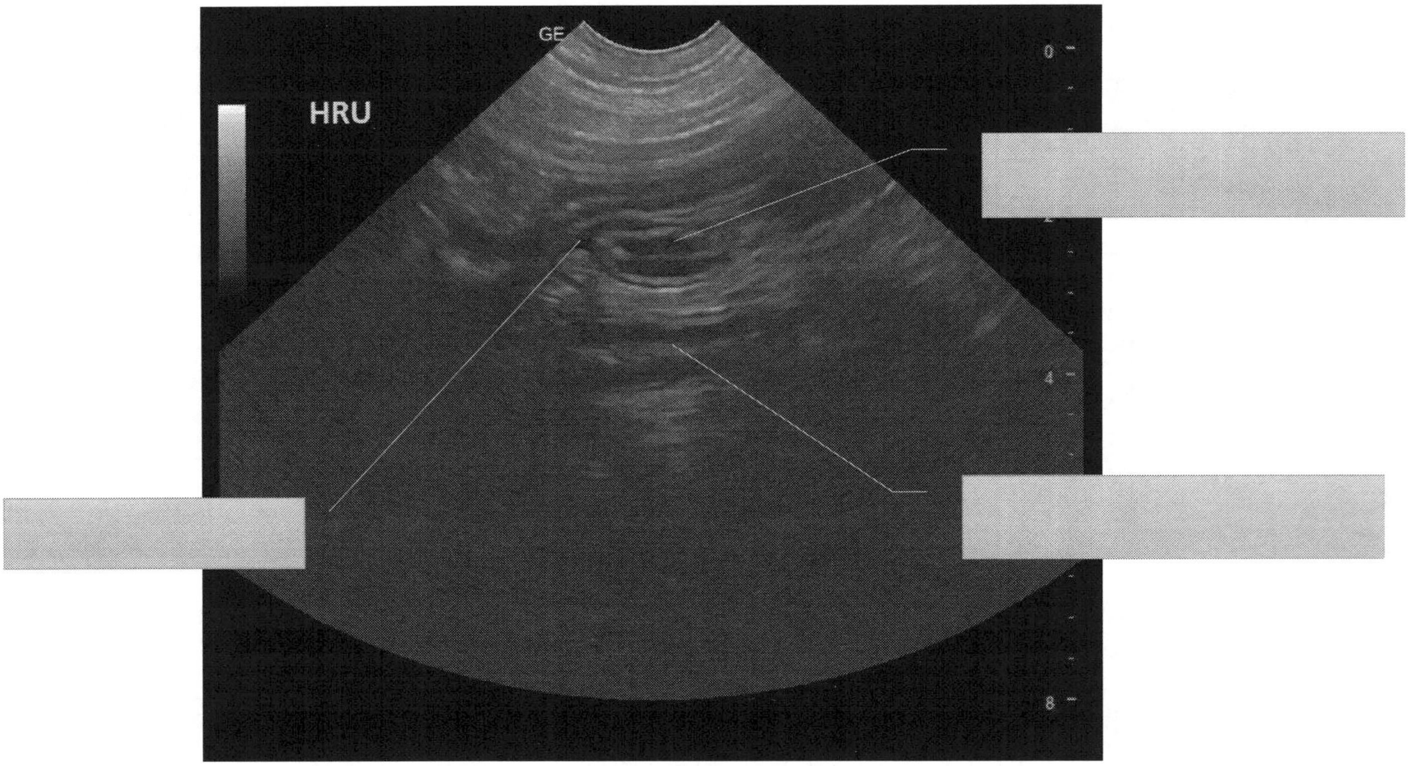

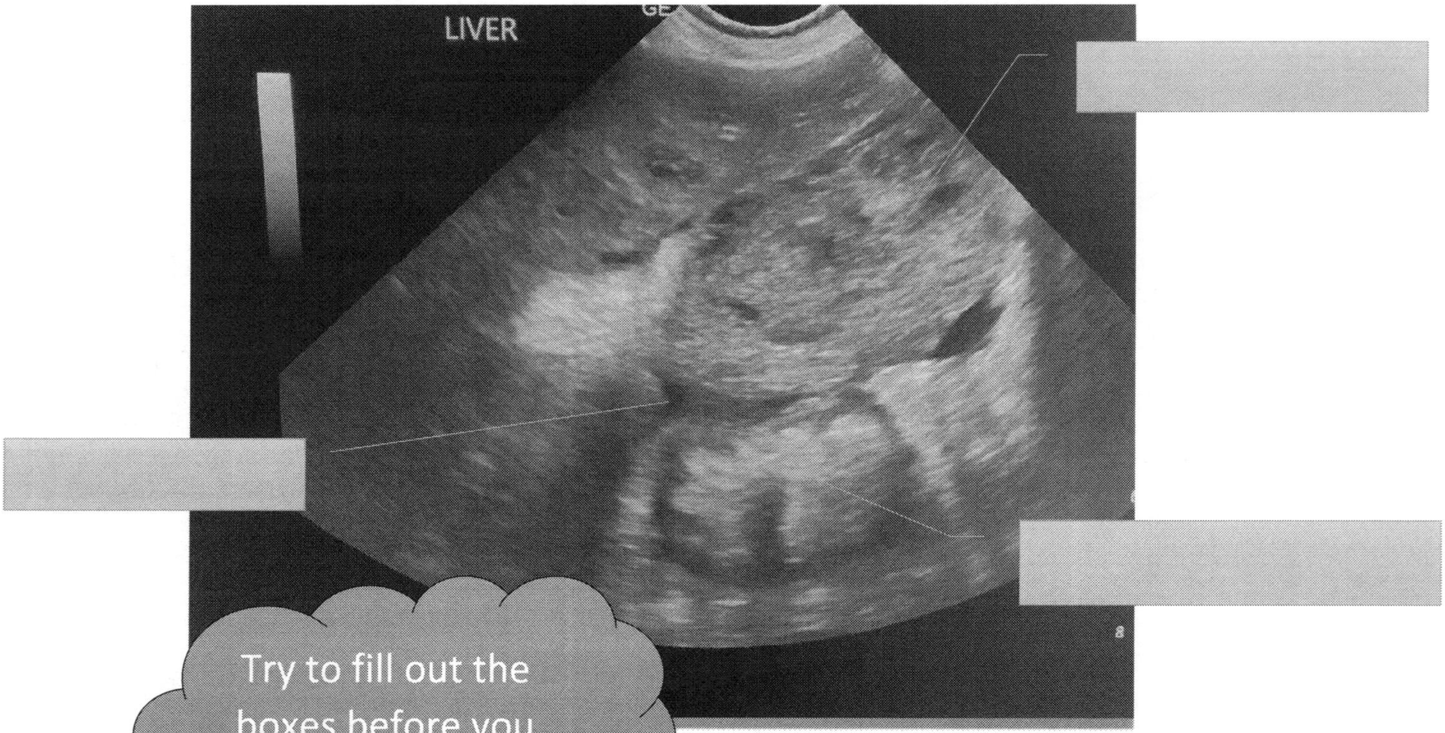

Try to fill out the boxes before you turn the page!

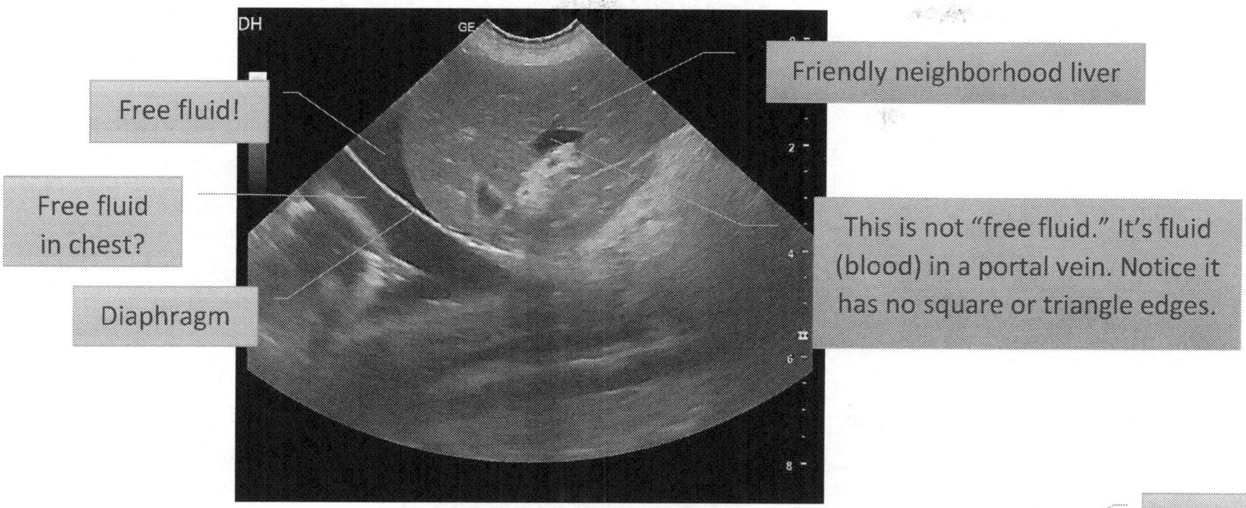
DH
GE
Free fluid!
Free fluid in chest?
Diaphragm
Friendly neighborhood liver
This is not “free fluid.” It’s fluid (blood) in a portal vein. Notice it has no square or triangle edges.

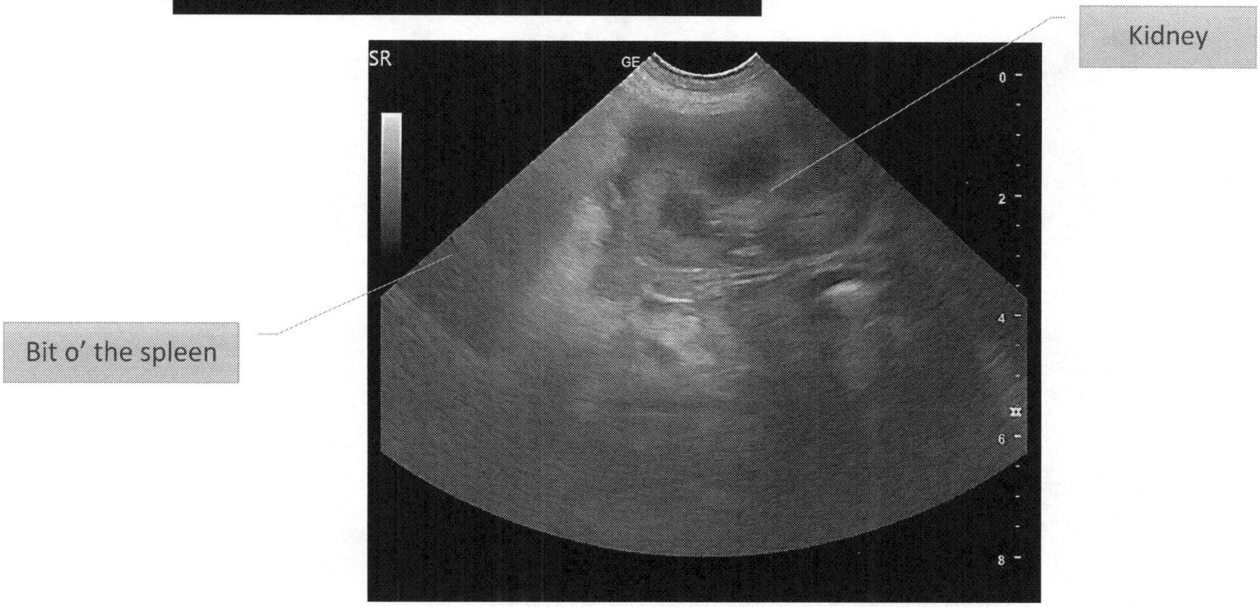
SR
GE
Kidney
Bit o’ the spleen

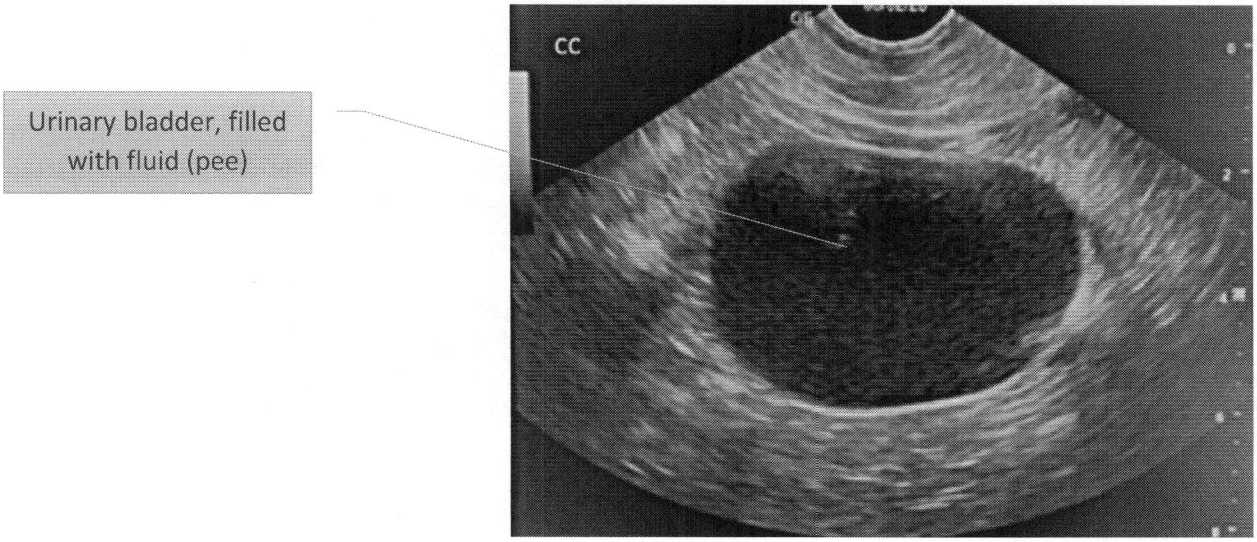
CC
Urinary bladder, filled with fluid (pee)

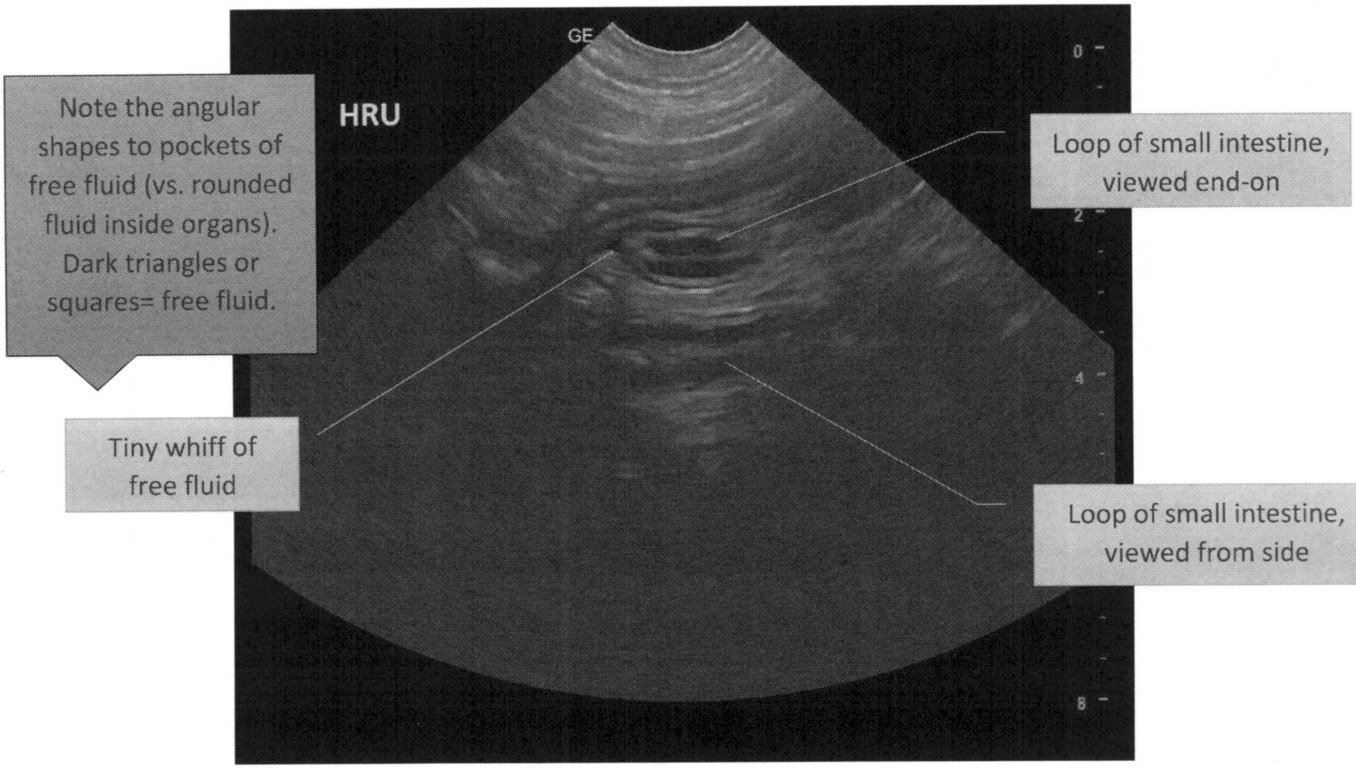
HRU
Note the angular shapes to pockets of free fluid (vs. rounded fluid inside organs). Dark triangles or squares= free fluid.
Loop of small intestine, viewed end-on
Tiny whiff of free fluid
Loop of small intestine, viewed from side

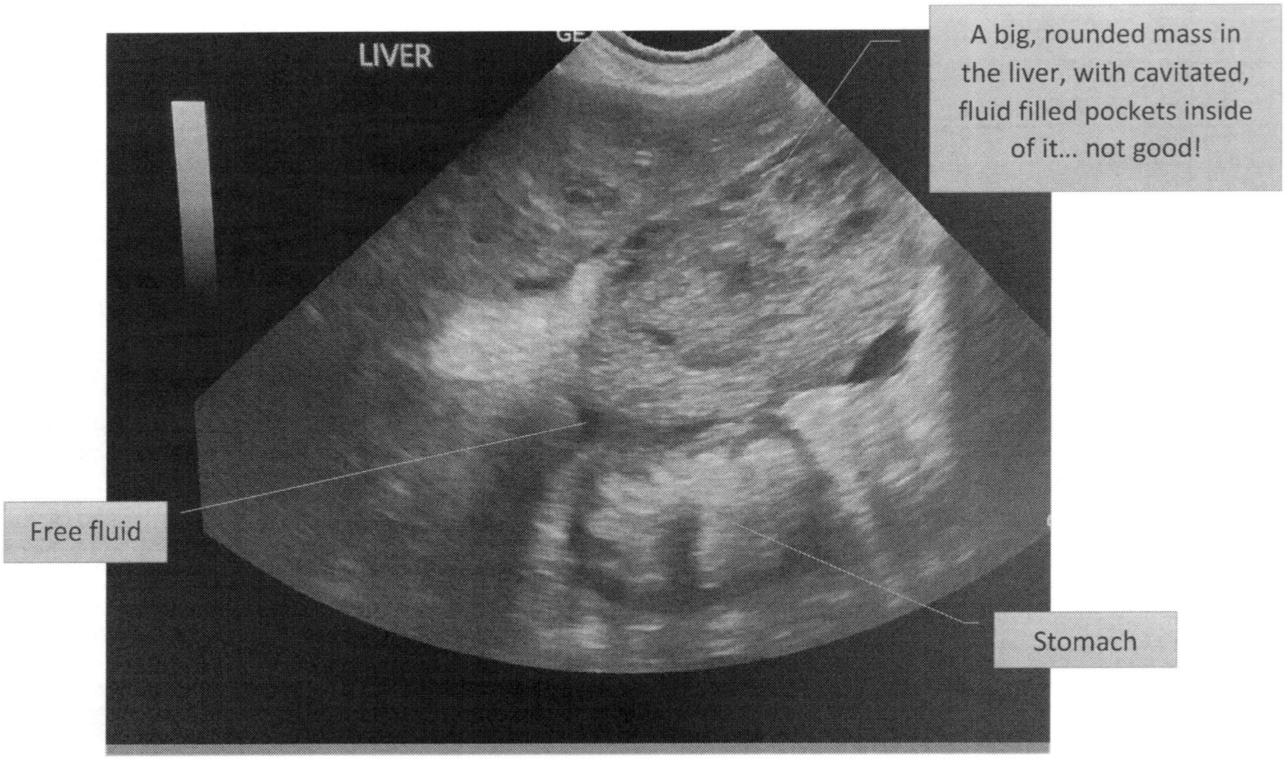
LIVER
A big, rounded mass in the liver, with cavitated, fluid filled pockets inside of it... not good!
Free fluid
Stomach

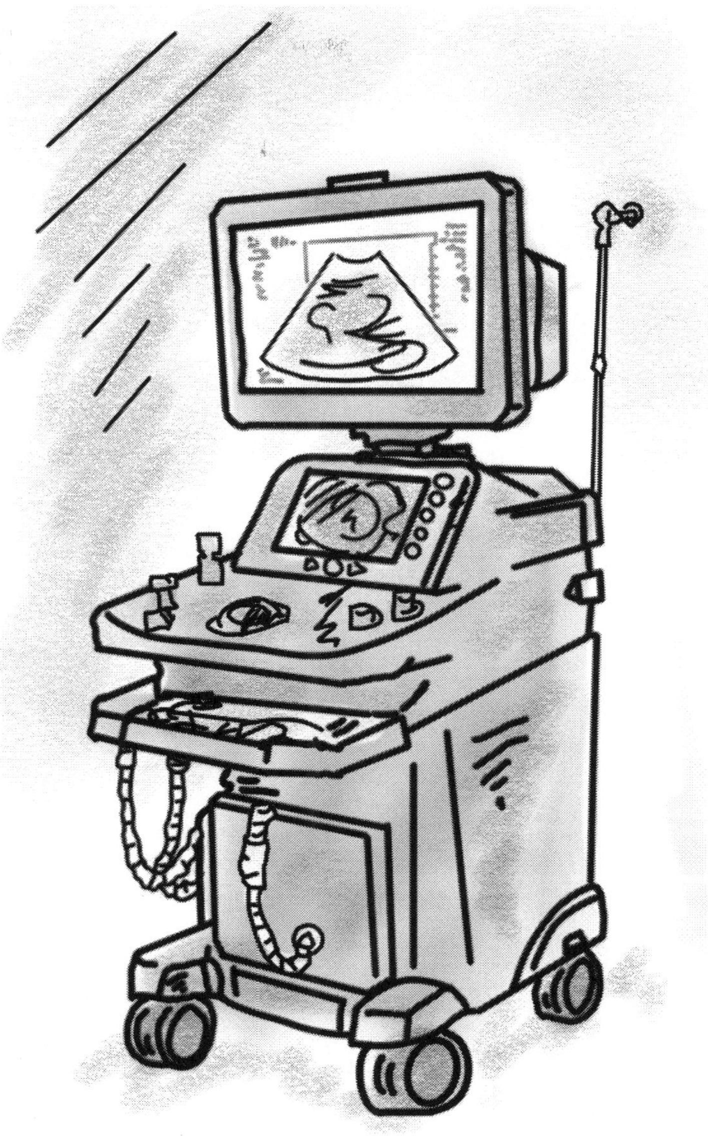

Whoa! There is indeed free fluid in this patient's abdomen! Free fluid is noted in the DH view, the HR view (also called HRU), and a little bit in the SR view near a kidney. This would give a fluid score of 3/4 (or 2.5/4 if you use the 0.5 scale to say there's only a little fluid near the kidneys).

So, plenty of free fluid. Now you definitely look at differentials like ascites, hemoabdomen, and uroabdomen. You can probably rule out things like GDV and food bloat and pain from this list, since they wouldn't usually cause lots of free fluid by themselves. You've learned a lot from this quick ultrasound! In fancy doctor words, we'd say an AFAST has a "high diagnostic yield."

But wait! There's more. The more focused views of this guy's liver look weird. There's a really rounded something on the back edge of the liver, and it's probably not a snowflake or a jolly old snowman either. It's mottled (spotty with dark and light areas) and very discrete (has edges you can follow). This could be a weirdly shaped liver lobe (which would be abnormal) or it could be a tumor. Uh oh!

What tests should you do to help investigate this further?

Go back to the list of possible tests and pick some more…

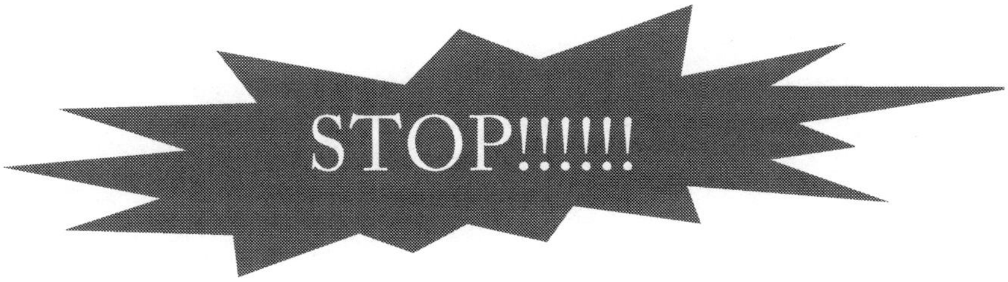

If you picked testing for ringworm, that is not a good choice. If you picked ultrasound you were not paying attention. We did that already! Though it would not be wrong to recommend a more detailed ultrasound than an AFAST. Sometimes (depending on a clinic's set up) a specialist will be called in for a more detailed diagnostic ultrasound.

But in the meantime, I would pick: **bloodwork** and **cytology** (of the fluid from your patient's belly). You can run a few simple tests (like the ones you do on the blood) on the fluid from the abdomen (that's usually called "**fluid analysis**" for obvious reasons).

You found fluid. Test it! Stare at it! Figure out what it is. Just don't lick it… You carefully poke a needle into a pocket of free fluid (after asking Monkfruit's owner, and giving a slight touch of sedation because he's a wiggly corgi). The stuff you get out looks like a clear yellowish fluid with some dilute blood. It doesn't smell like urine and is not straight blood. That's probably not good, is it? It's probably time to panic, but you're too tired… You hand the fluid-filled syringe to your trusty assistants and ask them to make you a slide to examine on the microscope, test the fluid, and run bloodwork while the slide dries.

While these are running, you decide to talk to Monkfruit's owner about what you've found so far. This is a bold move, since you don't have all your tests done yet. Part of the art of being a veterinarian is reading people and deciding how and when to communicate news. You have the impression that Piper Larsen will appreciate a more gradual approach to bad news and decide to talk about your findings as you get them so she can start to process them internally.

"So… Monkfruit's leaking inside, and you think you found a possible tumor in the liver?" She summarizes the conversation with an acuteness that proves her mind to be much neater than her exterior.

"Yes. That's a good way to summarize it."

She nods, taking this bad news calmer than you expected. "I work in the medical profession too," she says, "so it makes sense."

This is a phrase that can mean many things. "Ah!" you say, with a highly calculated vagueness that can also mean many things.

You leave the room and find more test results to look over. Remember, for some hints about reading bloodwork panels, you can check out the Appendices of this book. After all a good clinician is not someone who knows all the facts: it's someone who knows where to find the facts and how to piece them together to tell what they mean.

Da Bloods

Client: Larsen, Piper	Species: Canine	Sex: MC
Patient: Monkfruit	Breed: Welsh Corgi	
Patient ID: 03762		

Chemistry Panel

TEST	RESULT	FLAG	REFERENCE RANGE[iv]
ALT	128	H	8.2-57 IU/L
ALP	865	H	10.6-101 IU/L
GGT	10	H	1.0-9.7 IU/L
tBili	0.3		0.1-0.6 mg/dL
Glucose	84		62-108 mg/dL
Cholesterol	113		116-254 mg/dL
Total Protein	6.9		5.5-7.5 g/dL
Albumin	2	L	2.6-4.0 g/dL
Globulin	4.9	H	2.1-3.7 g/dL
Calcium	16.3	H	8.7-11.8 mg/dL
BUN	24		8.8-26 mg/dL
Creatinine	1.1		0.5-1.6 mg/dL
Phosphorus	2	L	2.9-6.2 mg/dL
Sodium	143		140-154 mEq/L
Potassium	3.2	L	3.8-5.6 mEq/L
Chloride	112		102-117 mEq/L

Client: Larsen, Piper	Species: Canine	Sex: MC
Patient: Monkfruit	Breed: Welsh Corgi	
Patient ID: 03762		

CBC

TEST	RESULT	FLAG	REFERENCE RANGE[V]	
WBC	20.3	H	6.0-17.0	$10^3/\mu L$
Neutrophils	10		3-11.4	$10^3/\mu L$
Monocytes	1.1		0.15-1.35	$10^3/\mu L$
Lymphocytes	23	H	1-4.8	$10^3/\mu L$
Eosinophils	0.6		0.1-0.75	$10^3/\mu L$
Hematocrit (HCT)	43		37-55	%
MCV	69		60-77	fL
Platelet Count	302		200-900	$10^3/\mu L$

What do you think about those results? It's easy to get lost in the details of a bloodwork panel, and helpful to "zoom out" and look at trends to get the overall picture. In Monkfruit's bloodwork we see several troubling trends stand out:

- Liver numbers (ALT, ALP, GGT) are high.
- Protein levels (Albumin) are wonky (an important technical term). Albumin is made in the liver. If the liver is failing, you might see low albumin.
- WBC (white blood cell) counts are really high, lymphocytes (a type of white blood cells) in particular. Globulin is made by lymphocytes. If something is making lymphocytes multiply like madmen, you might get high globulin counts.
- Calcium is really high. I'll throw in a free factoid (because I happen to have gone to vet school): a big cause of high calcium levels in dogs is cancer. This is called hypercalcemia of malignancy.

Can you think of something you've already found which could cause this stuff?

That's right! A big ol' tumor on the liver could affect liver function. If that lump on the ultrasound is a type of cancer affecting lymphocytes (i.e. lymphoma or lymphosarcoma) then it would make the lymphocyte counts really high and raise the globulin counts. This is going from bad to worse…

That was the bloodwork, what about the fluid in the abdomen?

Your lovely assistant Lolita gives you fluid analysis results.

- The total protein content of the fluid was 3.6.
- The PCV of the fluid was 12%.
- The creatinine of the fluid was 0.2 and the potassium level in the fluid was 2.9

"I see lots of cells under the microscope, but you'll have to tell me what they are," she adds (as you frantically try to scribble all the numbers she's spouting out onto the closest sticky note).

"Nice work Lolita!" You wisely decide not to follow up with, "What does that mean?" since you're the doctor and everyone expects *you* to tell them what it all means. What kind of fluid could this be? To answer that, you'll need to understand the common types of fluid a dog can get in the abdomen (i.e. some differentials for fluid in the abdomen), and how to tell them apart. And to do that, you'll need ***A TEXTBOOK!!!!!***

"Umm… Be right back!"

You scurry into your office.

Here (says your pal the textbook) are three different kinds of fluids you can find in an abdomen:

- **Ascites fluid** is described as either transudate, modified transudate, or exudate.
  - Transudate: total protein less than 2.5 mg/dL and few to no cells.
  - Modified transudate: total protein of 2.5-5 md/dL, and more cells.
  - Exudate: total protein greater than 4 mg/dL and lots of cells (with inflammatory cells especially).
- **Blood** in the abdomen from cytology will usually have a PCV (packed cell volume) that is about the same as the PCV (also called the HCT or "Hematocrit") on your blood panel.
- **Urine** in the abdomen will have a higher creatinine and higher potassium than the circulating blood on your panel.

So which of these three kinds of fluids is this? Time to solve this case. What do you think is going on?

And your diagnosis is?

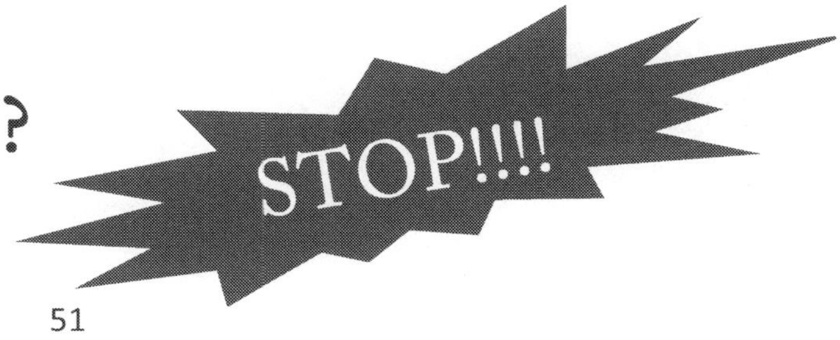

You got it on the first try! Well done. This here liquid's **ascites fluid**, more specifically a **modified transudate**. That's a kind of fluid you often see with (surprise surprise!) neoplasia (cancer).

So, what do the cells under the microscope look like? Let's take a peek!

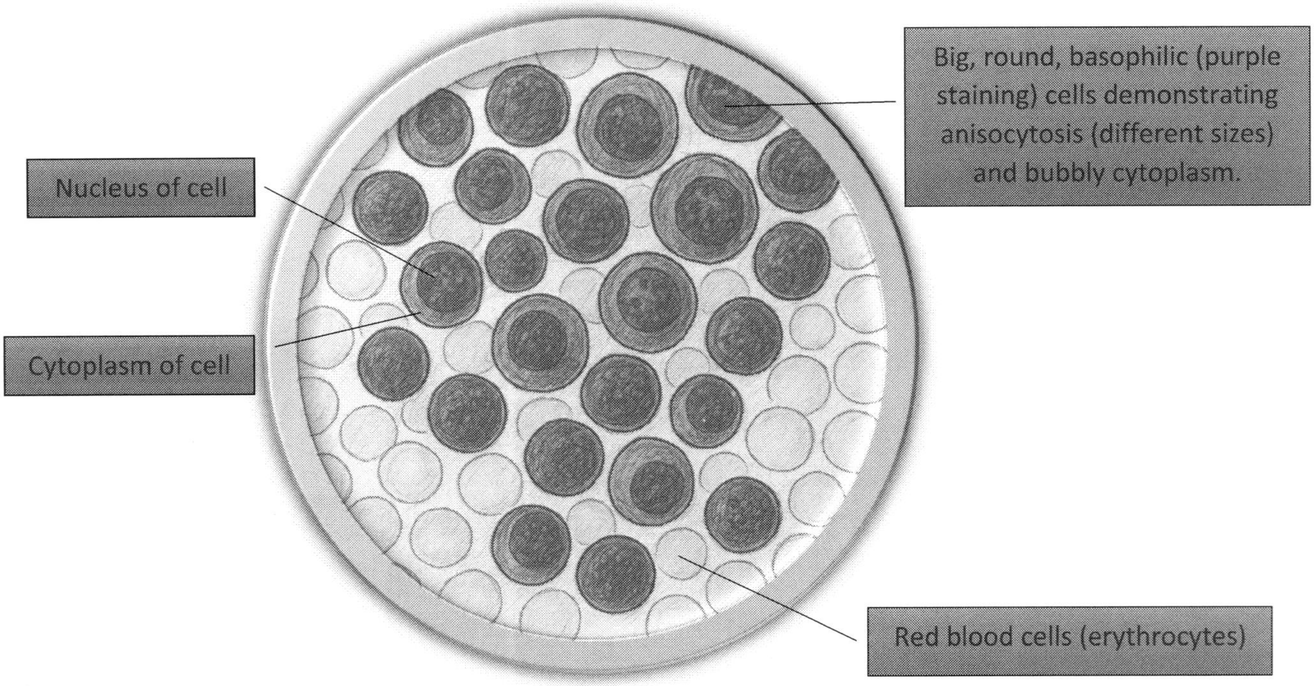

"BLOBS! AHHHH! Look at all these pretty little blobs in here, guys…" is what you definitely do not say to your technicians (not after that first time you said it as a new grad). Instead, you make wise "mmm-hmm" sounds and interesting noises.

Those pale round guys in the background are red blood cells. I like to remember they are about 7 microns in diameter, to help mentally size up other cells. The big blue round guys are lymphocytes. The smaller ones with the nucleus filling most of the cell (the nucleus is the circle inside the cell) are mature lymphocytes. The bigger ones with some bubbly open space between the nucleus (that bubbly space is called cytoplasm) are lymphoblasts. A lymphoblast is a type of immature lymphocyte (you know, the kind that constantly plays pranks on his friends and can't be trusted babysitting).

Keep in mind this is a black and white picture because I, your hungry author, am too poor to pay for color printing. Lymphocytes are usually blue with blood stains used in clinics, and red blood cells are usually reddish. If you tell enough of your friends to buy this book, maybe I can make another edition with color.

So… Now you have to go tell this client that her beloved corgi hound has **cancer**, which is probably **hepatic lymphoma**. Poor Monkfruit has a big cancerous tumor on his liver. You've collected enough evidence to have a high degree of confidence but can't be completely sure without biopsies (cutting out a chunk of tissue) and histopathology (sending said chuck of tissue to a lab). The one good thing is that you haven't found evidence of other tumors.

Lymphoma is a type of cancer that can come in several different forms. It is generally divided into B cell or T cell lymphoma. It can "settle in" lots of different types of tissue: including skin, abdominal organs, lymph nodes, bone marrow, and lungs. Some forms tend to spread around the body (metastasize) more readily than others. Its aggressiveness can be graded (by sending a sample of a tumor into a lab) to see how likely it is to spread. Its extent (how far it has spread in the body) is described by its stage. There are five stages in canine lymphoma. Prognosis is probably not great, but the stage and grade will tell us more about the chances of treating Monkfruit meaningfully. Usually high calcium is a bad prognostic factor. Lymphoma in the liver generally has a poorer prognosis than other types, unfortunately.

You explain all these things to Piper and those green eyes hid behind layers of grime get a bit soggy, but she holds it in with the stoicism characteristic of her Viking ancestry.

"What are our options from here, Doctor?" she asks.

That's a good question. And like so many conundrums of life, 'tis much easier when posed as multiple choice. What should you recommend?

Choose from this list of treatment options.

What is your treatment plan? (pick several)

a) Antibiotics

b) Diuretics

c) Euthanasia

d) Heart medication

e) Hospitalization and IV fluids

f) Nausea medications

g) Oxygen supplementation

h) Pain medications

i) Probiotics

j) Referral to a specialist

k) Surgery

l) Therapeutic adomnocentesis — Draining fluid from his belly.

m) Vitamins and Minerals

Remember that here in the nitty-gritty, blood-drenched, tear-stained trenches of the real world there is usually more than one acceptable way to treat a case.

Here's the options I would discuss: **f, h, j, and l… or c.**

To treat Monkfruit I would start with some **pain medications** (for abdominal discomfort), and **nausea medication** in the form of a maropitant injection (a medication to prevent vomiting, as well as help with discomfort). Keep in mind that this patient has liver dysfunction, which means that drugs metabolized in the liver (i.e. most of them) could last longer in his bloodstream.

After that I would feel out the client's goals very carefully to figure out where we go from here.

There are a couple of major options.

1. If the owner wants to treat Monkfruit's cancer, you should **refer to a specialist**, in this case a veterinary oncologist. This will be expensive, and some treatments (like chemotherapy) can be hard for Monkfruit to go through. If the tumor has not spread extensively, the oncologist might recommend surgery to remove the tumor. (By the way, surgery was not a bad pick off the treatment list, but in almost all cases it not be performed by you, but by the specialists.)
2. If she does not want to treat Monkfruit, then it would not be wrong to offer **humane euthanasia**. You've found a bad disease, suspect a poor prognosis, and the patient is suffering.
3. If she is on the fence, you could discuss **therapeutic abdominocentesis** just to make the patient more comfortable while his medications kick in. Be careful with this one. If you took out too much fluid from the abdomen, you could reduce his albumin levels dangerously and potentially drop his blood pressure enough to cause shock. The fluid is going to return at some point as well, so this is not a permanent solution.

Miss Larsen surprises you. She would like to see a specialist. You gladly give little Monkfruit some medications to help with the pain, nausea, and abdominal discomfort. You fill out an online referral form for an oncologist in a big clinic in Albuquerque, and wish Piper and Monkfruit all the best.

"Let me know how things go, and how I can help down the road," you generously say as she leaves.

It's 5 am now, and Greg Smith walks in the lobby as Piper Larsen walks out. He waves at her cheerily as she leaves. You and your technicians register surprise upon your countenances.

"That was the receptionist at my dentist's office…" he mentions. You had a feeling Piper's "medical experience" meant something along those lines.

"Mr. Smith, you weren't supposed to be here for another couple hours," Graham chides. Since this is

Abdominocentesis: inserting a needle into the abdomen to check and/or remove fluid.

an overnight clinic, you are open only in the "off hours" to handle emergencies when the other clinics are closed. You send any patients you've hospitalized to their regular daytime clinics when they open so you can go home.

"Yeah, but Angie is mad about Siegfried, and won't let me in the house. And I'm tired of hanging out at the Waffle Barn down the street. I tried to sleep in the car, but it's cold and that creepy…um…person is still in your parking lot. Can I visit Siggy for a bit?"

"Sure," Lolita sighs.

Graham asks you to go with them so Lolita isn't alone in the back with a client. "I'm gonna go ask Doug to sleep somewhere else tonight."

"You don't need me to come?"

Graham shrugs. "Doug's fine. He's a veteran. I'm more worried about fancypants Greg there…"

"In that case, why don't you offer Doug a cup of coffee?" you suggest, poking your head out the door a minute. "It is pretty cold out." It looks like snowflakes are drifting through the deep night sky.

Graham nods. "You've got a good heart, Doc!"

You mutter something about how 'tis the season for good cheer (since you've never been good at taking compliments) and shuffle down the hall. You make small talk with Greg Smith and try to act like you're not watching him for shady behavior. It's time for Siggy's vitals and Lolita reads you off his blood pressure, heart rate, respiratory rate, and temperature.

Oh yeah… When you hospitalize a patient in the ER you set up a treatment sheet that tells your technicians what treatments need to happen when and what to check on at certain times. Most places have a digital treatment sheet with special software that turns all red and angry (and sometimes beeps annoyingly) whenever treatments are missed. Some clinics still use paper forms.

Either way, write out a treatment and monitoring plan that will keep your team on the same page about these cases (since the more complicated, critical cases get hospitalized). Treatment sheets are even more important on nights when there are several patients hospitalized. If the clinic is set up well, technicians will run on "autopilot" doing treatments and recording vitals, which makes your job a bit like an orchestra conductor: you set up and tweak treatment plans to guide the nurses who do the hands-on work, all to make a lovely composition of happy animals.

"Are those good numbers?" Mr. Smith asks. You assure him Siggy's vitals are within normal limits. "What's she giving him in that IV line?"

"That's methadone. It's an opioid pain medication, sorta like morphine…" you explain.

The light in Greg's eye makes you uncomfortable. "Yeah? Siggy's getting the good stuff!" he laughs. "Not gonna make him an addict like some folks I know, is it?"

"Er… No. It won't."

"You, um…you have drugs like that around here, do you?"

Your sleep deprived mind becomes aware of alarm bells and red lights strobing at the periphery of your consciousness. "Every clinic's got some controlled drugs like methadone."

Fortunately, before you can blurt out more little details about where the lockbox is and who keeps the keys to these DEA controlled drugs that bad dudes would love to steal and sell on the street, the doorbell rings.

Another emergency calls!

Case #3

"GAAAAH! Little bugs! Little bugs!" The quiet of the night is split by harsh yells from the lobby. "Tiny little bugs! They're all over him I tell you!"

You walk Greg Smith to the lobby to find Graham and a shabby-looking guy wearing three old coats (who you deduce must be Doug) staring at an elderly man. Graham is trying to calm him, but he is hopping up and down with a small ball of fluff that you suspect to be a Shih Tzu. This hopping individual is red in the face and talking so loudly and excitedly that he sounds drunk. Graham loads him in a room and tells you that no, this new client is not drunk, he's just insane.

"Well…" you sigh. "That's better, I guess?" You will come to learn that long ER shifts tend to bring dumb words out of you. "What's he here for?"

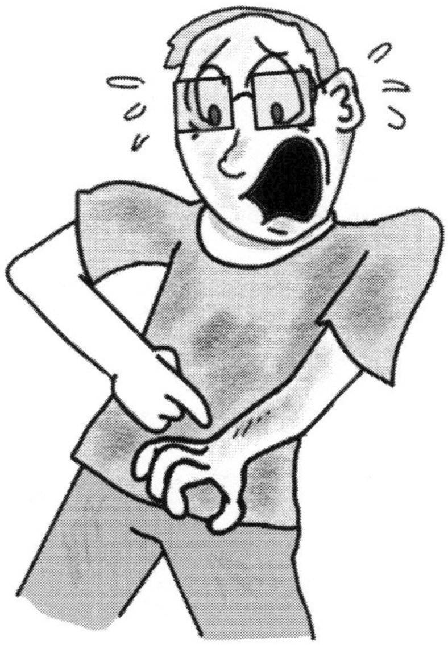

"Sounds like his dog has little bugs…" Graham grins.

You roll your eyes and fearlessly step into Exam Room 1. The first thing you notice about this worried-looking elderly gentleman is that he won't stop scratching his arms and legs. You shake his proffered hand with understandable reluctance.

"Nice to meet you d-d-doctor. My name is Harold Wibbly, and this is Ham. We have bugs…"

"Um… Can you describe these bugs?" You wisely slip on some gloves for the exam.

Scratch! Scratch! Scratch! "Th-th-they're like tiny white ants mostly. I first saw them on Ham on S-S-S-Sunday. But tonight I keep seeing them on me t-t-too. Those are ticks, right?"

"I don't know, Mr. Wibbly," you wisely avoid committing to a diagnosis before you've done an exam.

Step 1 – Organize the History

Signalment:

7 years old

Male neutered

Shih Tzu

Presenting Complaints:

Alleged bugs all over man and dog

Step 2 – Gather Clues

Physical Examination:

Abdominal palpation: Unremarkable. No splinting or tensing. No obvious distention or fluid wave noted. No mass or foreign bodies palpated.

Attitude: Bright, alert, and responsive.

Cardiac: No murmur or arrhythmia noted. Strong and synchronous femoral pulses.

Ears: Swollen canal noted AU (both ears). A moderate amounts of black, ceruminous, odiferous debris.

Eyes: NSF.

Integument: There is a small scab behind the right ear, and two small scabs on the patient's back. Otherwise no wounds or sores are noted, no rashes, no hair loss. Normal skin turgor. No visible ectoparasites that you can find. You do not see any "flea dirt" (little black specks of flea poop). You do not see any scabs that would be associated with ticks.

Lymph Nodes: NSF.

Musculoskeletal: NSF, weight bearing on all four limbs

Neurologic: BAR, normal menace response and palpebral reflexes noted OU, normal conscious proprioception on all four paws

Oronasal: Heavy dental calculus in general with inflamed gums.

Respiratory: Normal respiratory rate and normal respiratory effort (the patient is eupneic). All lung fields sound clear with your stethoscope.

Urogenital: Urinary bladder palpates normally

Vitals: Mucous membranes are pink and moist. CRT is less than 2 seconds.

Ceruminous: waxy; this refers to ear wax in particular.

Debris: a fancier way to say "gunk."

Eupneic: a fancy way to say "breathing normally" in a single word.

Odiferous: bad smelling.

There you have it! An organized history and signalment, and a physical exam performed… Now what are you going to do? Start by making a list of all the possible causes for Ham's presenting complaint.

Make a differential list for Ham's little bugs before you turn the page...

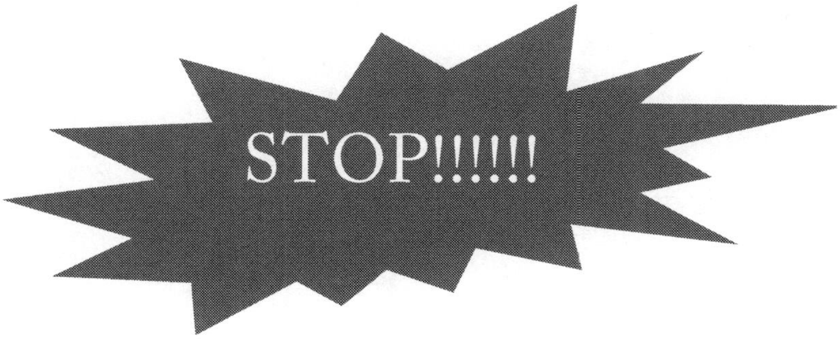

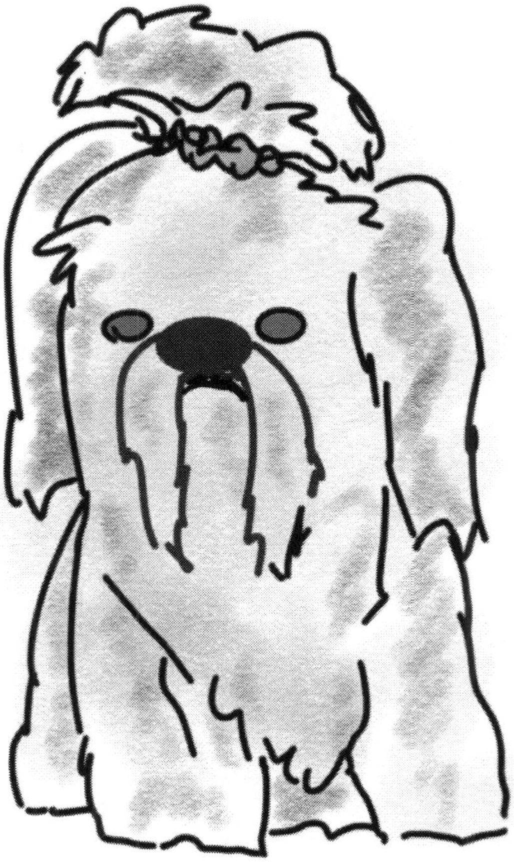

This is a tough one, since you don't exactly see anything wrong, and can't see evidence of the presenting complaint the owner describes. This is not an uncommon situation for veterinarians, probably because they work with a population of patients who can't speak for themselves and live with nervous people who love them.

But there are still several possibilities…

Differential Diagnoses:

- Visible ectoparasites (like fleas or ticks). These bugs are very small and good at hiding in the lush jungles of fur that grow on breeds like Shih Tzu dogs
- Microscopic ectoparasites (like mites or lice). These seem a bit less likely, since they're hard to see with the naked eye. But maybe Harold Wibbly has some kind of super vision?
- Insect hitchhikers. Could there have been some little bugs (sugar ants or some sort of lice or something) that crawled into Ham's fur and fell out on the way to the clinic?
- Skin condition. Exudative or suppurative skin condition that the owner is mistaking for parasites.
- Lunacy. Maybe your poor client is as nutty as a fruitcake. Maybe he's nuttier than a fruitcake, and is making all these little bugs up from thin air.

Congrats if you were able to think of some differentials!

You know what to do next…

Exudative: "goopy," a process that leaks fluid of some kind.

Suppurative: "nasty and goopy," a process that creates pus leaking from infection.

Decision time!

What tests do you want to run first?

Here's what you can do in your clinic:

- ✓ Basic bloodwork (a chemistry panel and CBC)
- ✓ Benchtop Ethylene glycol test
- ✓ Blood gas analysis
- ✓ Clotting times
- ✓ Cytology
- ✓ Fecal floatation and direct saline exam
- ✓ FeLV/FIV test
- ✓ Giardia test
- ✓ Heartworm test (with rickettsial diseases)
- ✓ Leptospirosis test
- ✓ Pancreatic lipase
- ✓ Parvo test
- ✓ Pregnancy test
- ✓ Radiographs (X-rays)
- ✓ Skin scraping
- ✓ Thyroid hormone level (T4)
- ✓ Ultrasound
- ✓ Urinalysis

What tests do you want to run?

____

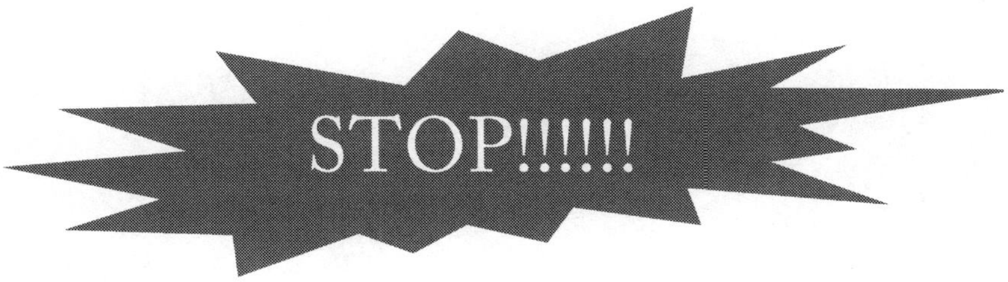

I, the all-knowing author of this book, would pick: **a skin scraping and maybe bloodwork**. If you picked **cytology** as well, then I say unto you a hearty and resounding "good job." Cytology is looking at cells on a slide. That's what we're going to do with our skin scraping (so technically a "skin scraping cytology").

Why bloodwork, you ask? Good question. I'm glad you asked that, you smart young vet you. There are some skin conditions that happen because of internal changes, such as liver disease or infection. Also, you're shooting in the dark, without any real reason for "little bugs" that you can find, and a general blood panel can tell you a lot about a dog's overall health.

You tell Harold all this. Then Graham tells Harold how much all this will cost. You find it helpful to distance yourself as much as you can from the financial aspects of a case to reduce the risk of cost overly affecting your medical recommendation and to reduce the risk of you being perceived as a salesman. That's why technicians usually go over the estimates in veterinary medicine. Harold says no to bloodwork, but is fine with you running a cytology of a skin scraping.

You scrape some skin near the scabs on this patient with a dulled sterile blade until a slight oozing of blood is visible. Then you put the samples on a slide or two with some mineral oil and a coverslip. You also do a spiffy thing called an acetate tape prep. That sounds fancy. But it just means you take some scotch tape and rub it over the patient's back before sticking it to a slide. This is a way to find certain types of bugs like sarcoptic mange, that like to move around over the fur.

You sit down to commune with a microscope. Tell me what you see…

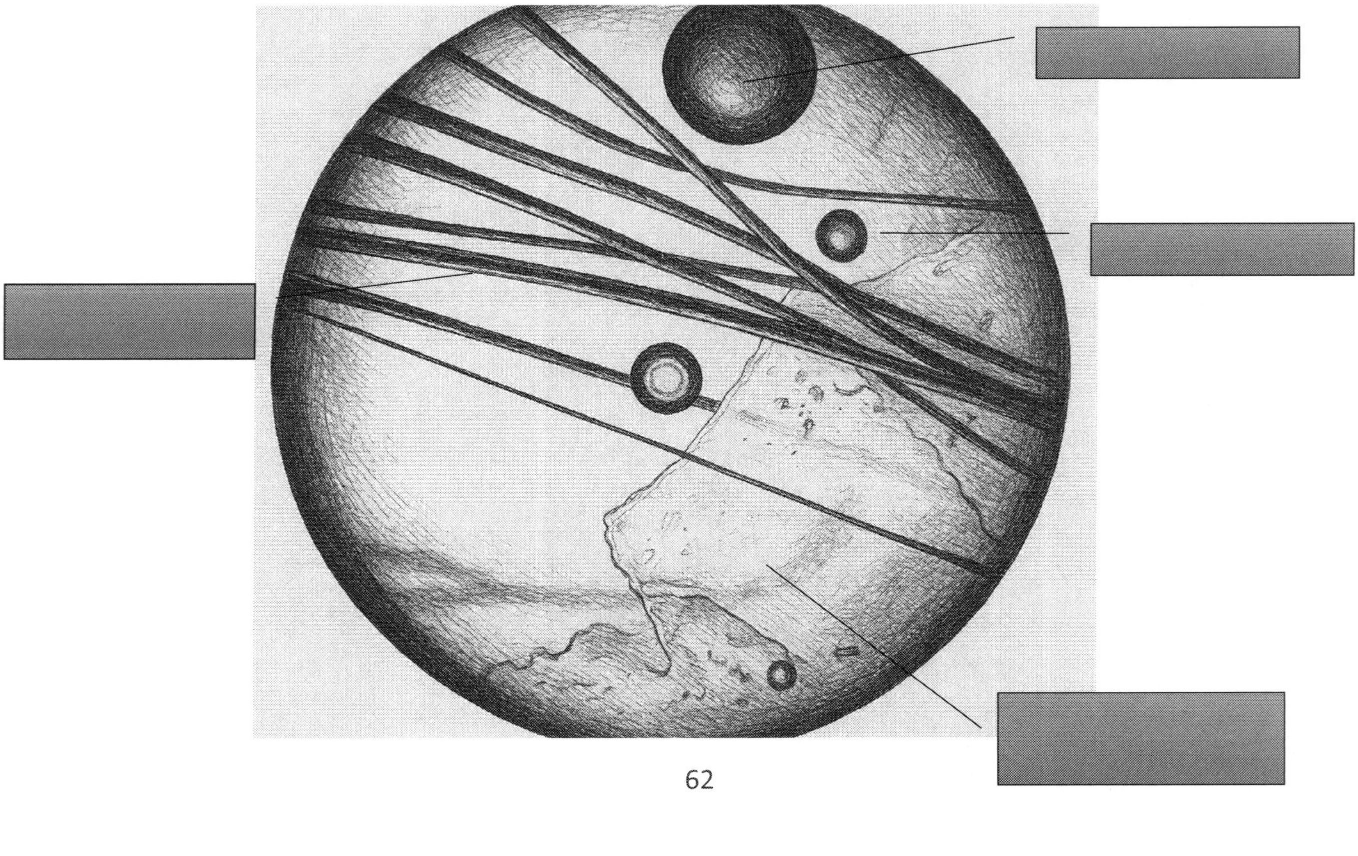

Here's what I see…

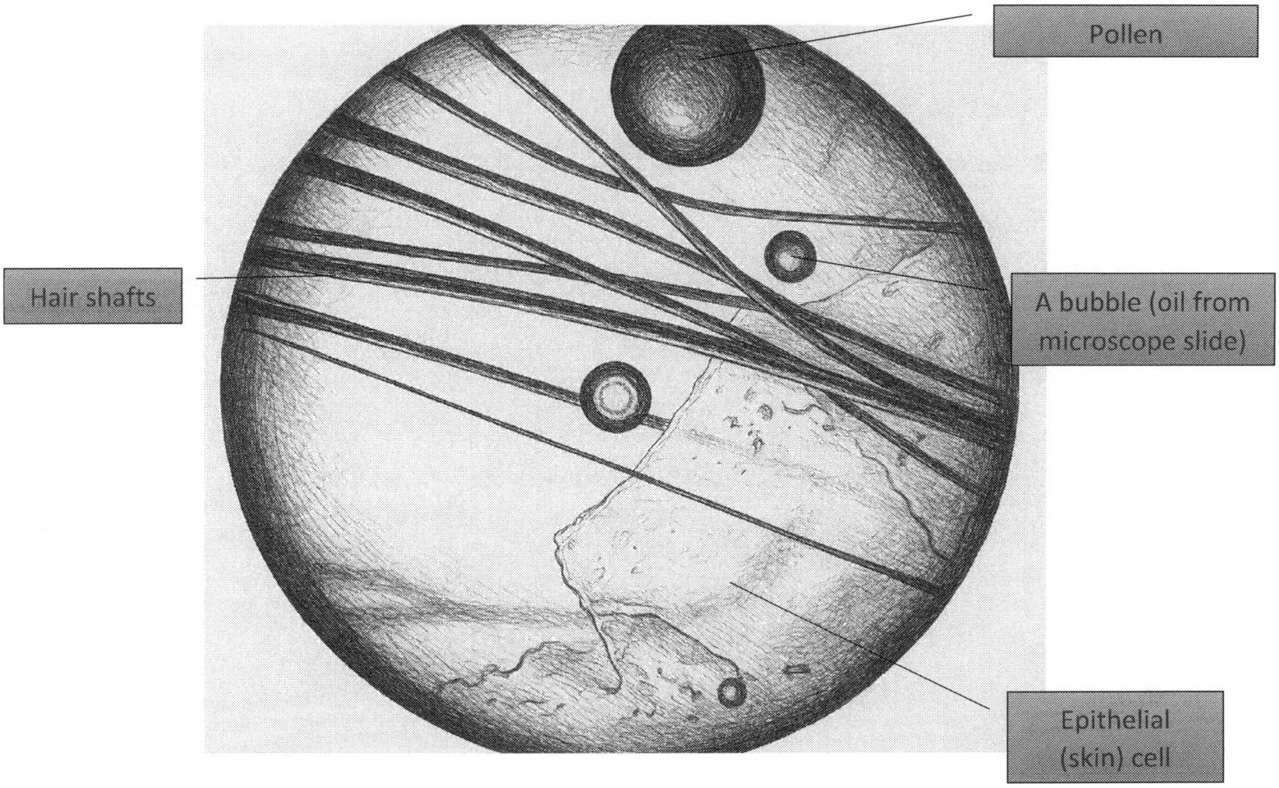

Hair, skin cells, some bubbles, pollen…

Those are normal things find on skin, aren't they? Consequently, they are not surprising things to see on a skin scraping. So "Nothing Interesting" is what you've found. Now go back to your differential list and cross off what you can. What you don't see are any mites or lice or signs of fleas.

And your diagnosis is?

What are you left with? What are you going to tell Mr. Wibbly these little bugs are?

____

STOP!!!!!

This is still a tough one. At this point your answer should be "I have no idea what these little bugs are." You do know some things the bugs probably are not. No fleas or ticks were seen on exam. No mites or lice were seen on cytology of a skin scraping. There are no signs of exudate or suppurative discharge from the scabs on this guy. So you've ruled those things out.

Mr. Wibbly did not approve bloodwork, so you can't completely rule out uncommon skin disease related to internal problems. But you haven't really found any real evidence of skin problems to start with. That leaves you with one more item on your differential list to call your most likely diagnosis:

Your client is crazy.

You remember reading about a condition called delusional parasitosis. This is a psychological disorder that involves a false belief that one is infested with "little bugs" despite healthcare professionals declaring otherwise. Morgellons Disease is a more commonly known form (which technically involves feeling phantom fibers in your skin). Your technician is grinning at you very annoyingly and you are tempted to blurt out "Darn it, Graham, I'm a veterinarian, not a psychiatrist!"

Instead, you diplomatically tell your client that you can't find any evidence of parasites. But since Ham is not on any flea and tick preventative, you're happy to write a script for a dose or two so he can cover that possibility. Then you wax even more diplomatic. "If you think these bugs are on you, Mr. Wibbly, I strongly suggest you see your own doctor… Just in case, you know." Now the psychosis diagnosis is squarely in the hands of the human-doctors where it ought to be!

Harold seems dissatisfied. But you can't make everyone happy. And one unexpected side effect of night-shift exhaustion is, when you're sleepy enough, you no longer care about making everyone happy.

You feel a bit envious of Siggy's owner, snoozing on the bench in your lobby next to… Wait. He's not there anymore. Doug is sipping gratefully on his coffee, but there is nobody else.

Noises come from the back of the clinic. SHHHHP! Clop! Clomp! Clop!

"Did Mr. Smith leave?" you yawn to Graham and Lolita, who are chatting at the front desk.

Tap! Tap! Tap! Clop!

"I guess so…" Lolita says. You become vaguely aware of footsteps and some clattering noises in the back of the clinic. "Er… If you and Graham (and Doug) are all here, and I'm here too, who is back there?"

Lolita steps briskly down the dark hallway and you follow. In the treatment area at the back of the clinic you find exactly…nothing. The flickering fluorescent light blinks at an empty room lined with kennels on one wall and lab equipment on the other. The slight *plop plip* of a leaky faucet in the central washtub treatment table is the only sound the fills the cavernous room.

"Um… Anyone here?" you ask the eerie shadows. The eerie shadows don't reply. The footsteps and the clattering are gone. "You heard those noises, didn't you?"

Lolita nods as she walks over to check that the safe which holds the control drugs is still locked (it is). "Maybe it was Sigbert?"

You walk through the alcove lined with cabinets full of drugs that serves as the clinic pharmacy, but still see nobody. Then you follow Lolita through the echoing shadows of the central hallway to the dog runs. You find Graham unhooking Sigbert's IV catheter from the fluid line. Mr. Smith is there too.

"Just checking out Sigbert," Graham comments. You're surprised to find it's already nearly 7 am, and you fumble around in proper doctor-pretending-he-can-still-tech fashion trying to help. Soon Mr. Smith is on the road to his primary care clinic, where your records have been emailed. When they open at 8 am you will call them to round (that means discuss the case).

But first you need to round with your technicians. "Was Sigbert's person in the back by himself?"

Graham shakes his head. "Naw, he came in the front door just a little bit after you two went back there. Said he was out smoking."

Huh. "Did you hear all those footsteps and clattering?"

Graham nods.

"Was someone else here?"

Graham and Lolita look at each other.

"What are you guys not telling me?"

"Nobody here but us, Doc," Graham answers cheerily.

"At least nobody with a body," Lolita adds.

"Um…"

They both laugh. "Pretty much all of us have heard weird noises on shifts before. Sometimes it's footsteps like this morning. Sometimes it's the jingle of a collar. But then there's nobody there."

"What are you saying?"

"It's the ghosts," Lolita blurts out, blunter than her compatriot.

"The what now?" You rub your ears.

"Every ER's got ghosts," Graham says matter of factly. You'll come to find that this is true as your career progresses. There is not an overnight clinic or 24-hour ER you work in that does not have rumors of ghosts. It's probably a function of gathering sleepy people with big hearts and good imaginations into a strange building to spend the night together. When that strange building is old and run down and creepy, the chances of ghost stories are multiplied a dozen-fold.

"They don't hurt anyone or anything," Lolita clarifies. "You just hear them sometimes."

"THEM? How do you know there's more than one?"

She shrugs. "I guess I don't. But different people have heard different things. Tonight we heard footsteps. About a month ago, I heard music by the surgery suite that stopped when I walked in."

"Yeah. They're not always human ghosts," Graham adds. "One night I heard a dog whining. Thing is, we hadn't hospitalized anything that night. When I went back, I couldn't find a thing."

"I mean, it makes sense. We see a lot of death here." At this point you'd rather not know more, but Lolita continues merrily. "And phantom doorbell rings are pretty common on my shifts too."

"Well… That could be pranksters, right?"

"Maybe…" They both shrug and stare at you seriously.

"The Christmas ghosts seem to be out though," Lolita adds. "The noises have been different lately." Graham shrugs. "No really! I've heard tapping on the walls and footsteps and shuffling: like Marley at a Christmas dance."

You shake your head and go to your office. You're too tired for this kind of thing. Napping around here just got harder, that's for sure.

Not long later, you finish your records and made your transfer call to Sigbert's primary care vet. Graham stops you on the way out the door.

"Oh, Doc! Do you mind signing the log before you go?"

"Captain's log?" you yawn, head filled with lines from your favorite science fiction show.

"Naw. Drug log."

"We used a couple of controlled drugs on the cases last night. I already filled the lines in, but the doctor on duty is supposed to double check and initial them." He hands you a notebook…

Controlled Substance Dispensing Log

Controlled Substance: Methadone Form: injectable Strength: 10mg/Ml Size: 10 mL

Date	**Animal/Owner Name**	**Amount Dispensed**	**Balance Remaining**	**Dr. Initials**

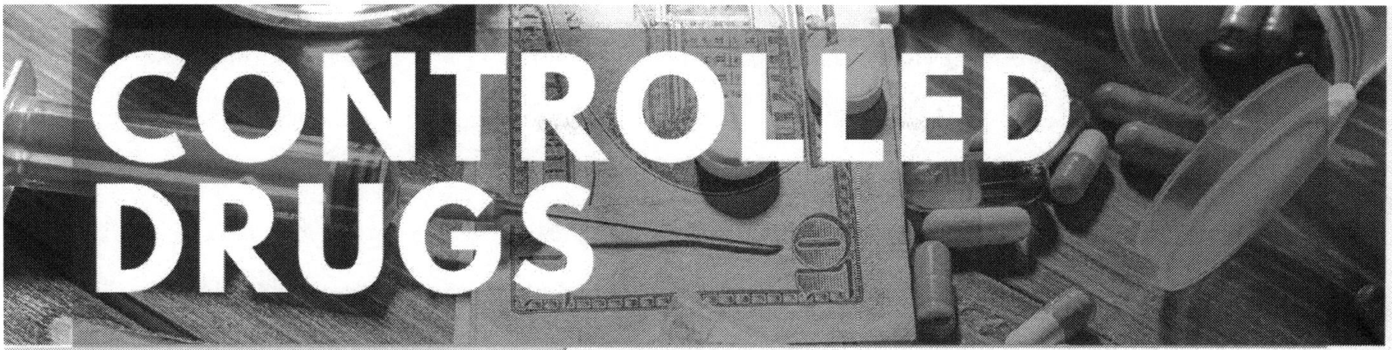

CONTROLLED DRUGS

1.15

MILLION

Deaths from drug overdose in the US since 1999

48.5M Americans over 12 years old (14.2% of population) suffer from a diagnosable substance use disorder

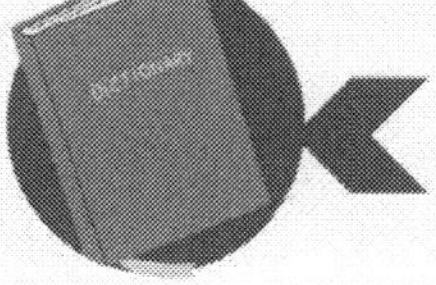

Definition

Drugs classified by the government as having potential for abuse are called controlled drugs.

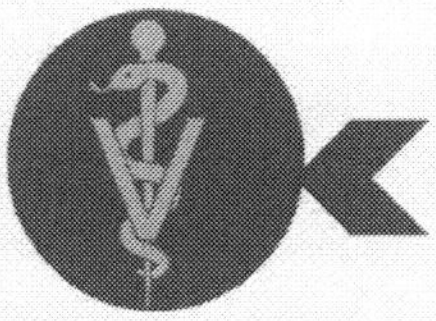

Some commonly used controlled drugs in vet medicine

Schedule II: fentanyl, hydrocodone, morphine
Schedule III: ketamine, codeine, buprenorphine
Schedule IV: diazepam, alfaxalone, butorphanol, phenobarbital
Schedule V: lomotil

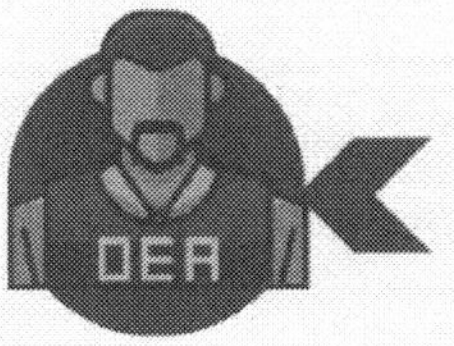

The DEA

The Drug Enforcement Administration (DEA) is the US agency responsible for enforcing laws about illegal drugs, and a special DEA number is needed to prescribe them.

DRUG SCHEDULES

Controlled drugs in the USA are classified into 5 different groups based on their risk for abuse.

Schedule I: highly addictive, no medical use (heroine, LSD, etc.)

Schedule II: Highly addictive, potential medical use (cocaine, oxycodone, etc)

Schedule III: Moderate abuse and addition potential (codeine, ketamine, etc)

Schedule IV: Low potential for abuse and addiction (Xanax, Valium, etc)

Schedule V: Lowest potential for abuse and addiction (cough syrups, etc)

Controlled drugs are very useful when used properly in medicine! They are destructive and deadly when used for fun.

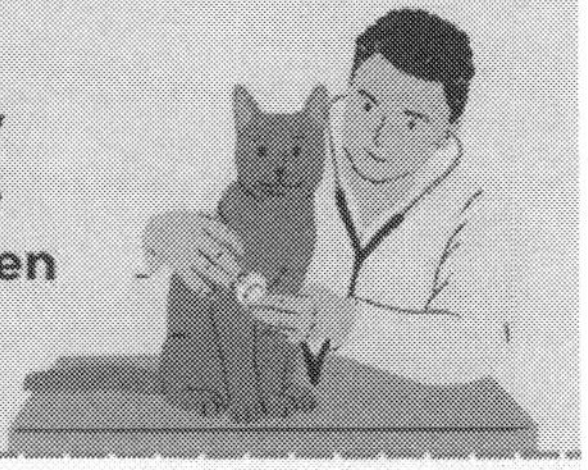

"Opiates are God's own medicine." - Sir William Osler, 19th century

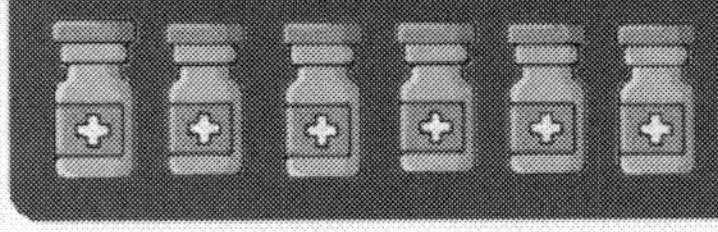

Statistical data obtained from NCDAS Drug Abuse Statistics. www.drugabusestatistics.org. 2025

A few pen strokes later and you're on your way home. Ah! The mattress never looked so good! You sigh as you get back at last to your bedroom. You take a quick shower and collapse for a well-earned rest.

Then you stare at the ceiling for a while.

One of the more challenging things about shift work is the havoc it plays on your biological clock. It's a common problem to feel exhausted after a long shift but to be kept awake by the stream of adrenaline, which perversely refuses to dry up in the morning. You get up and watch a show. You're into sci-fi musical comedies right now, and season 3 of Starship Beethoven just dropped. It tickles your funny bone, and you laugh along with Ensign Adagio as he dances across planetoid Phargon-7. You speculate on the identity of the mysterious alien who accosts Science Officer Coda in the middle of Holobay B.

What it doesn't do is put you to sleep. You sigh and walk to the kitchen to make a second breakfast. About halfway through a bowl of cereal, you remember you promised to drive Sam to his doctor's appointment.

You make your way to Mac and Carley Fugal's front door. Mac went to undergrad with you, before going to pharmacy school. After he married Carley they'd moved nearby, and it was nice to become friends all over again. What was even nicer is that they agreed to foster young Sam. But since they both work, you help as much as you could with Sam's appointments and school schedule.

"Hey there!" Samuel flashes a big grin as he buckles in the back seat. "Did you fix some dogs last night?"

"A couple, yeah." You proceed to tell harrowing tales of last night's adventures while driving to the hospital. Soon you and Samuel Melendez step into an overflow parking lot a full block away from the hospital. The sun shines brightly down through a dry desert atmosphere which seems to defy the Christmas songs blaring over your car radio the entire drive.

Little Sam chats merrily about his day, which helps the anxious thoughts you carry about your cases slide away. Most veterinarians have a very hard time letting a stressful case go. I have spent many wakeful nights (and days) second guessing my diagnosis and treatment decisions, stressing over whether they're helping my patient, and sweating about what my clients and colleagues must think of them. Almost invariably things turn out OK, but a vet's brain isn't trained to recognize that pattern. So it's really nice to have kids like Samuel in our lives, who remind us there are happy events and people who love us outside the clinic.

"Oh look!" Sam points to an odd-looking, twisted purple mess of a thing advertised on the waiting room TV. "It's a Squishwidget! Lots of my friends have those. Maybe I can get one when I'm grown enough to get a job."

You smile at the delight he exhibits at the creepy fangs drawn in yellow over the Squishwidget's bumpy surface. "You can squish it, and twist it, and even draw on it with a crayon!"

You can do all those things with a piece of paper too, you think. But you remember being a kid (so very, very long ago) and how exciting toys can be. Well, you know what to get your little buddy for Christmas. Then you notice the price tag. $47.99! You should have gone to school to be a toy maker! But since you didn't, it looks like you're gonna need to work another ER shift…

It doesn't take long for little Sam to get his injections. Soon you drop him back off with Carley, who thanks you for taking him to his appointment.

"Hey, how are the new night shifts going?"

"Had the first one last night," you yawn. "It was OK. Did a GDV surgery and met a ghost." That's the sort of comment you can't just leave floating in the air, and you are forced to give her more details. Christmas has traditionally been the time for swapping ghost stories after all.

"Crazy! Some of our friends are coming over for Starship Beethoven marathon Friday," she says. "Love to have you join us."

"Wow, I wish I could but I'm working another shift that night…" A serious downside to ER work, you're beginning to discover, is that you wind up working most of the hours your friends are partying.

A few days fly past. You finish a busy day at Noah's Haus Veterinary Clinic, just in time to run home and get your things for your second night shift at the ER. It's 5:30pm but rosy strips of sunset colors herald another fast-approaching winter darkness. There's a battered gray pickup in the parking lot when you drive up. A lanky guy in a black cowboy hat with a medium-sized dog nods at you from the bench in the lobby while you self-consciously walk past to deposit your backpack and laptop in the office.

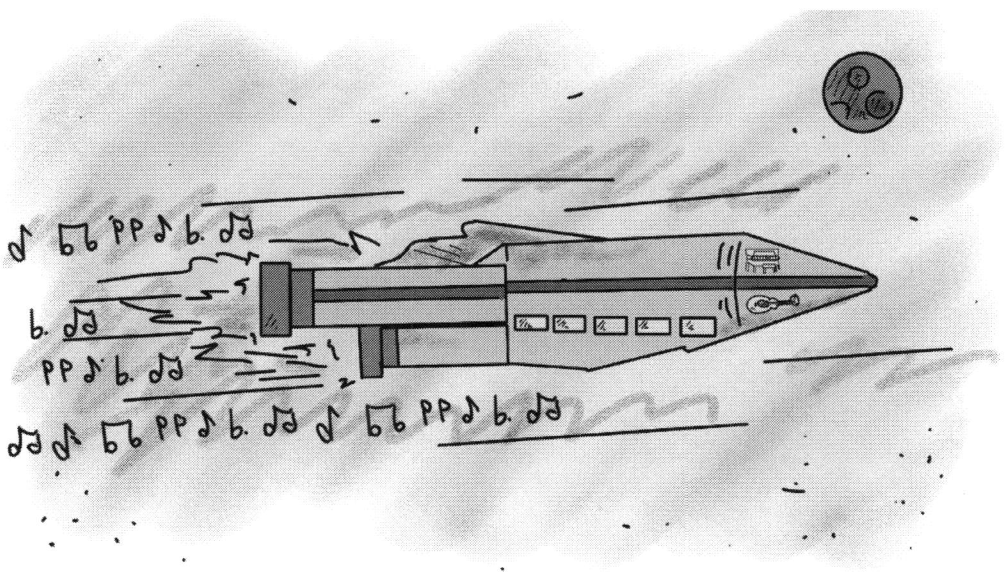

Case #4

Soon a middle-aged technician comes to tell you about the case. "Hi Doc, ready to work?" he grins at his own little joke as he knocks at the office door frame.

"Fred! Fred Kawalkovitch! I thought it was you at the front desk! Hi."

"Hi!"

"I didn't know you worked here too." Fred is one of the technicians from your daytime practice. He recently cut back on his days there, which made you sad. Fred may be the most efficient and knowledgeable technician you've ever worked with. He's also a confirmed geek who likes most of the things that get you excited, and is just fun to hang out with.

"Yeah. I've been pulling some shifts here and working less daytimes. Gives me time to work on some…er…other projects. So! I've got a snakebite case…" Fred proceeds to tell you the sad, sad tale.

Mr. James P. Chissum is here with his German Shepherd named Bullet. Bullet was out in the yard at his ranch house today and met with an unfriendly reptile (the kind with rattles on one end and fangs on the other, you know the sort). By the time James drove here, the pup's face had swollen significantly. No coughing, sneezing, vomiting, or diarrhea has been noted. She's been healthy before tonight. She's on a regular heartworm preventative and a flea and tick preventative, but no other medication. He already gave Fred permission for a pain injection if needed.

You nod with the consummate coolness befitting a nighttime, superhero, ER vet, and head into Exam Room 1 to see a swollen pooch. A firm handshake from a weathered cowboy starts off the proceedings.

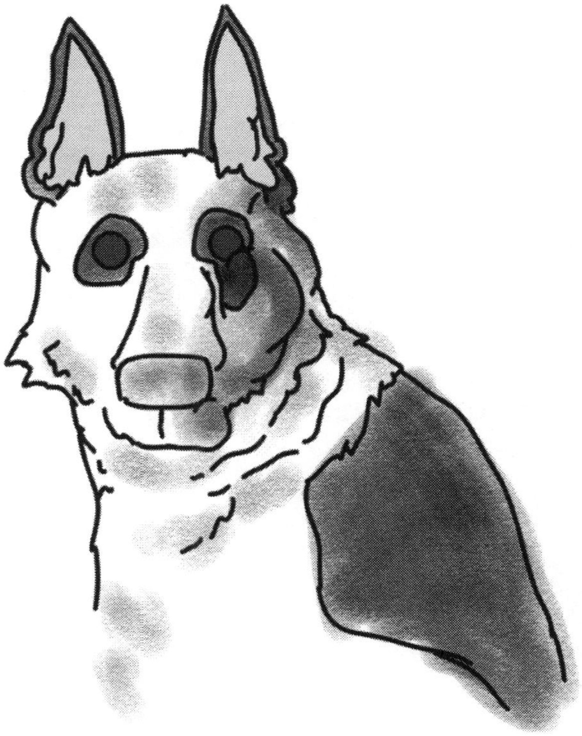

"Howdy! James P. Chissum. Glad to meet ya."

"Glad to meet you. This must be Bullet. Poor girl looks awfully swollen." You refrain from telling him you thought she might be a capybara or a large mutant guinea pig when you saw her in the lobby, since her head is roughly the width of her neck. Fred restrains the patient while you do your physical exam.

Step 1 – Organize the History

Signalment:

7 years old

Female Spayed

German Shepherd dog

Presenting Complaints:

Swollen face

Suspected snake bite

Step 2 – Gather Clues

Physical Examination:

Abdominal palpation: Unremarkable. Pliable with no splinting noted. No distention or fluid wave noted. No obvious foreign body or mass palpated.

Attitude: Quiet, slightly depressed, but responsive.

Cardiac: No murmurs or arrhythmia noted. Strong femoral pulse noted bilaterally.

Ears: Canals appear clear with no swelling or discharge.

Eyes: Clear OU.

Integument: There is severe swelling (edema) over the upper lips bilaterally, worse on the left than the right side. A trickle of blood is visible from a small mark on the left upper lip, and the patient seems very painful when the area is palpated. No bruising is noted on the skin.

Lymph Nodes: Palpate normally.

Musculoskeletal: Weight bearing on all four limbs.

Neurologic: Mildly lethargic, but otherwise alert and responsive. Normal cranial nerve exam and normal conscious proprioception on all four paws.

Oronasal: Bruising and petechiation on the left side of the gums. Drooling.

Respiratory: Increased respiratory rate with no increase in respiratory effort. No cyanosis or distress.

Bilaterally: including two sides.
Cyanosis: a blue or purple color to the mucous membranes (usually seen in the gums and/or tongue best) from lack of oxygen circulating.
Petechiation: tiny spots covering the mucous membranes, usually a sign of blood clotting problems.

Urogenital: NSF.

Vitals: MM pink and moist. CRT<2 seconds.

Whelpers…

This hyar is a bit tricky pardners, 'cuz the differential list seems pretty dang obvious. We know what caused poor Bullet to swell a few extra calibers already, don't we? But it's always good practice to mull over a list of differentials, even when the answer to a case seems plain as the swollen nose on your patient's fat face.

What do you think?

Imagine that you didn't hear any of the story leading up to Bullet's swollen face, and think of as many things as you can that could cause her symptoms.

What's your differential list?

"The formulation of the problem is often more essential than its solution, which may be merely a matter of mathematical or experimental skill."
—Albert Einstein[vi]

Differential Diagnoses for Bullet's symptoms:

- Crotalid envomonation
- Hymenoptera or insect envenomation
- Hypersensitivity reaction
- Infection (such as abscess or cellulitis)
- Neoplasia
- Peripheral edema (conditions such as low albumin or vascular compromise)
- Trauma (especially blunt trauma like getting kicked or hit by a car)

Crotalid envomonation is the fancy doctor word for snakebite, at least in America. That's because the types of venomous snakes in America belong to the crotalus genus, also known as "pit vipers." These are rattlesnakes (of various species), copperheads, and cottonmouths. The only exception is the coral snake (who is not a crotalid), but he doesn't usually cause swelling like the pit vipers do. He just nukes your nervous system and kills you.

Decision time!

What tests do you want to run first?

Here's what you can do in your clinic:

- ✓ Basic bloodwork (a chemistry panel and CBC)
- ✓ Benchtop Ethylene glycol test
- ✓ Blood gas analysis
- ✓ Clotting times
- ✓ Cytology
- ✓ Fecal floatation and direct saline exam
- ✓ FeLV/FIV test
- ✓ Giardia test
- ✓ Heartworm test (with rickettsial diseases)
- ✓ Leptospirosis test
- ✓ Pancreatic lipase
- ✓ Parvo test
- ✓ Pregnancy test
- ✓ Radiographs (X-rays)
- ✓ Skin scraping
- ✓ Thyroid hormone level (T4)
- ✓ Ultrasound
- ✓ Urinalysis

What tests do you want to run?

Even though you pretty much know what happened,

what tests might still be helpful to run?

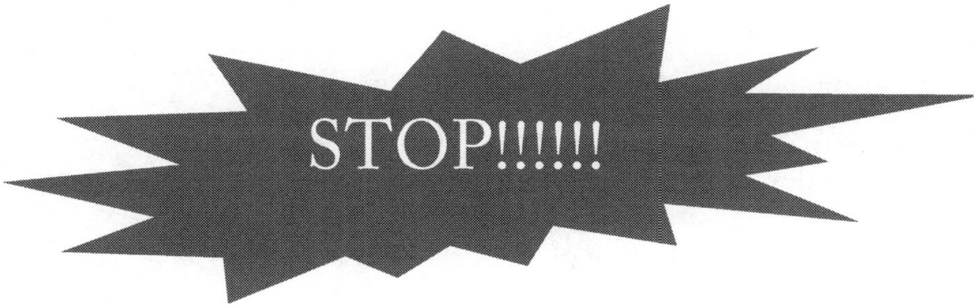

> "Take nothing on its looks;
> take everything on evidence.
> There's no better rule."
>
> -Charles Dickens, *Great Expectations*[vii]

As you consider these lists of possible tests to run within your mind's bunkhouse, your new rancher friend decides things for you.

"So I have the snake that bit ol' Bullet, if you want to see it, Doc." Mr. Chissum offers.

Staring at the snake that bit your patient is a pretty accurate test! You've seen a case or two in the past where the snake was killed and brought in with the patient to help identify it.

"Sure!" you reply with a naïve grin.

A few minutes later you hear rattling and shouting from the lobby. You find Mr. James P. Chissum holding a white bucket with a LIVE rattlesnake inside. There's no lid on the bucket. The snake is about three feet long and looks really, really annoyed about being lugged around in a bucket. He's coiled up, and rattling, and striking at the sides of the bucket.[6]

"Oh! Wow! Um… Yeah… Look at that," you find yourself stuttering as you peek into the bucket from far across the room. "That's a rattlesnake, sure 'nough! Why don't you take it back outside."

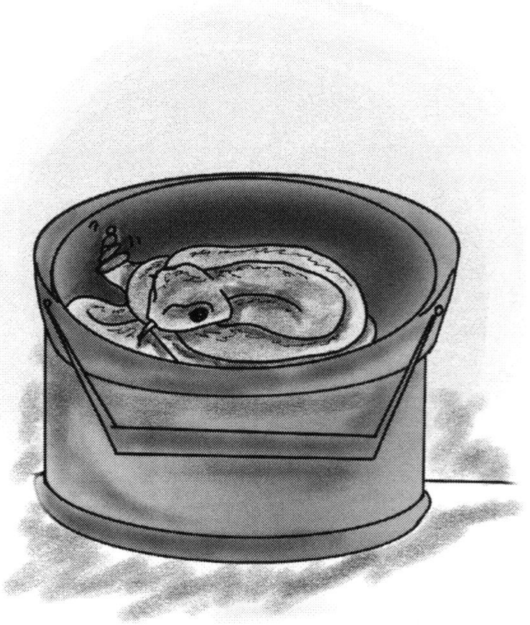

"Ah named 'im Fast Eddie," Chissum grins, pulling his hand back just before the snake strikes the upper rim of the bucket.

"Yeah? Looks, um, looks like an Eddie. Why don't we take Eddie outside, huh?"

"Doubt mah wife'll let me keep 'im though," Mr. Chissum laughs.

Not if she's halfway sane, you think. Fred and Lolita (who just came in) stare in silence during this bizarre turn of events. At least you have a definite diagnosis. Eddie's head width matches the two little puncture wounds on Bullet's swollen face nicely. Now it's time to figure out what to do about it.

After your client deposits his angry snake bucket back in his truck (hopefully not in the front seat) and comes back, you go over your recommendations.

Wall, Pilgrim, even though you're dang sure this is a rattler bite, yer still gonna run a couple of tests to see how bad the bite is. I would pick **clotting times** and a **CBC**. That's because snake venom can mess with platelets and clotting factors and cause serious coagulation (blood clotting) disorders that lead to shock.

[6] Just for the record, this exact thing did happen to me once at an ER I worked at. Sometimes truth is stranger than fiction!

Ah, clotting times! Don't be embarrassed if these look new. Many daytime clinics don't routinely run them. But they are quite useful to the ER clinician for many cases.

Here's what you get.

Client: Chissum, James P	Species: Canine	Sex: MN
Patient: Bullet	Breed: German Shepherd	
Patient ID: 02696		

Clotting Times

TEST	RESULT	FLAG	REFERENCE RANGE
APTT	214	H	84-72 seconds
PT	35	H	11-17 seconds

Clotting times are measurements of two parts of the coagulation cascade. Coagulation involves platelets. But it also involves a complex list of proteins in the blood that interact with each other in a complicated string of cool chemical reactions to encourage blood to clot.

- aPTT: Activated partial prothrombin time (aPTT) measures the effectiveness of clotting factors VIII, IX, XI, and XII (in the set of reactions called the intrinsic pathway) and factors I (fibrinogen), II, V, and X (involved in the common pathway).
- PT: The prothrombin time (PT) measures the effectiveness of clotting factor V, VII, X (which controls the chemical reactions called the extrinsic pathway).

Confused? The clotting cascade confuses every normal human being on the planet! But the takeaway is, these are numbers that time how long it takes blood to clot. If the numbers are high, that means clotting factors are missing and blood is not clotting normally.

What kinds of things can cause this to happen? Good question. Now you're thinking with differentials! Here are some possible reasons for prolonged clotting times and the pesky high flag:

- DIC (disseminated intravascular coagulation: a deadly condition where the blood starts making micro-clots inside a patient in response to too much inflammation).

Coagulation: blood clotting.

- Genetic clotting disorders (like hemophilia).
- Poison (like rat poisons) or venom (like pit viper venom) that attack clotting factor proteins.
- Rapid fibrinolysis (a fancy word for breaking down clots, in conditions like allergic reactions).
- Really bad liver disease (because the liver makes clotting factors).

Coagulation

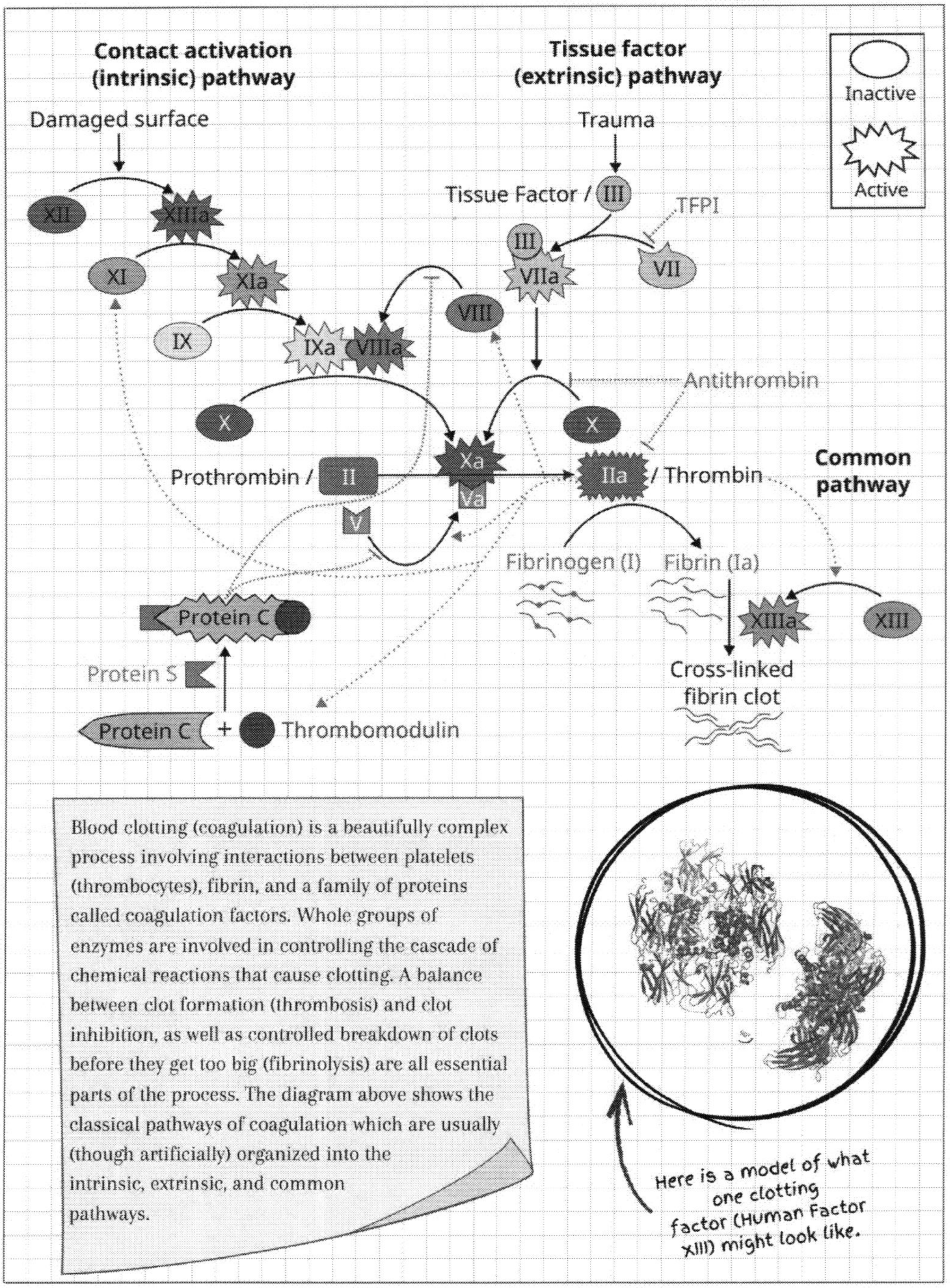

Diagram By Jonathan Dyre - File:Coagulation_full.svg, CC BY-SAh 3.0 https://commons.wikimedia.org/w/index.php?curid=136455001

Client: Chissum, James P.	Species: Canine	Sex: MN
Patient: Bullet	Breed: German Shepherd	
Patient ID: 02696		

CBC

Test	Result	Flag	Reference Range	
WBC	18	H	6.0-17.0	$10^3/\mu L$
Neutrophils	12	H	3-11.4	$10^3/\mu L$
Monocytes	1.23		0.15-1.35	$10^3/\mu L$
Lymphocytes	2		1-4.8	$10^3/\mu L$
Eosinophils	0.6		0.1-0.75	$10^3/\mu L$
Hematocrit	56	H	37-55	%
MCV	67		60-77	fL
Platelet Count	181	L	200-900	$10^3/\mu L$

So, you have elevated clotting time, meaning there's enough venom in this guy to mess up his blood clotting and potentially cause shock. The venom has also affected platelet numbers (but not yet to a dangerous level), and caused inflammation (elevated white blood cells, of which neutrophils are the first to go up). Hemoconcentration (increased red blood cell counts) is common with snake venom as well.

Wall, pardner, you've established that this ain't no "dry bite." In fact, it sounds kinda serious…

VIPER VENOM

CLINICALLY RELEVANT FACTS ABOUT PIT VIPER VENOM

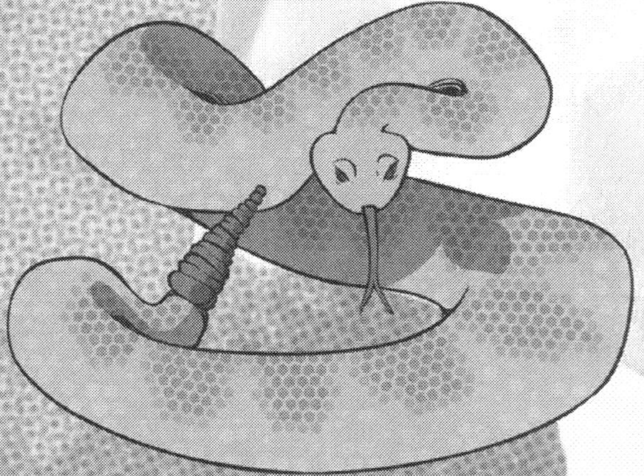

1 Ranking

North American crotalids (pit vipers) can be ranked by bite severity.

1. Rattlesnake

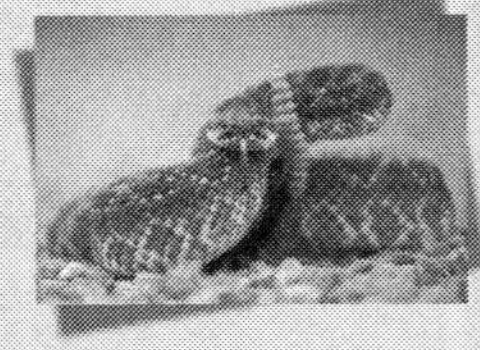

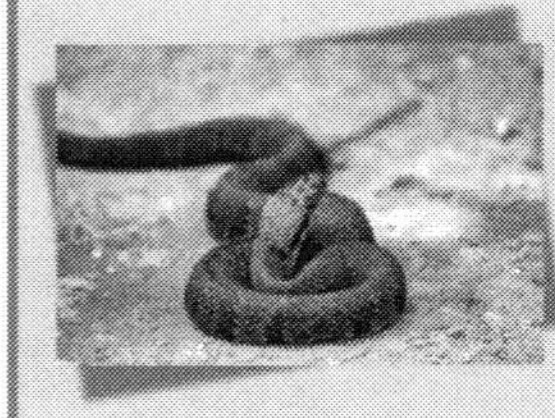

2. Water Moccasin

3. Copperhead

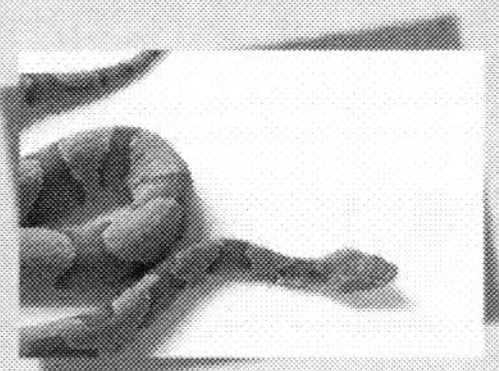

2 Venom Fractions

Venom has more than 50 enzymes that include myotoxins (hurt muscle), cytotoxins (hurt local tissue), and cardiotoxins (hurt the heart and vessels). Some neurotoxins are present as well, with a higher amounts in the Mojave rattlesnake.

3 Venom Delivery

1. Larger snakes deliver higher volume of venom
2. Young snakes deliver more potent venom
3. Dying snakes deliver more venom

4 Diagnostics

Useful tests to monitor how severe a bite is might include coagulation tests, a complete blood count, cytology, and electrolyte measurements.

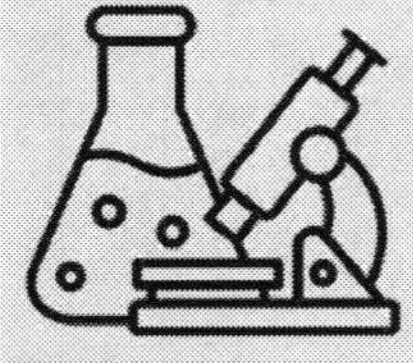

What are ya gonna do for this snakebit beasty?

a) Anti-arrhythmic medication (drug to fix an abnormal heartbeat)

b) Antibiotics

c) Antivenin

d) Benadryl or Diphenhydramine (an antihistamine drug for allergic reactions)

e) Diuretic medication (drugs that get fluid out)

f) The hoochie-coochie (after which, you will turn yourself around)

g) IV fluids

h) Monitor vital signs overnight

i) Pain medications

j) Steroids

k) Suck on the fang marks to schluck out all the venom

l) Surgery

Check out the fact-packed poster on the previous page to help you decide on treatments. Think about the bad things the venom does to your patient, and how you might want to counteract those things.

Then, pick some treatments from the list…

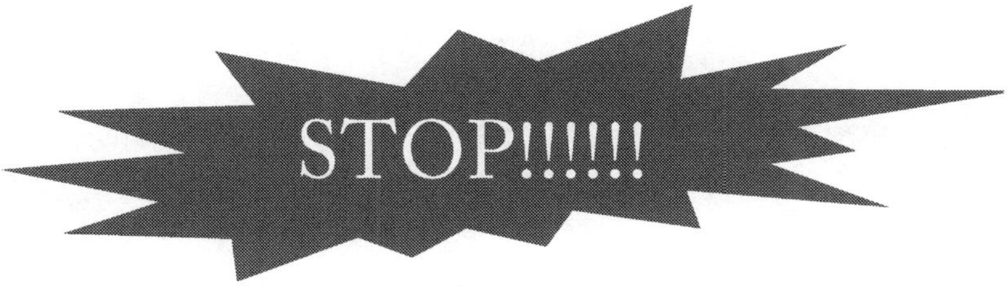

Antihistamine: a drug to treat allergic reactions.

I would pick: **c, g, h and i.**

Though option f *is* what it's all about, I would not pick it in this case.

Snake venom attacks tissue and really hurts, so **pain medications** are helpful, usually strong opioid pain meds. It's also a good idea to recommend **IV fluids** and **monitoring for the night**. Venom from crotalid snakes like angry ol' Eddie attack the circulatory system, potentially affecting the heart and blood pressure and causing shock. IV fluids will help keep the blood pressure stable, help protect the kidneys, and keep the patient hydrated. The first eight hours is typically when systemic signs (signs all around the body) will be seen from a snakebite and is the most important period to watch a patient closely. Some signs, like swelling, can last for days!

Finally, I would consider **antivenin**. This is really the only drug we can give that will treat the underlying problem (the venom) directly. What is antivenin? Good question! This is a substance that binds to snake venom and neutralizes it. Antivenin is technically in the family of medicines called immunizing agents, which boost the immune system to fight against something (in this case snake venom). Antivenin is usually made by isolating special immunoglobulins produced in the body of a larger animal and purifying it out of their blood stream to be injected into snakebite victims. The antivenins we use in the United States are generally made from injecting either horses (equine origin) or sheep (ovine origin) with venom, then purifying the immunoglobulins their body makes. Administering antivenin to your patient involves giving a dose intravenously over a certain time frame (generally around an hour) along with the IV fluids. Severe allergic reactions can happen with antivenin, and the patient needs to be monitored very closely. You usually want to give antivenin within 24 hours of a snake bite.

Some treatments that would have been used years ago were steroids, allergy medications, and antibiotics. Steroids were a common treatment for snakebites to reduce inflammation. More recent studies have shown that they can increase mortality (i.e. cause more dogs to die) and they're generally considered contraindicated[7] for snakebites. Allergy medications like diphenhydramine were also commonly given, but more recent studies have shown them to be ineffective (unless you think there's an allergic reaction). Antibiotics are another treatment that was commonly given. It makes sense, right? A nasty snake mouth full of bacteria just injected fangs into your patient's skin... Some cases of snakebite do get infected. But more recent research has shown that most don't get an infection, and experts recommend waiting to give antibiotics to these cases only if infection happens.

[7] A fancy word that means "no, no! Just don't do it, man!"

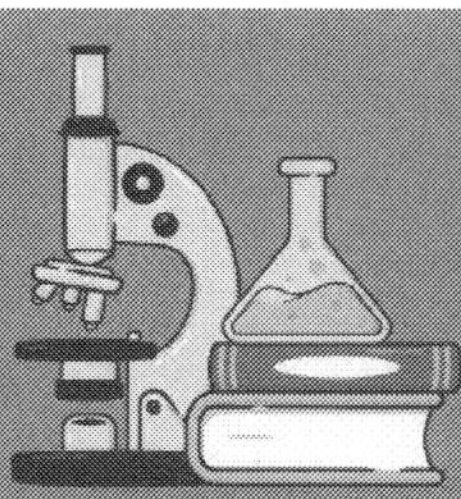

ANTIVENIN

SNAKE VENOM IMMUNIZING AGENT

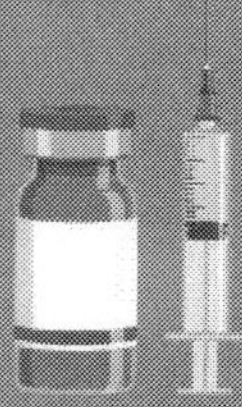

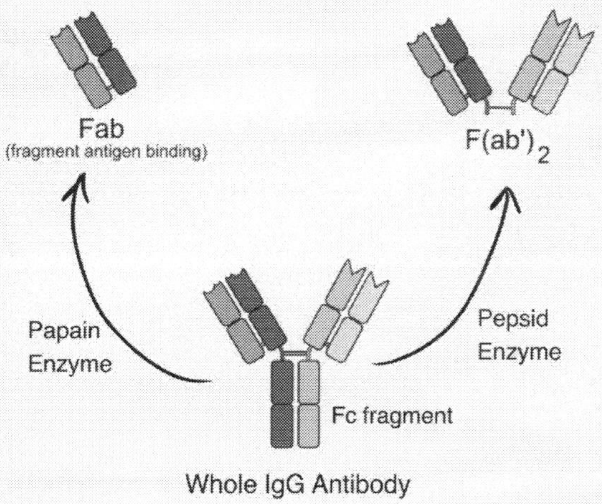

Removing the Fc portion of IgG when making antivenin can speed the neutralization of venom, clear antivenin from the body faster, and decrease the chance of allergic reaction.

WHAT'S ITS STRUCTURE?

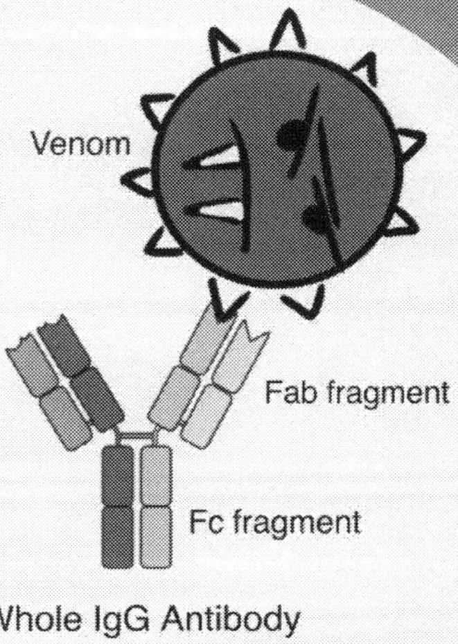

IgG molecule binds (at the Fab fragment) to proteins on venom molecules, which neutralizes the molecules while the body clears the venom.

HOW DOES IT WORK?

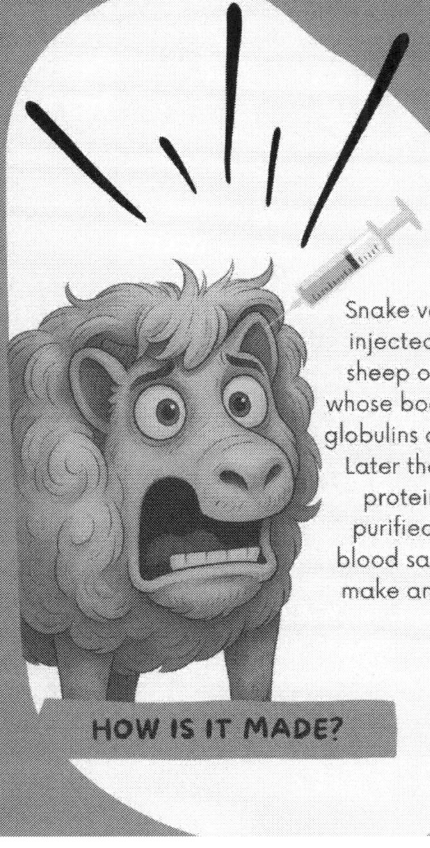

Snake venom is injected into a sheep or horse, whose body makes globulins against it. Later these IgG proteins are purified out of blood samples to make antivenin.

HOW IS IT MADE?

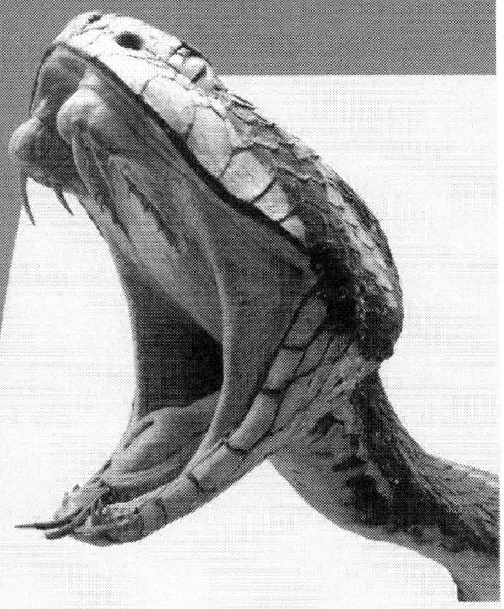

Snakebite cases are a good example of one aspect of medicine that is both wonderful and frustrating at the same time: treatments constantly change as we do better research. That means you can expect the great medicine you learn at vet school (through all that time and money and effort) will be totally different (and sometimes obsolete) 10 years or so into your career. Fun times!

You review your plan with Mr. Chissum. He expresses surprise that you can't just give some antivenin and send Bullet home, but he approves your plan. Bullet is much happier with pain medications and fluids. You give antivenin and will recheck CBC and clotting times in about six hours.

Whew! An hour or so later you settle back into your office chair and get ready to wait out the night. The night, however, seems to have more patience than you do. Before long, you are drooped over the journal article you've dutifully been trying to read as the quiet hours tick on and on. You lay down on the day bed (and wonder why it's called that, when it only gets slept on at night). Your sagging eyelids sag more.

Hours later you wake up with a start to the sound of knocking. You stumble across the room and open the office door to find…nobody there.

"Um…" you eloquently express your confusion, then walk up front to look for your technicians. It's strange how creepy an empty clinic feels at night, and you peer a bit nervously at every shadowy corner in open treatment room and hallways. Fred Kawalkovitch is leaning back in an office chair, reading and humming a Harry Nilsson song. Lolita is scrolling on her phone in the front lobby.

"What's up, Doc?"

"Did you guys need me? Someone knocked on the door."

Fred puts down his book (entitled *Dave's Phat Book of Physics*). "Nope. Nothin' going on here, Doc. Bullet's fine. She's not down to recheck clotting times for another two hours."

SHHHHP! KNOCK! KNOCK!

The sound echoes faintly in the back of the clinic. Lolita looks up from her phone, and stares meaningfully at Fred. Without a word you all walk to the back. Knocking and thumping sounds come from the vicinity of the doctor's office.

"Um… Is that a voice?" you whisper. For just a moment you thought you heard murmuring.

The sounds seem loudest in the pharmacy, but the pharmacy is empty.

"Hello?" Fred calls out. Nobody answers. The knocking stops.

"Did you hear like a creaking sound?" Lolita asks. You and Fred shake your heads.

Back across the treatment area, you open the doctor's office door and find nobody inside. Everything is completely silent, save for the low hum of the blood machines in the lab on the other side of the wall and a faraway whimper of Bullet in the dog runs.

"I think it was coming from inside Short's office. Let's go meet a ghost, huh?"

Fred crosses the doctor's office and opens a door on the other side. An empty room with a computer desk and some boxes of textbooks and supplies lies just beyond. There's no closet and the room is piled with junk. The practice manager and current owner of the clinic (Dr. Celia Short) uses this room as a business office and for storing stuff. It's all quiet, as quiet, in fact, as the grave.

Fred walks through the back door, which is set in the south wall of Dr. Short's office and opens to a crummy little fenced in yard at the back of the clinic. You and Lolita follow (feeling it would be less creepy to find whatever horrible phantasm is about tonight than to stand alone in the dark clinic). A quiet New Mexico moon shines down on a few square meters of desert dirt, an overgrown prickly pear cactus, a mesquite trees, a pile of scrap wood, and too much trash.

"Well, whatever it was it seems to have gone to bed," Fred comments, and you all walk inside. You wind your way together into the front lobby. No more knocking sounds are heard.

"Why don't we check Bullet's clotting times early, huh?" You are a bit embarrassed at the frightened squeak in your voice.

"Sure! Sure!" You three go together to get the job done. Happily, Bullet's clotting times are still normal, and you continue the plan of fluids and pain medications.

After that there's nothing for it but to head back to the office alone…in the dark… You wouldn't want to look like a coward by hanging out in the lobby. There isn't too much time left on your shift. You'll be OK, right? You sit and pretend to watch an episode of Starship Beethoven while nervously looking over your shoulders. Eventually you wander up front to find Lolita and Fred.

"Where are all the sick dogs and cats?" you ask.

They laugh. "They all stayed safe at home tonight."

"Is that normal?"

They shrug. "It's an ER. There is no normal. Anything you want to add to your discharges on Bullet?"

You look over your notes. A few minutes later, Mr. Chissum arrives to pick up Bullet. A few more minutes and you're headed home. Your mind feels rested and your heart is light with the realization that you are being paid a good wage for a job that lets you nap. Tonight, you learned the ER is that magic unicorn of a clinic where you get to work out the details of a case and really practice the medicine you learned in school, unlike your overly booked daytime job that allows about 13.7 minutes per case. And at the ER there is the lovely bonus of time to relax in between the few cases you do see!

"ER medicine is the best!" you say happily as you make breakfast and get ready to start your day.

You arrive the next night at the ER, ready to settle in for another relaxing shift. Maybe you'll watch a show tonight, do a little online shopping, and catch up on your reading in between seeing the case or two that come in.

A sudden cluttering and muttering in the business office on the other side of the wall nearly makes you jump out of your skin. It's the same room where the thumping and knocking sounds of your friendly clinic ghost came from on your last shift. You screw up your courage and open the door separating the doctor's office from the little room. You sigh with relief at the sight of a familiar face.

"Doctor Short! Hi there!"

Doctor Celia Short is not all that short (she stands about 5'8" in her purple flats), has faded blond hair, and worry lines along her middle-aged brow. She's been a veterinarian for 25 years and manages the ER. When you saw her last (to finalize the employment agreement) she seemed happier. Now, red rings stand out below her bloodshot eyes, and her left hand trembles just a little.

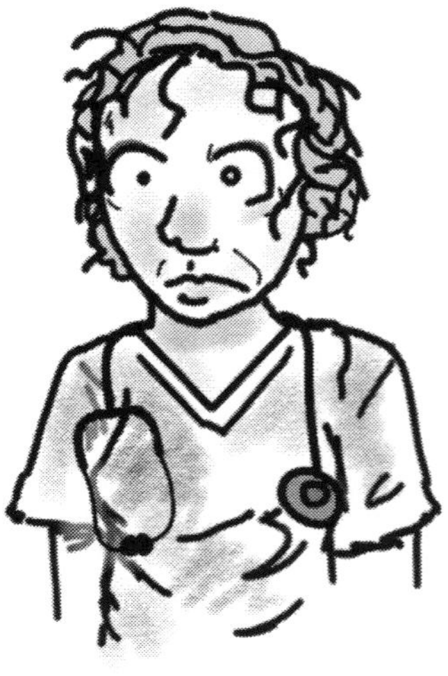

"Hello, doctor. How's the night going?"

"Fine. Fine. Just got here. Everything OK?"

She looks harried and distant. "Mostly… There's just a lot to do, you know. I'm behind in inventory and have to take a bunch of papers to the CSR. Got a meeting with the Vetraxis rep this afternoon, and I can't find the order forms I was going to show her. Don't ever manage a practice if you can help it…"

"Sounds like good advice!" you chuckle. "Sorry you're stressed."

"It's not doing my stomach any good." She sighed and put a hand on her stomach. "If you get a chance, be a Vetraxis rep instead. I'm sure they make tons of cash for way less work than we do. Commercial labs and pharmaceuticals: that's where the real money is! In fact, the old owner of the clinic made a ton after investing in Vetraxis in its early days…"

This pleasant conversation is interrupted by the sound of the doorbell. You bid your boss a good evening and retreat into the office to get ready for your night while your techs get whatever is here checked in. A few minutes later, you open the door to the dreaded sound of knocking.

CASE #5

Graham stands at the door with a clipboard. "Got a 2-year-old Lab that looks sick enough we brought him straight back to Treatment."

You nod with an outward calmness that doesn't match the sudden panic rising inside and follow him to the treatment area. Graham talks and walks, one of his many skills.

"This is Superfly. His owner is Doctor Crimshaw, who started this clinic."

Now you are more nervous. You've learned to feel anxiety about treating patients whose owners are in a medical field. They usually know more than you, or at least sound like they know more than you. Then again, you generally feel that most people know more than you…

"Superfly was fine until today. He's never had any health problems and is not on any medications other than heartworm and flea and tick preventatives. She found him collapsed in the yard about 20 minutes ago, weak and panting."

As you've got in the habit of doing, you are already starting to form a list of differentials as your technician gives you the history. You walk and take stock, one of your many skills.

You find a beautiful young yellow lab laying on his side on the wet table in Treatment. He is panting and looking very, very sick. Your anxiety-ometer rises yet another notch. This dog looks to be in critical condition. And everyone here (including your boss, and apparently the woman who built this clinic) is expecting you to fix him.

"Any toxin exposure?" You remember dudes on ER shows tend to ask that question a lot.

"Nothing specific that the owner knows of, though she does keep saying she has bad neighbors. She did find two piles of vomit near the patient. No diarrhea, coughing, or sneezing. No history of trauma. No seizures have ever been seen in this dog. He is fully vaccinated."

A friendly young lady with a nose ring and pink hair is finishing taking a temperature on Superfly. "He's got a fever of 103.7. And I think this is bloody diarrhea on the thermometer."

She extends her hand (not the one holding the bloody diarrhea thermometer). "I'm Lemon, by the way. Got in a little late tonight, and haven't met you yet."

You shake her hand, wonder inside if she said her name is Lemon or if you are hearing weird stuff around here again, and try to smile while feeling you need to do something about this dog quickly.

OK. How are you going to fix Superfly? Well… Let's start with a physical exam.

Step 1 – Organize the History

Signalment:

2 years old

Male neutered

Labrador retriever

Presenting Complaints:

Collapsing

Weakness

Panting

Vomiting

Step 2 – Gather Clues

Physical Examination:

Abdominal palpitation: No splinting or tensing noted. No obvious organomegally or mass palpated. No obvious distension or fluid wave noted.

Attitude: Weak, recumbent (can't stand), obtunded but slightly responsive.

Cardiac: Tackycardia noted (fast heart rate of 150 bpm). No heart murmur noted, steady rhythm. Femoral pulses are weak and thready.

Ears: The concave pinna is red looking. No swelling or exudate noted in the canals.

Eyes: Episcleral injection noted, but otherwise the eyes appear clear.

Integument: No lacerations or bruises or signs of trauma noted. There are some small hives pushing up the hair on his head and neck.

Lymph Nodes: All palpate within normal limits.

Musculoskeletal: No significant findings.

Neurologic: Obtunded and recumbent. Normal palpebral reflexes and menace response present OU.

Oronasal: WNL.

Remember, WNL means "Within Normal Limits."

Concave pinna: inside of part of the ear flap.
Episcleral injection: redness to the white bit of the eyes.
Obtunded: "out of it." Superfly is spacey, dude, like totally psychedelic.
Organomegaly: fun way to say "organs that are too big."

Respiratory: Panting but no increased respiratory effort. No cyanosis noted. Pulmonary auscultation is within normal limits.

Urogenital: No significant findings.

Vitals: MM are pale and tacky. CRT over 3 seconds.

"Looks bad," you mutter. Your technicians nod and look at you expectantly.

"So…. We should probably do something about this dog quickly, right?" Lemon says.

She's right. Your mind races. First, you need some idea of what you're treating…

Differential Diagnoses:

- Anaphylaxis (allergic) reaction
- Anemia
  - With associated differentials like internal bleeding/hemoabdomen, immune mediated anemia, cancer, or infections that attack blood cells.
- Congenital problems
  - Like a portosystemic shunt that has not been diagnosed yet.
- Heart disease
- Heat stroke or heat stress
- Hypovolemic shock
  - This is more of a sign, with its own list of differentials. It could also go along with DIC (disseminated intravascular coagulation): a "hypercoagulable" state that cause tiny clots in the blood vessels and makes organs fail).
- Infection
  - There are bacterial ones, viral ones (like distemper), or fungal ones (like histoplasmosis).
- Neurological disorders
  - Such as epilepsy or brain tumor or stroke.
- Spinal cord problems
  - Like intervertebral disc disease or embolism.
- Toxicity
- Trauma

That's a pretty good list!

This dog is in shock and not fully responsive, which means he could die before you have time to narrow down your list. Your mind still races. What would you put as the top three most likely possibilities on this list right now?

STOP!!!!!!

List the three most likely differentials based on the clues you have now (physical exam, history)…

____

____

____

It's so hard to choose. They're all just so lovely…

We're going to cheat and throw in hypovolemic shock for free (not one of the three). That's because it's more of a sign than a differential, and because I already gave it away. The weak pulse (a sign of low blood pressure), pale gums, delayed capillary refill time (CRT) and obtunded nature of this patient all point to poor perfusion through his body (i.e. hypovolemic shock). When your techs get a blood pressure, it will probably be low.

Graham takes the Doppler blood pressure headphones off. "Blood pressure's low, Doc. I think he's in shock."

There ya go!

My three top differentials at this point would be:

- Anaphylaxis
- Neurological disorders
- Toxicity

"A problem well put is half solved."
—John Dewey[viii]

Perfusion: flow of blood to organs.

What do you do next?

Pick a couple options…

a) Run some tests

b) Run and hide

c) Jump ahead to treatments

d) Start making an estimate

e) Go talk to Superfly's owner

Choices, choices, it's always about the choices…

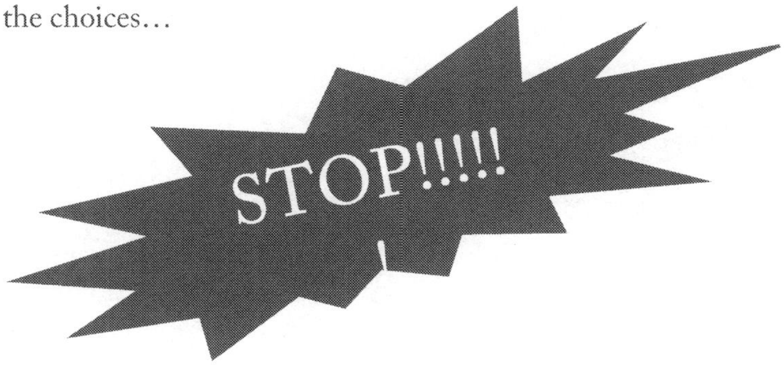

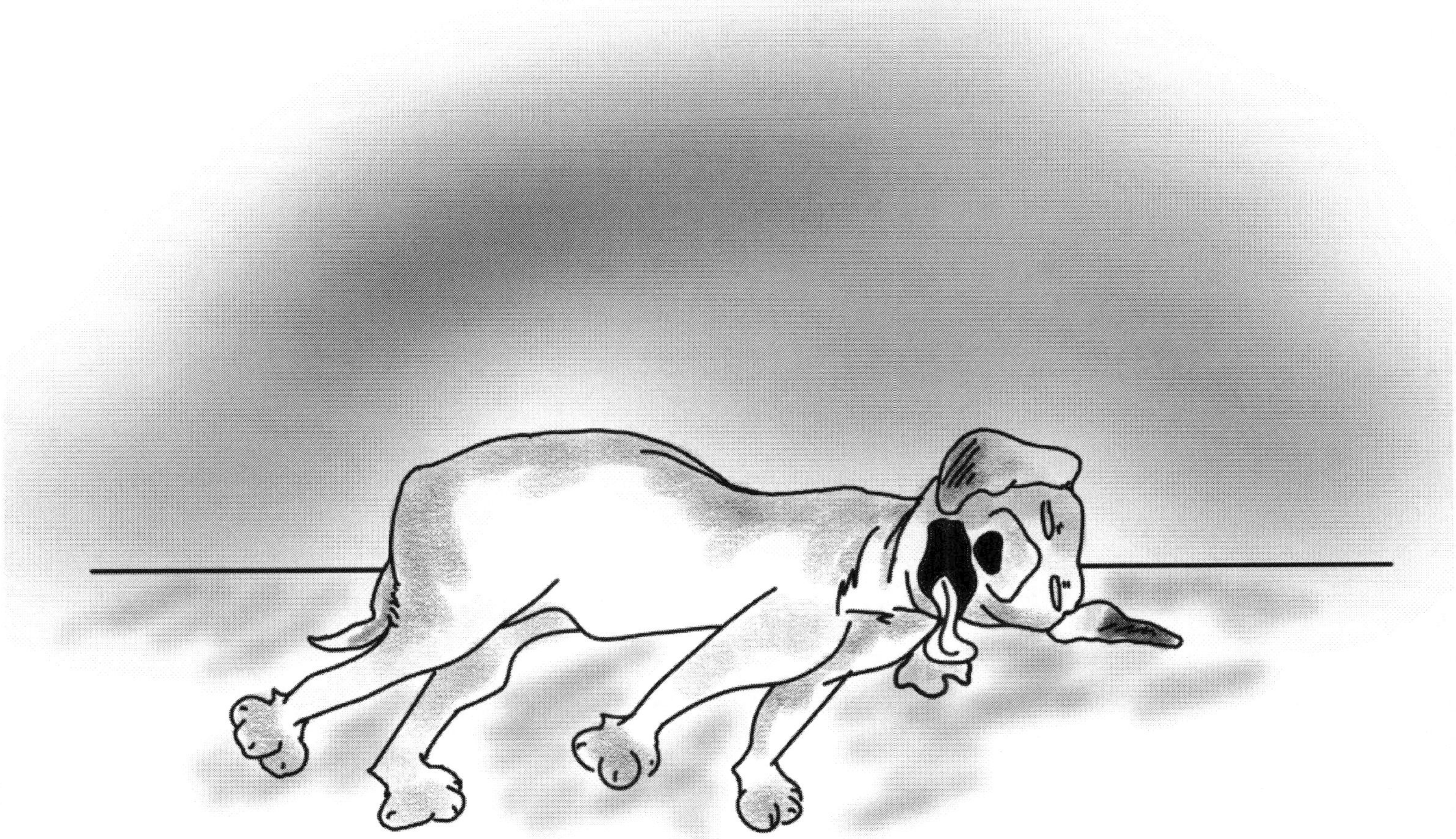

I'd recommend **starting some treatments, then talking to the owner**. Because this is an unstable patient in shock, time is limited. You don't have the luxury to wait for a bunch of test results or to painstakingly go over estimates.

"Set a catheter, and get some fluids started…" you tell your technicians. You give them a bolus dose of plasmalyte to give over the next 20 minutes, and ask them to recheck the blood pressure after that. That's the first thing you can do to treat shock. "I'll go talk to his owner."

In Exam Room 2 you find Dr. Debbie Crimshaw, the human in charge of Superfly. She looks about 107 years old. You introduce yourself, shaking her hand very carefully, hoping not to break it by accident.

"Nice to meet you, young man. Have you figured out what's happening with Superfly?"

"Not yet, Dr. Crimshaw. But I place toxins, anaphylaxis, or neurologic disorders at the top of my differential list." There's a proud tone in your voice, as you pull out some big words for this fellow veterinarian.

She gives you an appraising, critical look—much like the look Skylarkin Forte infamously cast upon Captain Hammer in S4E2 of Starship Beethoven (just before she broke out singing "You Young Fools Are Tools" and tap danced across the bridge). "Yes. It's probably a toxin. My neighbor is not a nice person, you know, and might have thrown something over the fence."

"Ah. Do you suspect a particular toxin?"

"Hmmmm?" You repeat your question. "Oh yes. It's probably a toxin. My neighbor is not very kind, and might have thrown something over the fence. She used to be a technician here, you know. But I fired her."

"Ah…" You begin to suspect that this may not be an easy conversation.

"I used to work in this building," Dr. Crimshaw pleasantly gabs. "Had it built for my practice back in the 1970, the summer after Woodstock. What a groovy time," she sighs. "You youngsters are so uptight today, not as hip as we were then…"

"Yes, I heard. Now about Superfly, I think he's in shock and…"

"Oh, poor Superfly! Do you think he's been poisoned, young man? I have this neighbor, you know…"

You cut her off as politely as you can. "You mentioned that, yes ma'am. I certainly think a toxin is possible. We should do some tests. But first we are treating him for shock, or he could die. I've already started Superfly on IV fluids."

She looks surprised. "You started fluids on Superfly? Is he sick?"

"Um…" You may need an escape route. "He is very sick."

She looks around the exam room, suddenly more distracted. "Did I leave something in here? I left something here last time I was in." She starts rummaging through her purse.

"I don't know, Dr. Crimshaw. But I should get back to Superfly."

"Poor dog! Do you think he could be poisoned? I have this neighbor who is not very kind, you see. She might have thrown something over the fence."

"I am going to check on Superfly real quick, OK? I'll send a technician in with a plan as soon as I can."

You beat a hasty retreat. A quick assessment of Superfly shows that you can now feel his pulses and his gums are light pink. Better. He's stable enough to recommend some tests now…

Decision time!

What tests do you want to run first?

Here's what you can do in your clinic:

- ✓ Basic bloodwork (a chemistry panel and CBC)
- ✓ Benchtop Ethylene glycol test
- ✓ Blood gas analysis
- ✓ Clotting times
- ✓ Cytology
- ✓ Fecal floatation and direct saline exam
- ✓ FeLV/FIV test
- ✓ Giardia test
- ✓ Heartworm test (with rickettsial diseases)
- ✓ Leptospirosis test
- ✓ Pancreatic lipase
- ✓ Parvo test
- ✓ Pregnancy test
- ✓ Radiographs (X-rays)
- ✓ Skin scraping
- ✓ Thyroid hormone level (T4)
- ✓ Ultrasound
- ✓ Urinalysis

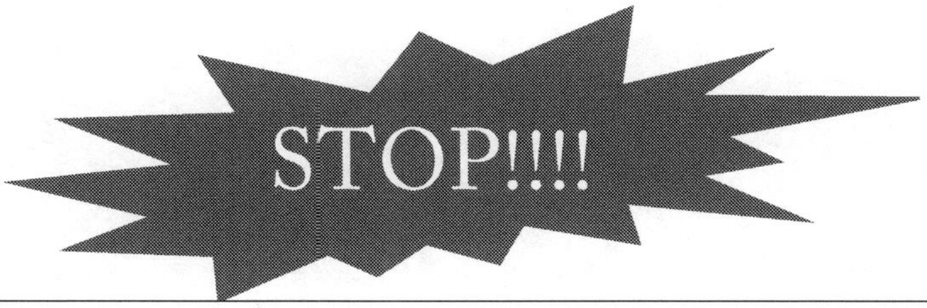

What tests do you want to run?

Bolus: a single large dose.

Plasmalyte: an IV fluids solution with electrolytes in it and a nicely balanced pH.

I would probably pick: **basic bloodwork**, **clotting times**, **ultrasound**, and **radiographs** to start with. On a case like this (collapsed and can't walk) the AFAST ultrasound would be helpful. You've already met this ultrasound and know its main function is to look for fluid pockets in the abdomen (where they shouldn't be). You pull out your super-groovy ultrasound machine and put the probe on the belly of your sick Labrador.

There, before your astonished eyes, wedges appear filled with wiggly lines and splotches!

"Hey guys! Check out all these vibin' lines and splotches!" you definitely *do not* say to the technicians who look over your shoulders expectantly.

Instead, you peer wisely at the screen as your nimble hand moves the probe from spot to spot on Superfly's belly. Remember, ultrasound is a real-time diagnostic: you see movies of the patient's abdomen as you look with the probe. The following images are only a few samples of what you see on the screen (that you wisely save in the computer to put in the patient's record).

What do you see? How many of these tags can you fill in?

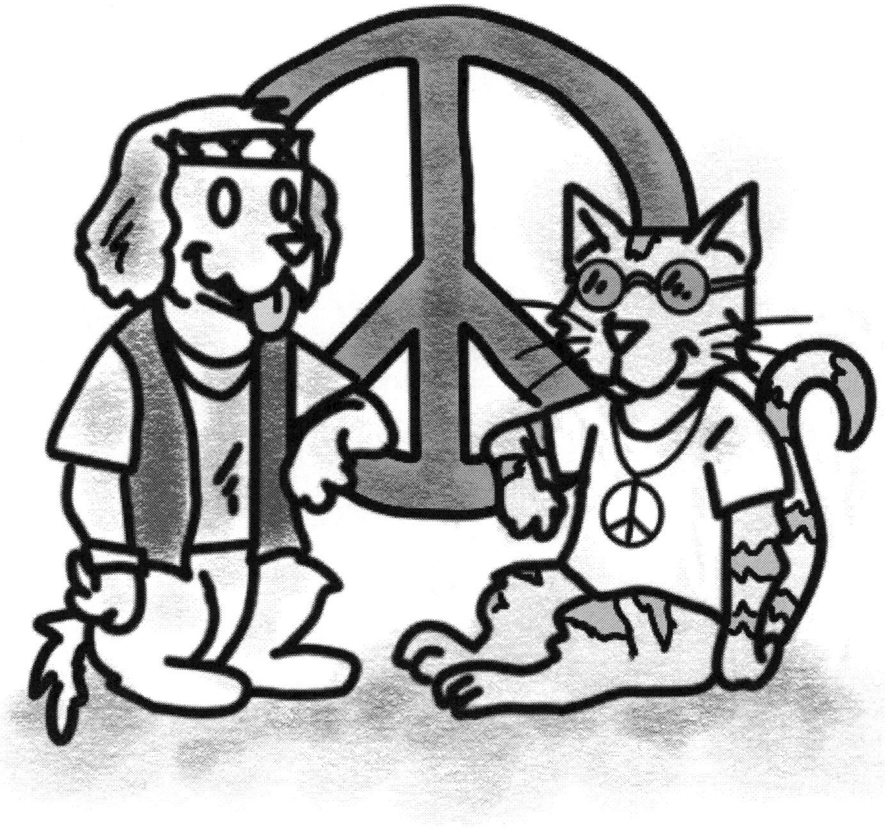

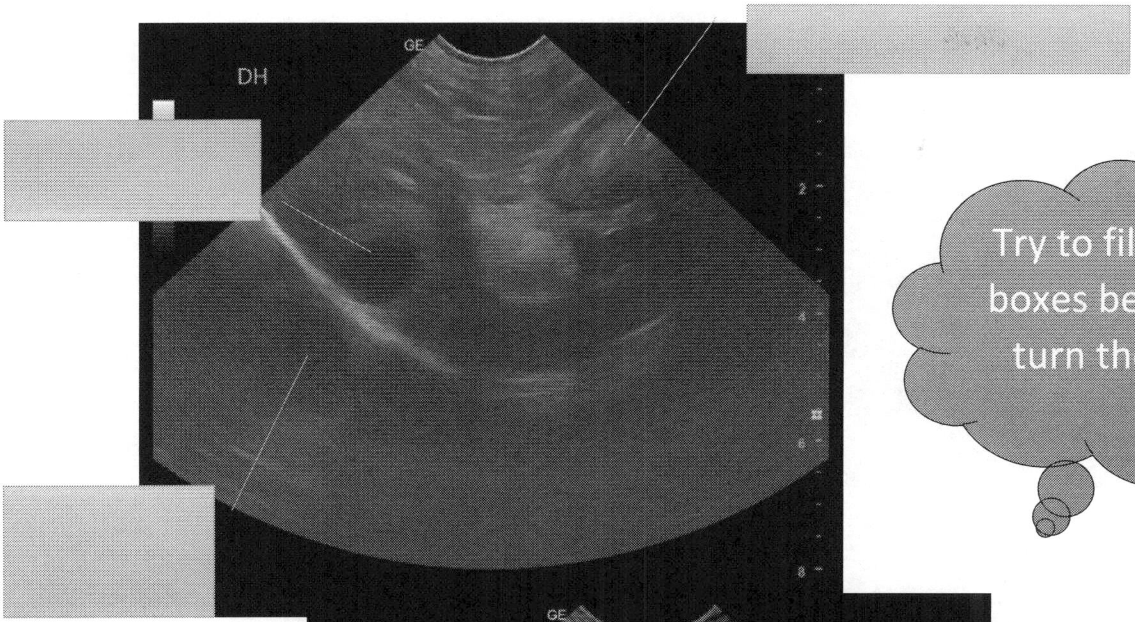

Try to fill out the boxes before you turn the page!

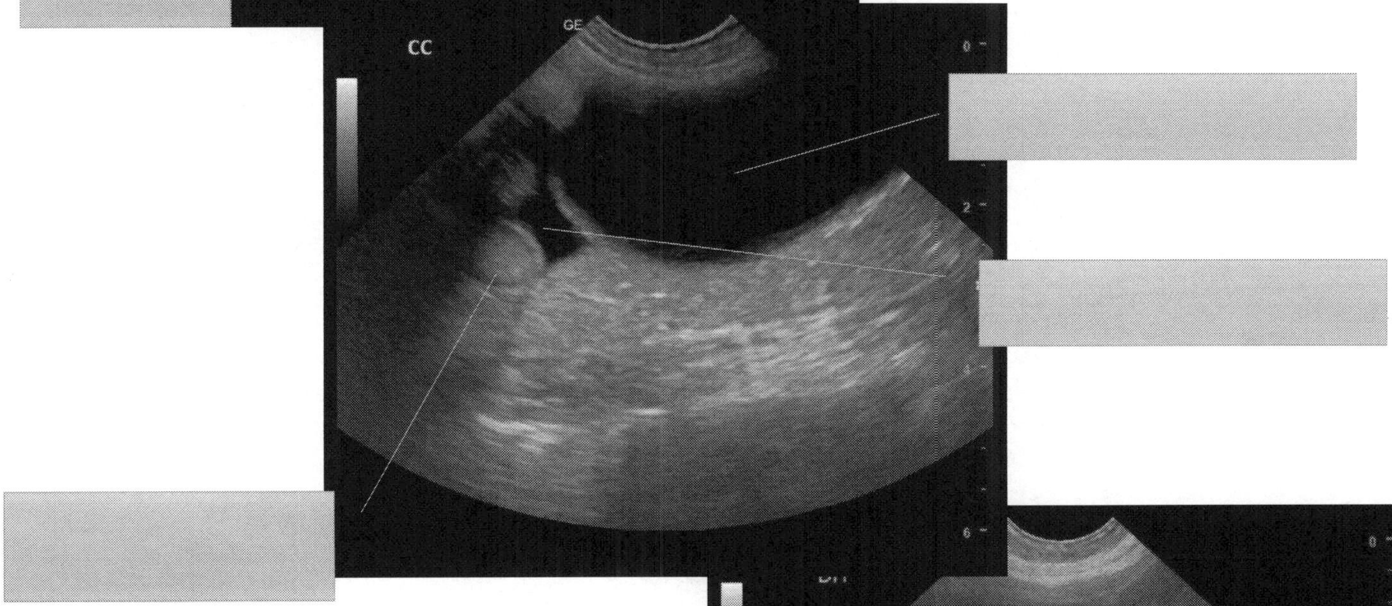

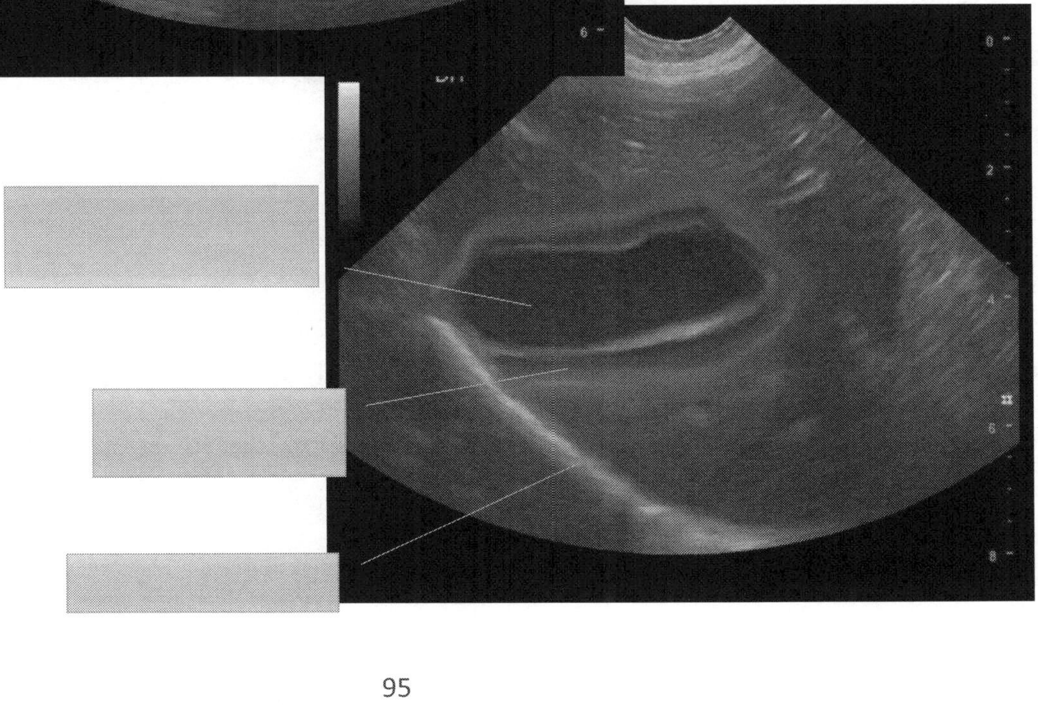

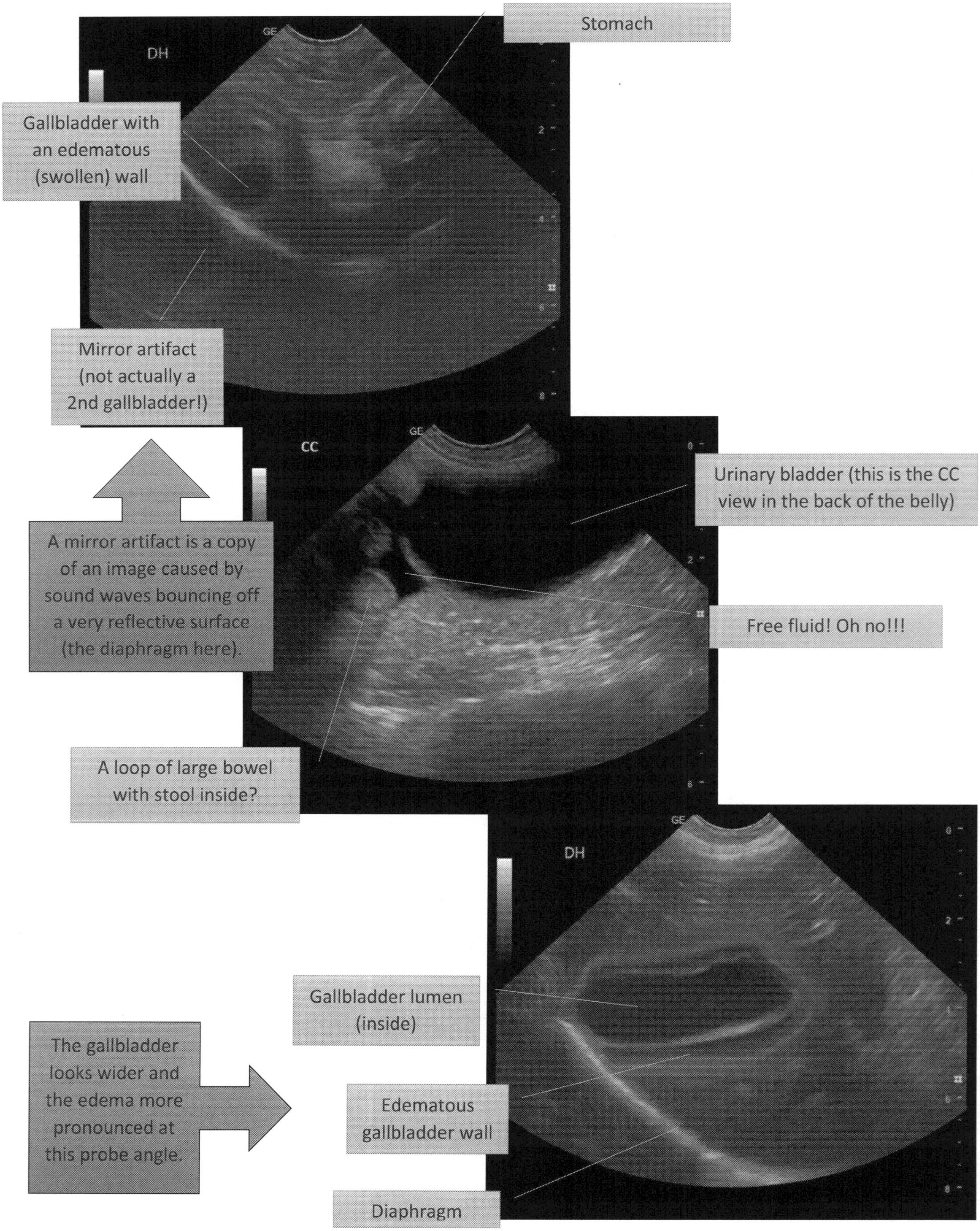
Stomach
DH
Gallbladder with an edematous (swollen) wall
Mirror artifact (not actually a 2nd gallbladder!)
A mirror artifact is a copy of an image caused by sound waves bouncing off a very reflective surface (the diaphragm here).
CC
Urinary bladder (this is the CC view in the back of the belly)
Free fluid! Oh no!!!
A loop of large bowel with stool inside?
DH
Gallbladder lumen (inside)
The gallbladder looks wider and the edema more pronounced at this probe angle.
Edematous gallbladder wall
Diaphragm

Superfly's ultrasound findings so far look something like this:

> AFS = Abdominal Fluid Score. Recall from earlier this is a score made usually by giving a 1 for fluid in each of the 4 main views of AFAST.

- A funky ring around the gallbladder.
- Some far-out, distended portal veins (which you forgot to save a pic of).
- Couple of mellow and totally uncool pockets of fluid in two views (AFS=2/4).

What's the overall picture?

Well, portal veins will get distended with liver congestion. When all those trippy little hepatocytes (liver cells) get swollen, fluids start flowing all mellow and chill as they backup, and that makes portal vessels distend. That gallbladder ring is what we in the biz call a "halo sign" and it means there is edema (swelling) of the gallbladder wall. You generally see a gallbladder halo sign with one of two things in dogs and cats: anaphylaxis or specific kinds of heart disease.

Fluid pockets in the abdomen can arise from several differentials like:

- Inflammation (from infection or allergic reactions)
- Bleeding
- Conditions that change the fluid balance in the blood vessels and organs. This might be low albumen protein causing pressure differences in blood, or heart failure causing backup of fluid.

Put all that together and we have an overall picture of abdominal inflammation. There's a trippy, hippy dippy inflammation causing this outta sight swelling of the gallbladder and oozing of little pockets of fab fluid into the abdomen. That inflammation is probably causing Superfly's fever. Can you dig it, Jack?

You manage to schluck out a little bit of fluid from a small pocket in Superfly's belly and it looks like good old-fashioned blood. That would be fine… If it were in his veins.

While you've been cruising around the patient's belly with an ultrasound probe, Graham was busy getting permission for some bloodwork and going over estimates with Dr. Crimshaw. He assures you there is no problem with approval as apparently the old doctor is loaded with cash. Lemon runs the blood they had drawn when Superfly came in as a critical patient. Good ER techs often get samples right away on critical cases, so tests can be run as soon as they're approved. Now Lemon hands you a couple of pages filled with bloodwork.

Look it over and…

A) Find some overall trends.

B) Decide what differentials you can rule off your list of possibilities based on the bloodwork.

C) Decide what your top differential is with this new information.

Client: Crimshaw, Debbie	Species: Canine	Sex: MN
Patient: Superfly	Breed: Labrador	
Patient ID: 02698		

CBC

TEST	RESULT	FLAG	REFERENCE RANGE	
WBC	20.5	H	6.0-17.0	$10^3/\mu L$
Neutrophils	13	H	3-11.4	$10^3/\mu L$
Monocytes	1.13		0.15-1.35	$10^3/\mu L$
Lymphocytes	2		1-4.8	$10^3/\mu L$
Eosinophils	0.8	H	0.1-0.75	$10^3/\mu L$
Hematocrit	59	H	37-55	%
MCV	67		60-77	fL
Platelet Count	47	L	200-900	$10^3/\mu L$

Hepatocytes: liver cells.

Client: Crimshaw, Debbie	Species: Canine	Sex: MN
Patient: Superfly	Breed: Labrador	
Patient ID: 02698		

Chemistry Panel

TEST	RESULT	FLAG	REFERENCE RANGE[ix]	
ALT	756	H	8.2-57	IU/L
ALP	102	H	10.6-101	IU/L
GGT	5		1.0-9.7	IU/L
tBili	0.3		0.1-0.6	mg/dL
Glucose	210	H	62-108	mg/dL
Cholesterol	123		116-254	mg/dL
Total Protein	5	L	5.5-7.5	g/dL
Albumin	2	L	2.6-4.0	g/dL
Globulin	4.5	H	2.1-3.7	g/dL
Calcium	9.2		8.7-11.8	mg/dL
BUN	27	H	8.8-26	mg/dL
Creatinine	1.7	H	0.5-1.6	mg/dL
Phosphorus	5		2.9-6.2	mg/dL
Sodium	159	H	140-154	mEq/L
Potassium	2.9	L	3.8-5.6	mEq/L
Chloride	116		102-117	mEq/L

Client: Crimshaw, Debbie	Species: Canine	Sex: MN
Patient: Superfly	Breed: Labrador	
Patient ID: 02698		

Clotting Times

TEST	RESULT	FLAG	REFERENCE RANGE
APTT	214	H	84-72 seconds
PT	21	H	11-17 seconds

Hoo boy! That's a lot of abnormal readings. This is one sick puppy! When there are so many abnormals on a bloodwork panel, it's easy to throw your arms up and just say, "Guess he's just doomed."

Stop and take a breath, take a step back, and look for big patterns.

We need to figure out a diagnosis, so we know what to treat…

A) Find some trends.

- Hemoconcentration (high hematocrit, meaning concentrated red cells in the blood) despite some blood leaking out in the abdomen.
- Inflammation (elevated globulins and white blood cell counts)
- Signs of dysfunction in more than one organ (liver and renal values are elevated). The ALT is especially high.
- Prolonged clotting times (from something using up clotting factors)

B) Decide what differentials you can rule off your list of possibilities based on the bloodwork

- Central nervous system disease (like stroke, brain tumor, or epilepsy) seems less likely since it wouldn't explain organ dysfunction, clotting problems, and abdominal bleeding
- An infection would usually cause more changes to the white blood cell counts on your CBC. There aren't many infections that will affect both the liver and kidneys and cause bleeding in the abdomen at the same time.
- Trauma is possible, but it wouldn't explain fever (and there's no signs on PE of it)
- Intervertebral disc disease (slipped disk causing paralysis) wouldn't affect bloodwork like this.

C) Decide what your top differential is with this new information

- To me, the top differential is… ANAPHYLAXIS! A whole-body allergic reaction.

ANAPHYLAXIS is severe (life-threatening) over-reaction of the body to an allergen. It is a whole-body allergic reaction.

ANAPHYLAXIS causes inflammation throughout the body, as it shunts white blood cells and inflammatory chemicals like histamine all through the blood stream. This affects multiple organs, and very famously raises the ALT in particular.

ANAPHYLAXIS causes halo sign to appear in the gallbladder.

ANAPHYLAXIS can cause hemoperitoneum (bleeding from the lining of the abdomen into the belly).

ANAPHYLAXIS causes fever due to the acute, massive inflammation.

ANAPHYLAXIS uses up clotting factors through rapid fibrinolysis (breaking up clots) caused by chemicals normally released during inflammation. That prolongs clotting times.

ANAPHYLAXIS causes very acute signs in an otherwise healthy dog. You see these cases come in with stories like, "My dog was fine, and then suddenly got all wobbly, then collapsed and is breathing fast!"

It fits the picture. Superfly is in shock from anaphylaxis! If it quacks like the infamous Moon-duck of Phargon-4 (Starship Beethoven S5E3), it probably is the infamous Moon-duck of Phargon-4.

Now what are you gonna do about it?

What is your treatment plan? (pick several)

a) Abdominocentesis
b) Antibiotics
c) Blood transfusion
d) Curare extracted from South American Dart frogs
e) Diphenhydramine
f) Epinephrine
g) IV fluids
h) Nausea drugs
i) NSAID anti-inflammatories
j) Plasma transfusion
k) Pump his stomach
l) Steroids
m) Yunnan baiyao

An herb that stops bleeding.

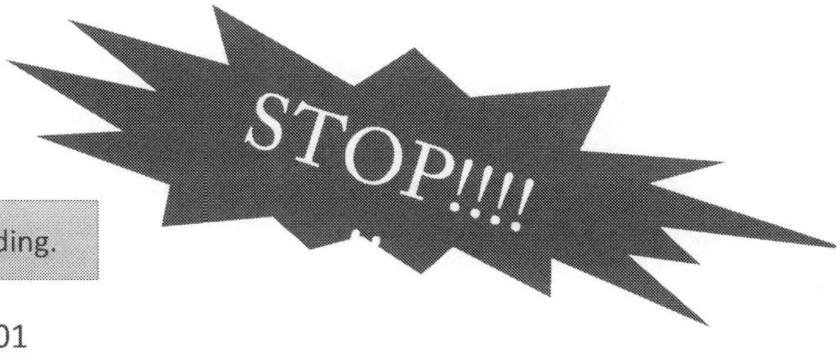

Did you choose any of the following treatments? I would pick: **e, f, g, h, j, and l**.

IV fluids are definitely important to treat the low blood pressure from shock. Good thing you've already started them. **Epinephrine** is super important for anaphylaxis patients. It is a catecholamine hormone that inhibits release of histamine (a major chemical released by the body to promote inflammation in allergic reactions) and does other useful things like opening the airways and constricting blood vessels to improve blood pressure. **Diphenhydramine** is another drug that inhibits histamine (an antihistamine). **Steroids** are often used for cases of anaphylaxis and allergic reactions to help reduce inflammation and dampen the immune system's overreaction to whatever allergen started this mess. **Nausea drugs** and other GI supportive drugs will help treat the gastrointestinal side effects in anaphylaxis and shock. **Plasma transfusions** can be needed in anaphylaxis cases that are severe or are not responding to treatment. Plasma is the liquid part of your blood (NOT the stuff the sun is made from). Giving donated plasma IV over a period of time will help blood pressure by treating shock and adding back in those clotting factors being used up. That's why…

"Freaky deaky! This looks bananas!" You turn to find old Doc Crimshaw standing behind you in the treatment area.

"Ack! You're not supposed to be back here!"

"I'm not? But I own this clinic! Or wait… Did I sell it? What time is it?"

"Um… 9:30 I think."

"Did I take my insulin yet? I need to take my insulin. It's on my phone…"

You scroll down the list of medications on the screen she hands you, then realize what you're doing and hand it back. "I don't know, Dr. Crimshaw! But that sounds important. Maybe you can call someone?"

"Well it should be right here. Every day I draw up a syringe for the morning and one at night and keep them with…Hey! That looks like Superfly! Why's he look so sick? I've got this neighbor…"

"Yes, you mentioned that, ma'am. Come with me and we'll talk about the plan to treat Superfly while my wonderful and efficient staff takes care of his treatments." Fortunately, you have already written out orders for drugs and IV fluids that Graham and Lemon can get done while you explain everything.

"Oh yes. Just let me get my notebook from the closet in the manager's office so I can write your suggestions down, young man…"

You gently, but firmly, redirect Dr. Crimshaw back to the exam room. She seems to be on board with your treatment plan and seems to agree with the diagnosis. That is, until she asks again if you think it's a toxin… You decide to content yourself with her agreement of your treatment plan and run with that.

It's a good call, especially since the doorbell rings and you have new things to worry about.

Case #6

"AAAAAAH! MY CAT CAN'T BREATHE! HELP HER! AAAAAAAAAAAAH!"

Subtle sounds of distress gently waft through the clinic. You sprint to the lobby. You find a state senator smashing the little bell on the front desk with one of his chubby hands and holding a gasping cat in the other. The bureaucratic appearance of his flannel pajamas (which are printed all over with judge's hammers and legal textbooks) is not the only clue to his profession. Senator Joe Dertoni is a regular client at your daytime job at Noah's Haus Animal Clinic, where you've treated more than one of his family pets.

The senator shakes your hand and beams a big, political smile (while still yelling in terrified tones at the top of his lungs). "THANK HEAVEN IT'S YOU, DOC! MY CAT, SWEETY LUMPKINS IS PRESENTING HERSELF AS UNDERWELL!!!!!"

You return the handshake and deftly slide right in to take the gasping cat from his arms. You still have much to learn, but you do know that gasping and open-mouth breathing is a bad sign. "I see that, Senator. Why don't you lower your voice a couple of hundred decibels, and I'll run her to the back to start some oxygen therapy while we figure this out?"

He mops a sweaty brow. "Very well, very well. Mistakes were made as to the range of my voice, in the heat of the moment and..."

"That's perfectly fine, Mr. Dertoni. Someone will be right with you," you say, as you run this poor cat (whose tongue is starting to look very blue) to the treatment area to start some oxygen.

"Oh look! A blue kitty. Very psychedelic..."

"Dr. Crimshaw! You are not supposed to... Oh, never mind. Come with me." You and Dr. Crimshaw traverse the rest of the hallway into Treatment and soon have the dyspneic kitty in some oxygen. You will note the preposition "in," not "on"... The cat is *in* a Snyder cage, a type of oxygen cage with clear doors and temperature controls. Dr. Crimshaw nods over your shoulder as you explain what you know about the new emergency (which is essentially nothing) to your technicians.

"OK," Graham is great at keeping his cool, an invaluable quality in the ER. "Lemon will help you with an exam, while I get some history and check him in. Maybe Dr. Crimshaw can sit with Superfly? His blood pressure is back to normal."

You note the Labrador sitting up and looking remarkably better, and perform another quick exam.

"Oh, Superfly! What are you doing here, man? Groooovy!" Dr. Crimshaw sits with Superfly.

You take two seconds to gather yourself, then stare at the blue cat in the Snyder cage. He is already looking just a bit better (breathing fast, but with a closed mouth now).

You do a cautious, cage-side exam. It would be nice to wait for a formal history, then do an exam. But severe respiratory emergencies like this one get bad fast, and you must assess the patient quickly and make the best diagnosis you can to start treatments to keep her from dying. You'll probably end up doing multiple exams as you watch her response to treatment. Here's what you know so far:

Step 1 – Organize the History

Signalment:

6 years old

male neutered

Domestic Shorthair cat

Presenting Complaints:

Dyspnea (difficulty breathing)

Step 2 – Gather Clues

Physical Examination:

Abdominal palpation: No significant findings. Tense in general, but no specific areas of pain or splinting. No obvious abdominal distention, fluid wave, or masses palpated.

Attitude: Bright, alert, and responsive (BAR).

Cardiac: No murmur noted. No arrhythmia noted. Decent femoral pulses palpable.

Ears: Canals appear clear with no debris noted.

Eyes: Mild conjunctival inflammation (the pink, squishy bit around the eyeball is swollen) with some serous discharge bilaterally.

Integument: Normal skin tenting (not dehydrated). No wounds or draining tracts. No obvious hives or rashes or other problems noted.

Lymph Nodes: WNL

Musculoskeletal: NSF. Weight bearing on all four limbs. No obvious fracture or luxation.

Conjunctival: a transparent membrane lining the inside of the eyelids and stretching across the sclera to the globe.
Serous: clear; a serous discharge is a watery secretion.

Neurologic: NSF. Alert and responsive patient. Normal menace reflex and palpebral.

Oronasal: No nasal discharge noted. No obvious obstruction or foreign material in mouth or throat.

Respiratory: Harsh lung sounds bilaterally with some fine crackles (more on the right than the left thorax). Cyanosis noted.

A crackling sound in lung tissue while listening with the stethoscope. Possibly caused by fluid inside lung tissue, inflamed airways, obstructive airway diseases, or lung tumors.

Urogenital: NSF. Urinary bladder palpates soft and moderate in size.

Vitals: Mucous membranes are blue/purple, moist. CRT<2s.

You gather all this information with admirable efficiency, goaded on by your blue and gaspy patient. You don't want to stress out a dyspneic cat since they can decompensate and die in respiratory compromise like this. Graham appears with a history from the client. Poor kid looks a bit overwhelmed. That's often the look people have after talking with Senator Dertoni.

"He said Sweety Lumpkins has been clearing her throat like a delegate engaged in a filibuster. He said he didn't want to bring her in at first because of something called 'front-loading' could cause a 'gaffe' and overextend his CFO's projected budget." Graham was squinting hard at the words he'd recorded.[8] "Evidently she has been doing something called a 'wedge issue campaign' by having a runny nose for some time and heavy breathing on and off. Tonight was the first time he'd seen her gasping for breath. Then, something about how he trusted this visit would not deplete the 'hard money' committed to other endeavors. I told him we'd make an estimate and hoped I answered the right question. Did I answer the right question??"

You pat Graham on the shoulder condescendingly. "You did fine, son. An intern working for a PAC couldn't have done better. Now make up a projected report of expenses while I make a differential list."

"Huh?"

"An estimate!" you laugh. "Go start an estimate for ___________." (blank to be filled in by you).

Graham scampers off while Lemon keeps an eye on Superfly and Dr. Debbie Crimshaw, and you slink into a hallway to think through what you know. Sometimes in an emergency setting the physical exam and history are taken out of order. But you've collected enough data to build a magnificent differential list.

What are you gonna put on that list?

Make a differential list before turning the page.

Decompensate: deterioration of organs.

[8] The emergency clinic recently started using an AI scribe program to record and organize histories. Many clinics are using similar technology. They help doctors write notes, records calls and conversations, and can make handy charts for discharging patients.

My differential list would look a bit like this:

- Bronchitis — Inflammation of the little airways in the lungs. This can be caused by A) infection of the airways or B) allergies (we call allergic bronchitis "asthma").
- Congestive heart failure — With differentials like cardiomyopathy or valve disease or heartworm.
- Diaphragmatic hernia — A defect in the diaphragm (the muscle separating the thorax and abdomen), caused by trauma or birth defect.
- DIC (Disseminated Intravascular Coagulation) — A "hypercoagulable" state that cause tiny clots in blood vessels, making organs fail and causing shock.
- Hypoalbuminemia — Low protein that can cause shifted fluid.
- Neoplasia
- Pericardial effusion — Fluid in the sack around the heart, with differentials like neoplasia or congestive heart failure.
- Pleural infection — With differentials like bacterial or viral or fungal disease).
- Pneumonia
- Pneumothorax — Air trapped in the space between the lungs and body wall, with differentials like trauma or lung defects called bullae that can rupture.
- Pulmonary embolism — Strokes in the lungs.
- Toxicity — With differentials like acetaminophen or baclofen).
- Trauma — With differentials like pulmonary contusions or pleural fluid).

That's a lot of possibilities, ain't it?

And just to fully intimidate you, realize that this is still an abbreviated differential list. There are entire books filled with long, detailed differential lists for all kinds of medical problems. Bodies are beautifully complex (whether human, cat, or guinea pig): and that means there's a huge array of things that can go wrong.

OK, so you have a pretty good idea of the more likely causes of Sweety Lumpkin's symptoms. Quite a few of them have potential to be catastrophic and fatal. How are you going to narrow down that list, so you can target appropriate treatments to help this suffering kitty?

You've come this far. You know the drill.

Go to the next page and pick some tests…

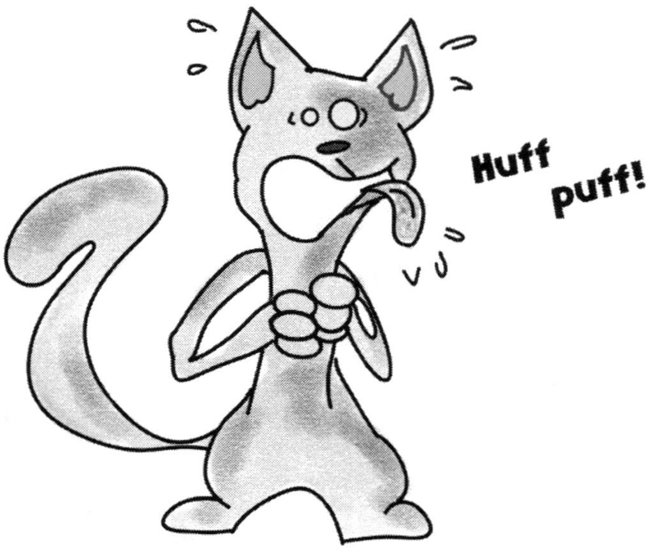

Decision time!

What tests do you want to run first?

Here's what you can do in your clinic:

- ✓ Basic bloodwork (a chemistry panel and CBC)
- ✓ Benchtop Ethylene glycol test
- ✓ Blood gas analysis
- ✓ Clotting times
- ✓ Cytology
- ✓ Fecal floatation and direct saline exam
- ✓ FeLV/FIV test
- ✓ Giardia test
- ✓ Heartworm test (with rickettsial diseases)
- ✓ Leptospirosis test
- ✓ Pancreatic lipase
- ✓ Parvo test
- ✓ Pregnancy test
- ✓ Radiographs (X-rays)
- ✓ Skin scraping
- ✓ Thyroid hormone level (T4)
- ✓ Ultrasound
- ✓ Urinalysis

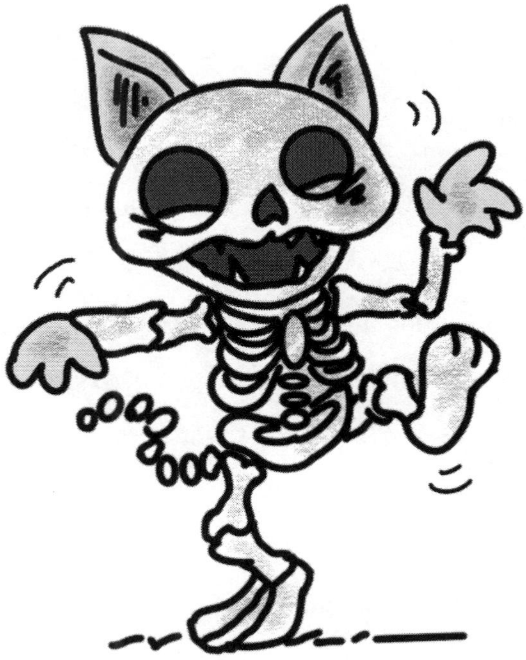

What tests do you want to run?

STOP!!!!!!

I'd probably pick: **bloodwork, radiographs**, and an **ultrasound** (specifically a TFAST scan).

Looking at that list of possibilities, those are the tests that will rule out the most items quickest.

But beware! BEWARE! **BEWARE!**

Dyspneic cats have been known to die during attempts to hold them down for tests. They can get more panicked, which makes them gasp more, which makes them panic more, which makes them gasp more, which makes… You get the idea. You do not want to start down that road. So, what are you gonna do?

I'd recommend starting with a brief TFAST ultrasound. TFAST stands for Thoracic Focused Assessment with Sonography for Trauma and is a method to rapidly look at a patient's chest with an ultrasound. TFAST is technically used more for assessing trauma patients for things like pneumothorax or internal bleeding. There are special names for other methods used to quickly look for diseases in the chest not related to trauma. But outside the ivory towers, and down in the grimy, blood-drenched trenches of the clinics, we generally use the term TFAST for an ultrasound of the thorax.

A TFAST, in skilled hands like your own, can show a lot with minimal stress to the patient. It can be done inside the oxygen cage (or with flow-by oxygen held to the patient's nose). Then after the patient has been in oxygen for a while and looks more stable (maybe after you've given some butorphanol to help calm her down and make her more stable: hint, hint…) you can work on those more stressful tests like radiographs and bloodwork.

Remember, you're putting the ultrasound against the chest now. Think about what types of structures might be in the chest. Look over the poster on the next page, and try to imagine what these friendly streams of soundwaves are trying to show you?

"Soundwave? What's the matter, Soundwave, ol' buddy?"
"Boing! Boing!!"
"Are you trying to say Timmy's stuck in the well again?"

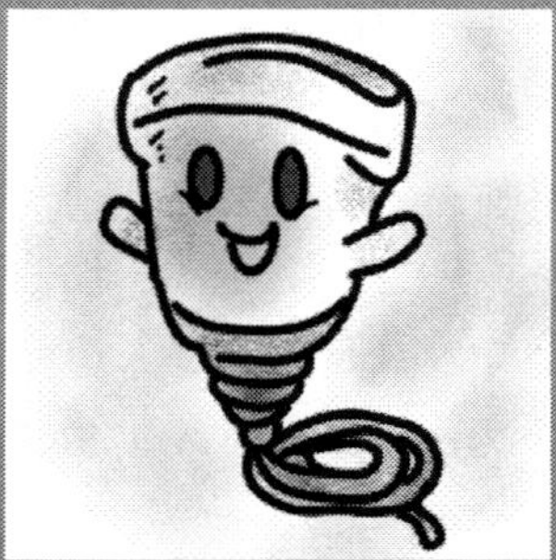

TFAST LUNG EXAM

Thoracic Focused Assessment with Sonography for Trauma

I generally start in the caudodorsal lungs here and work my way diagonally to the axilla, checking out lungs as I move...

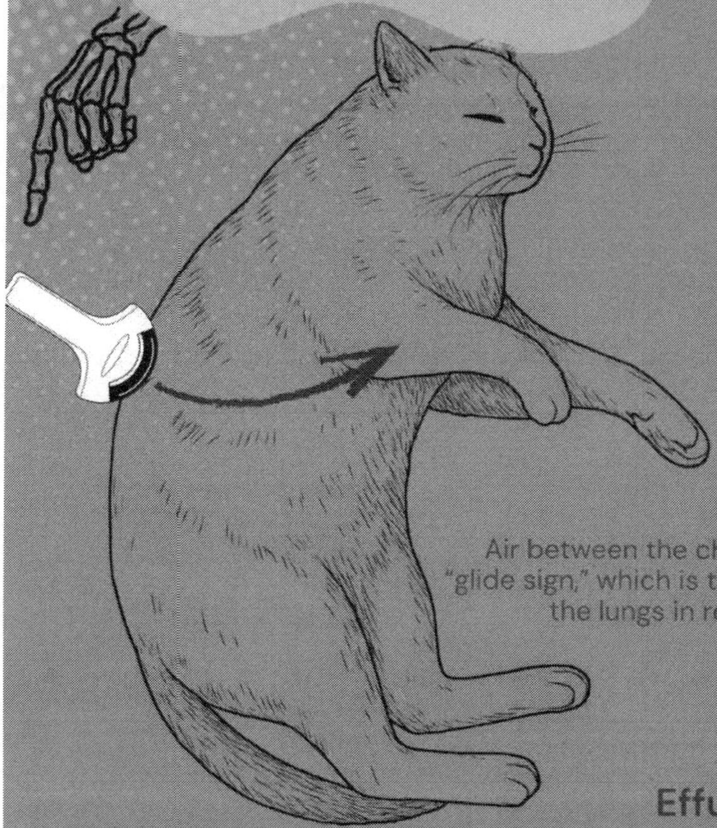

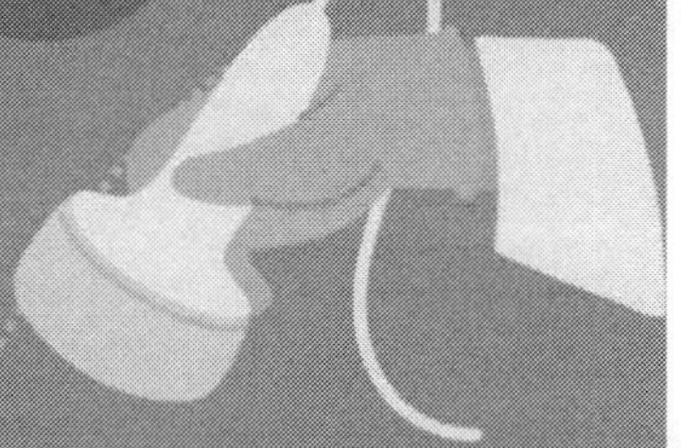

Major signs of of disease in the lungs to look for....

Pneumothorax

Air between the chest and lungs hides the "glide sign," which is the natural movement of the lungs in relation to the chest wall.

Effusion

Fluid trapped between the lungs and chest wall, (pleural) or inside the heart sac (pericardial) looks like a black gap on the screen

Pulmonary Edema

Fluid in the lung tissue will cause B-lines, verticals streaks of gray that flicker horizontally from the probe

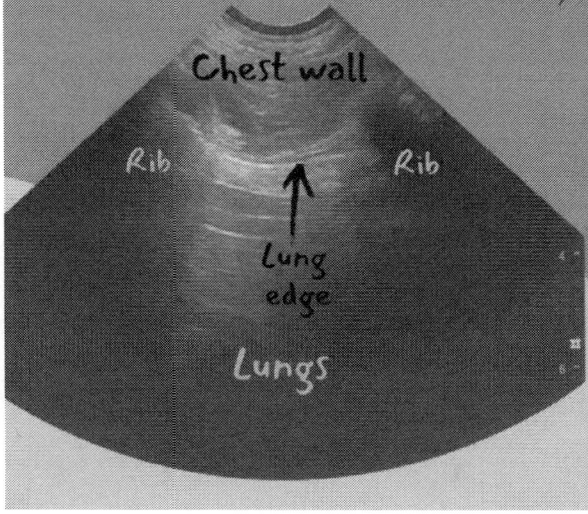

Solid Stuff

"Shred sign" (a hazy breakup in the normal lining of the lungs) or "tissue sign" (a solid gray look to lung tissue) are signs of problems like tumors or pneumonia

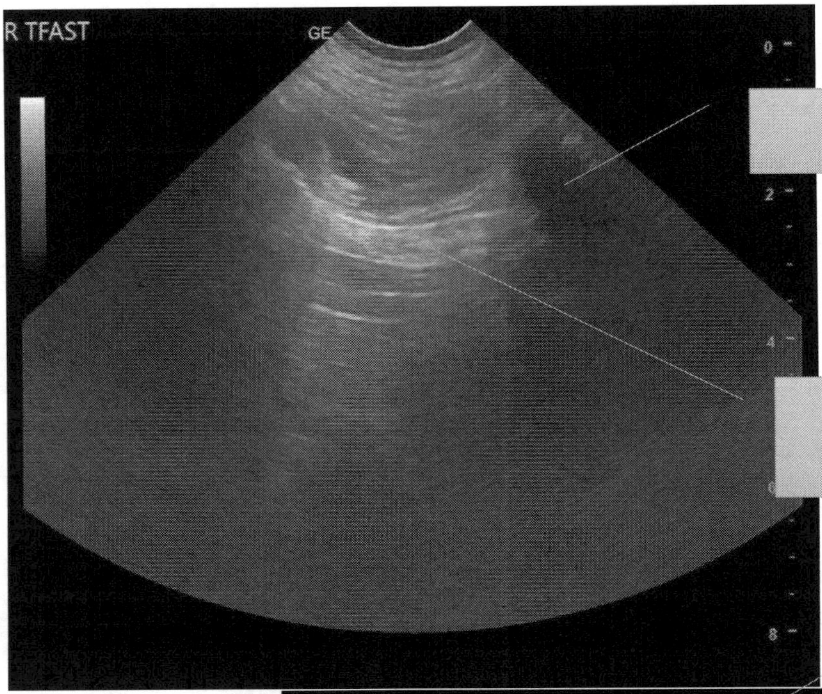

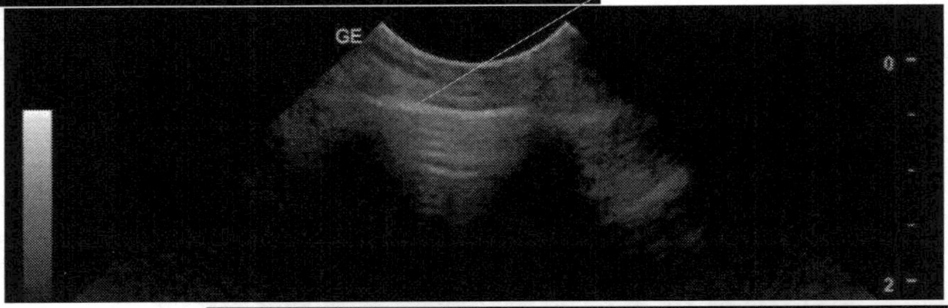

This image is from a linear probe, which shows more detail but less depth

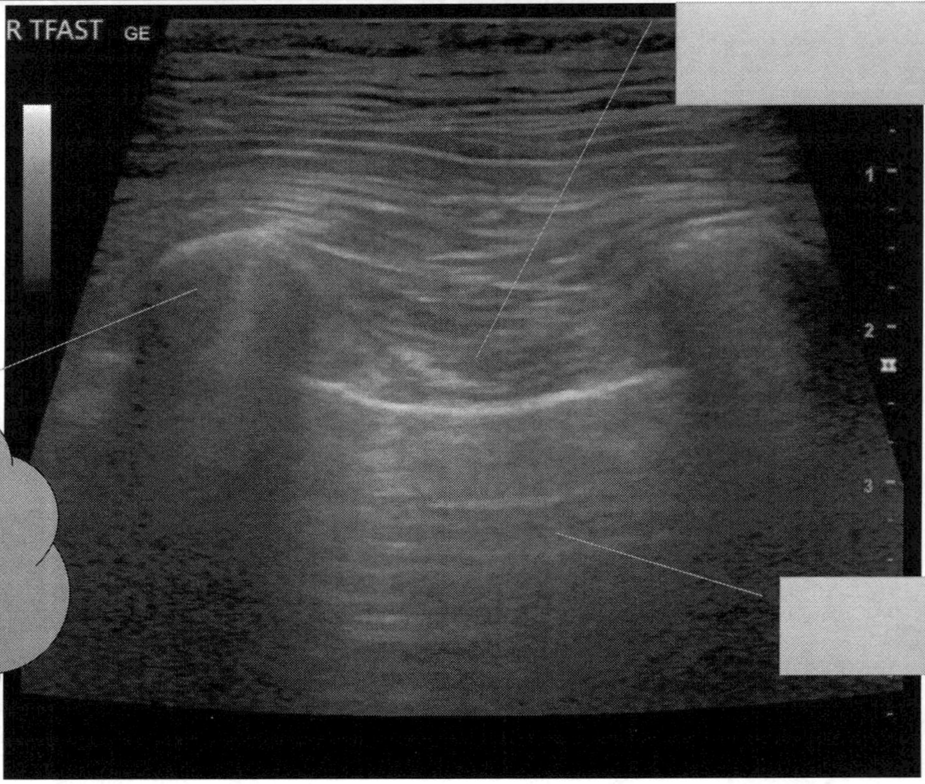

Try to fill out the boxes before you look at the next page!

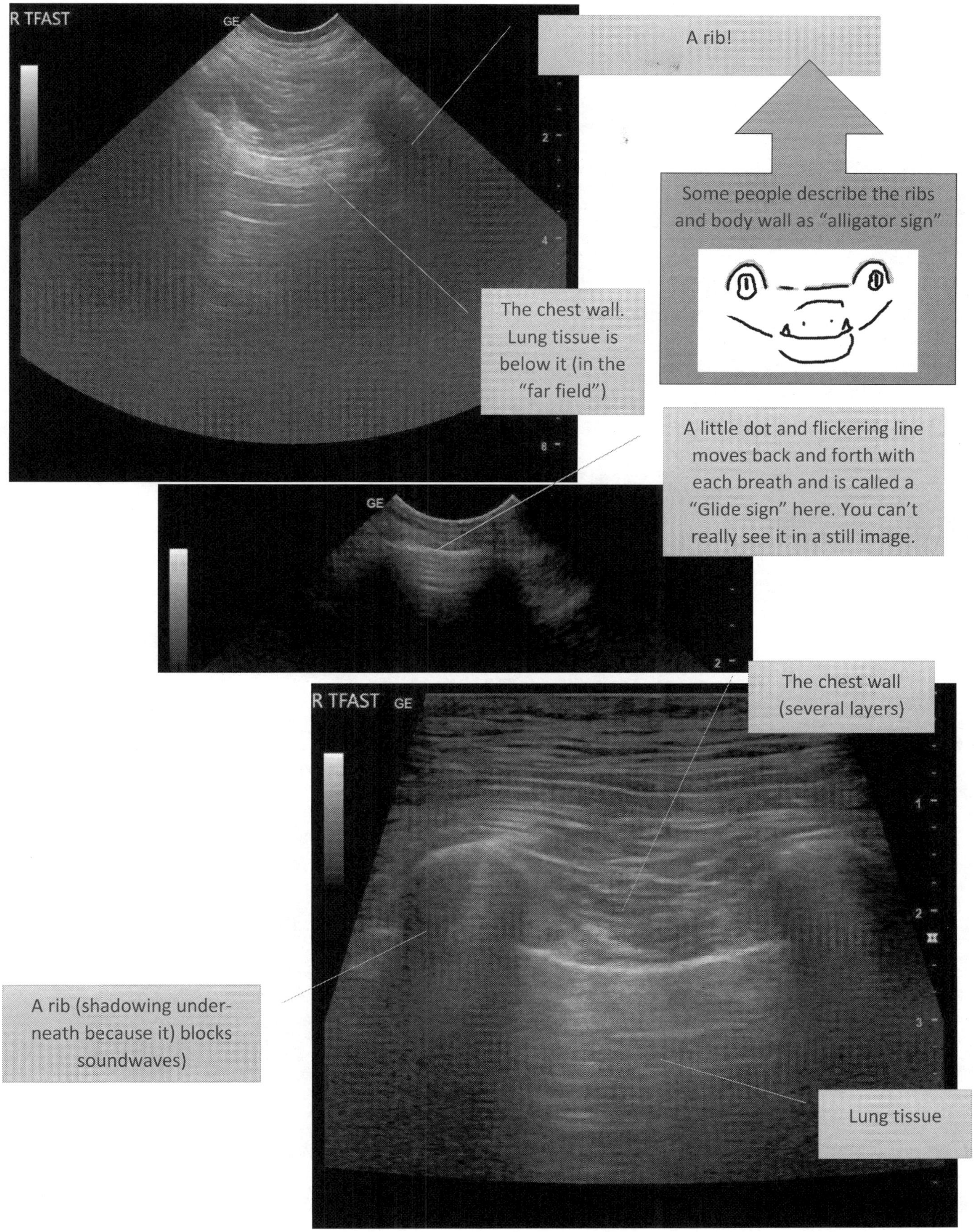
R TFAST
A rib!
Some people describe the ribs and body wall as "alligator sign"
The chest wall. Lung tissue is below it (in the "far field")
A little dot and flickering line moves back and forth with each breath and is called a "Glide sign" here. You can't really see it in a still image.
R TFAST
The chest wall (several layers)
A rib (shadowing underneath because it) blocks soundwaves)
Lung tissue

Here's examples of **BAD THINGS** you are looking out for, but do not see in this cat…

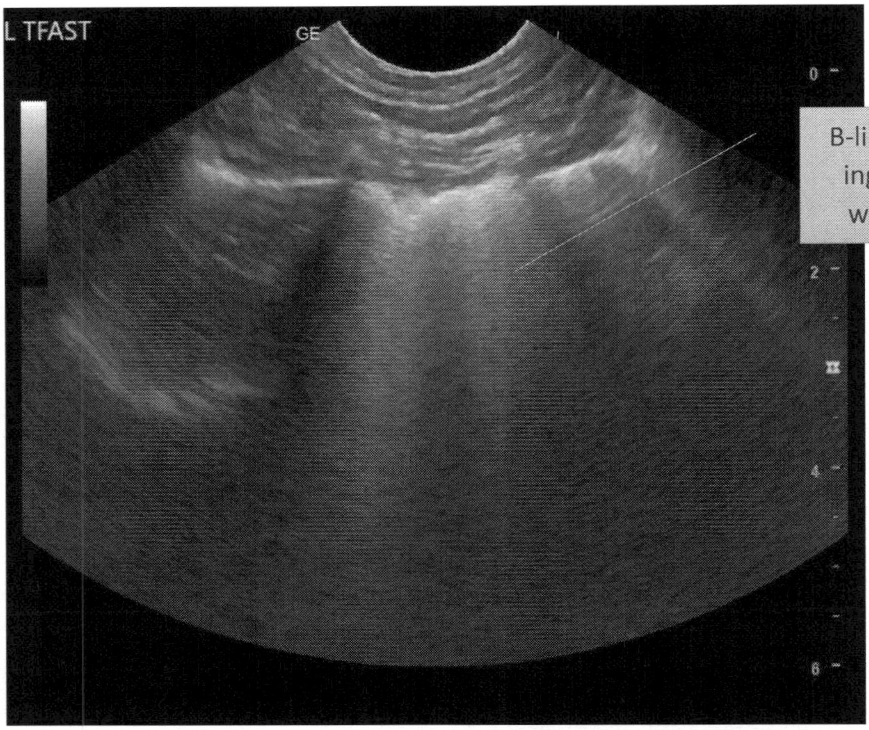

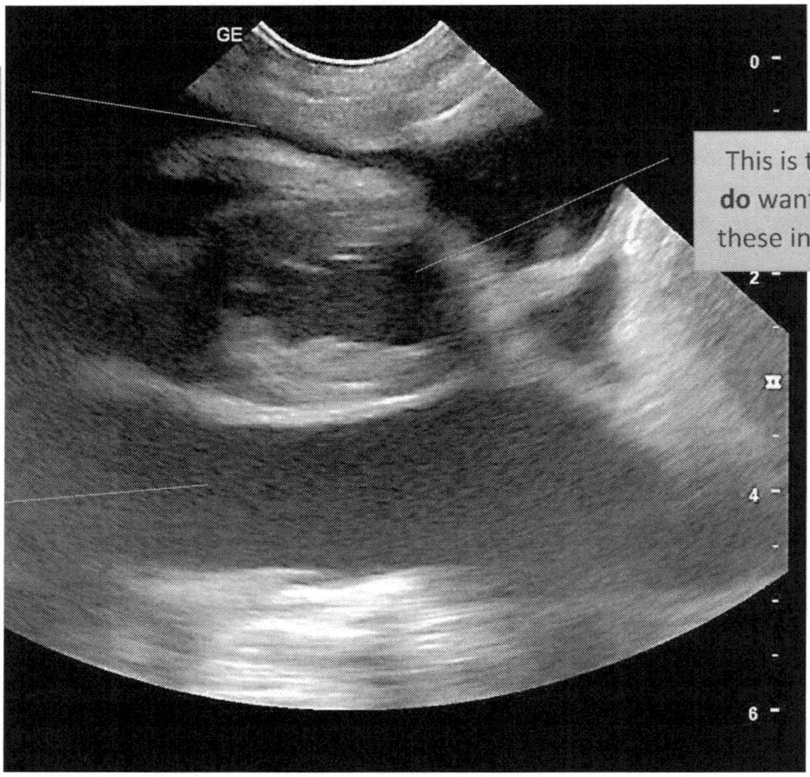

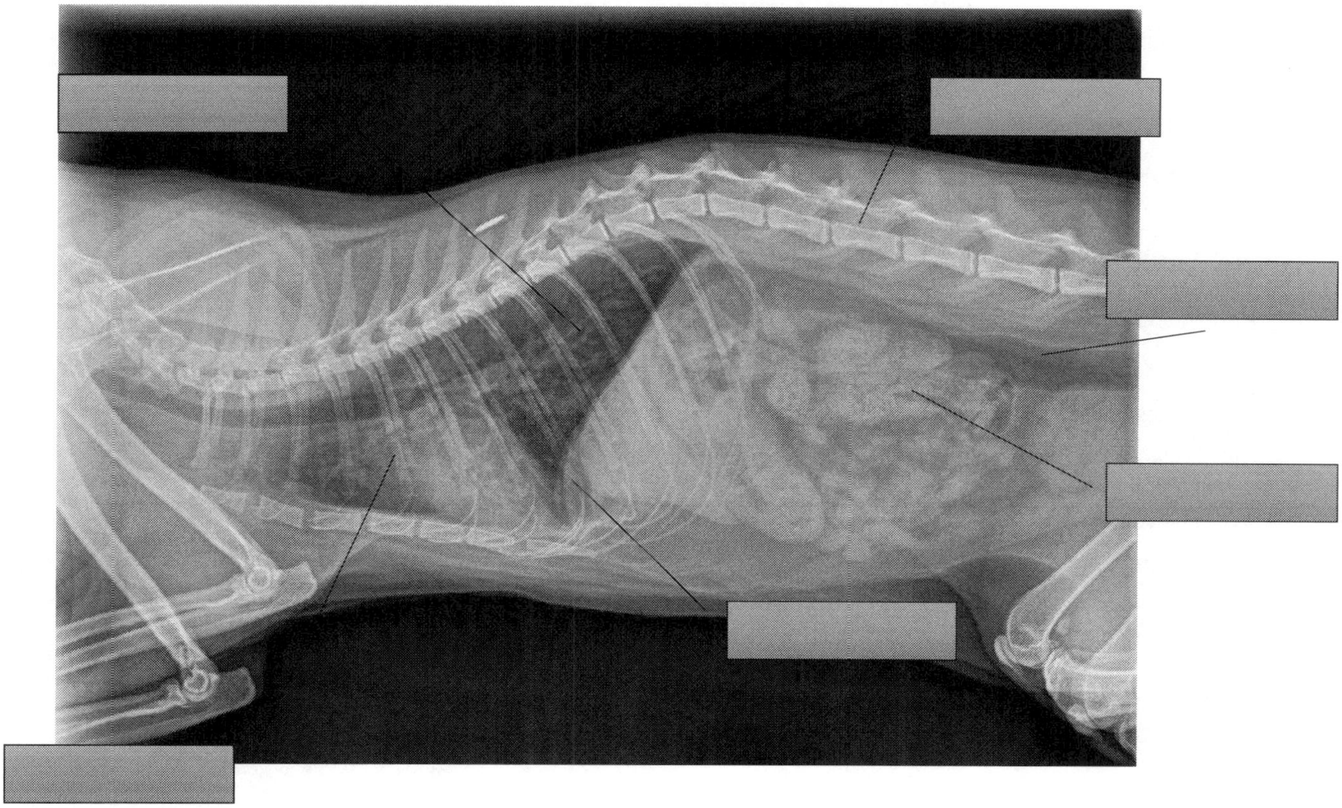

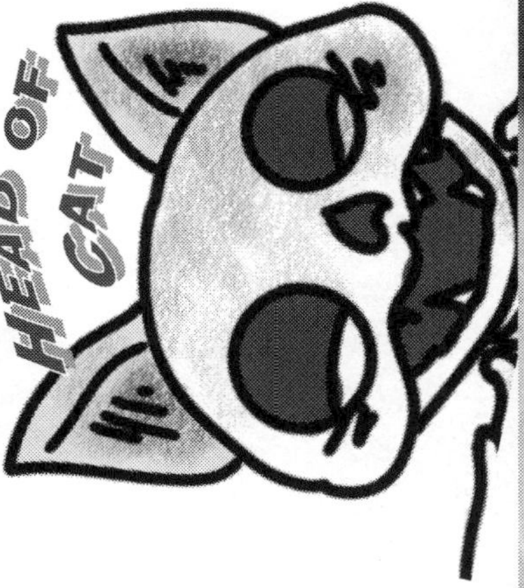
HEAD OF CAT

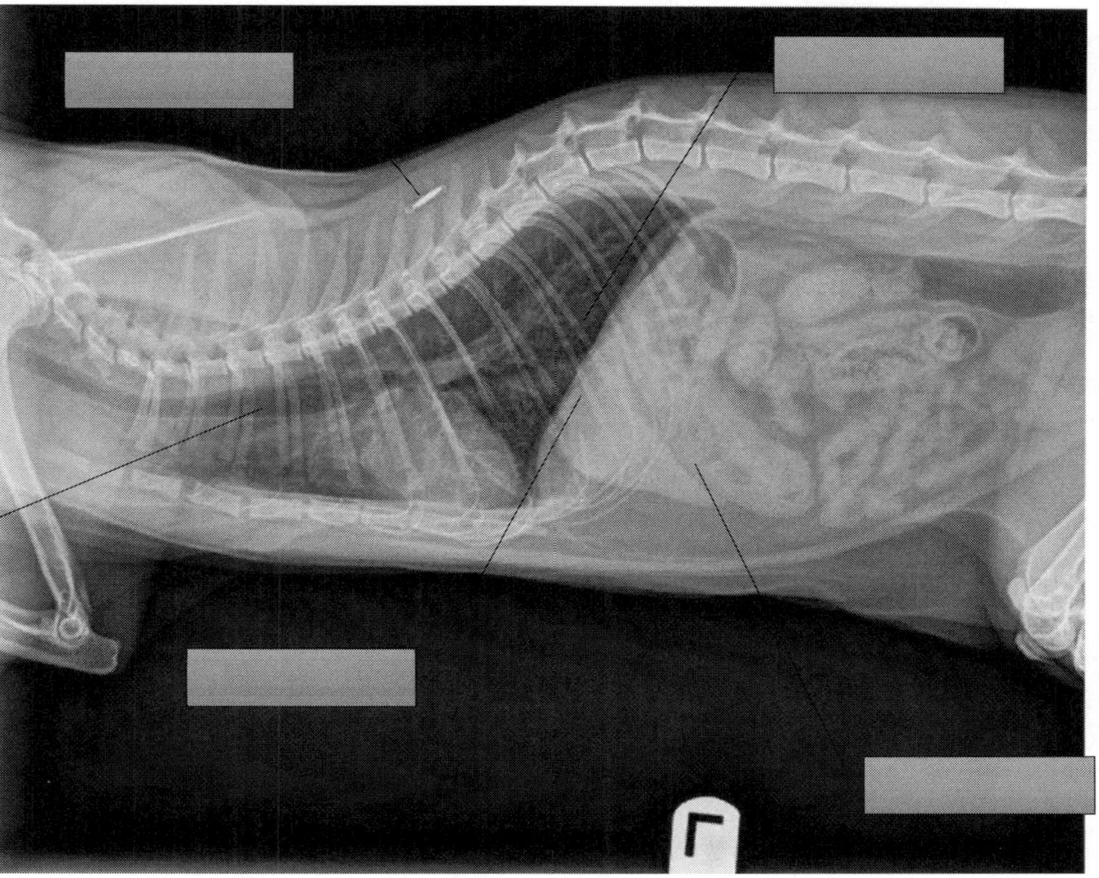

HEAD OF CAT

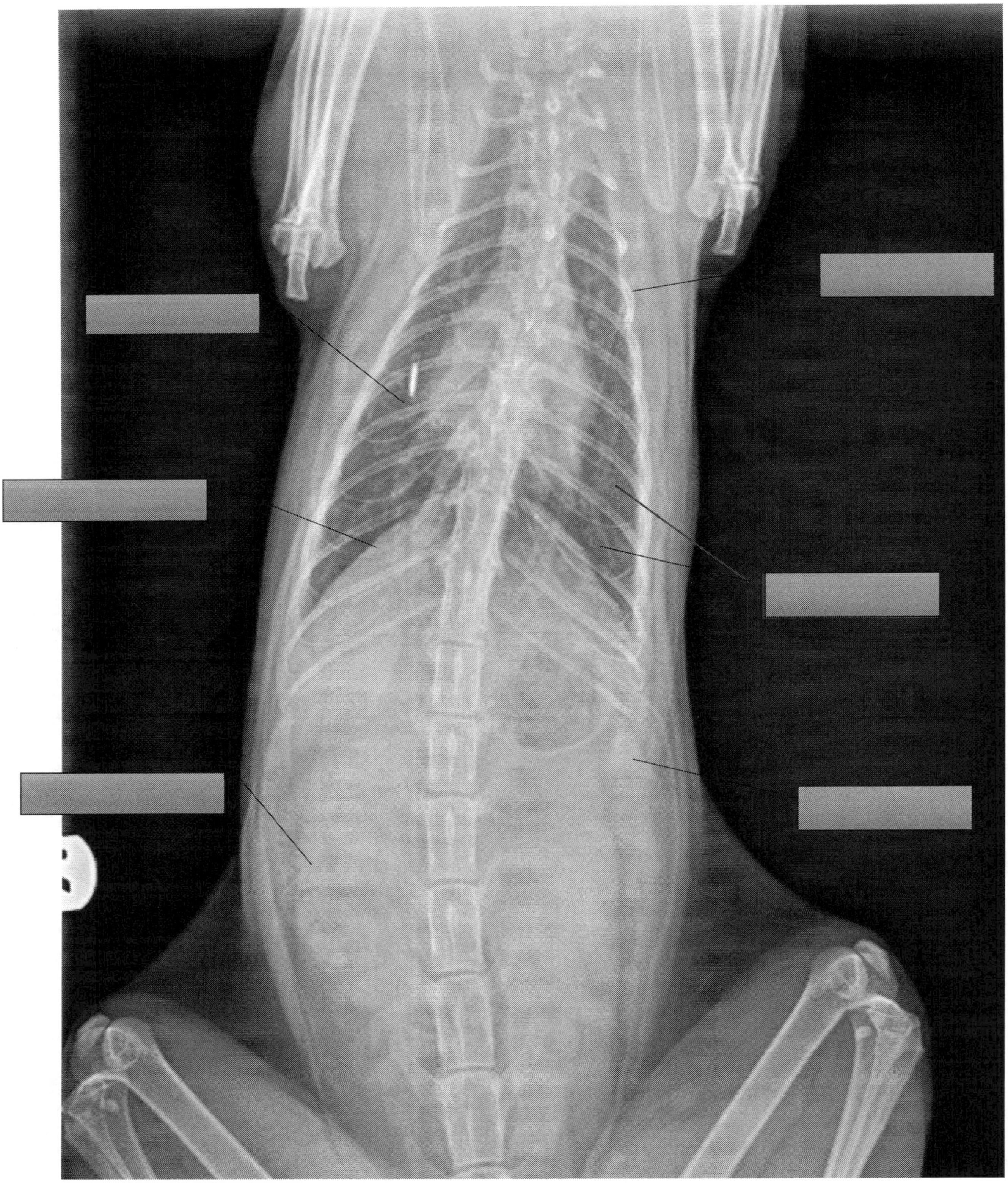

TAIL OF CAT

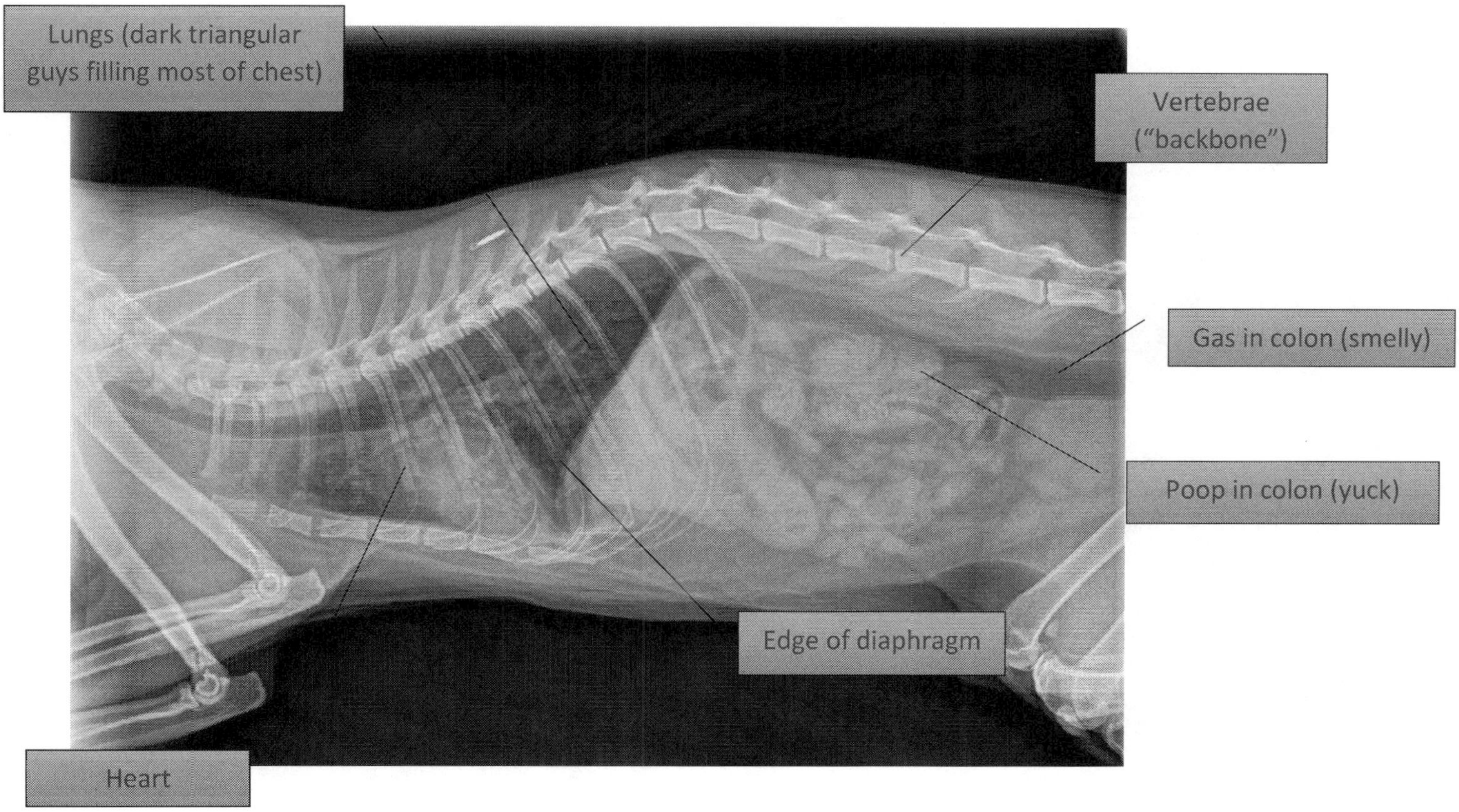
Lungs (dark triangular guys filling most of chest)
Vertebrae ("backbone")
Gas in colon (smelly)
Poop in colon (yuck)
Edge of diaphragm
Heart

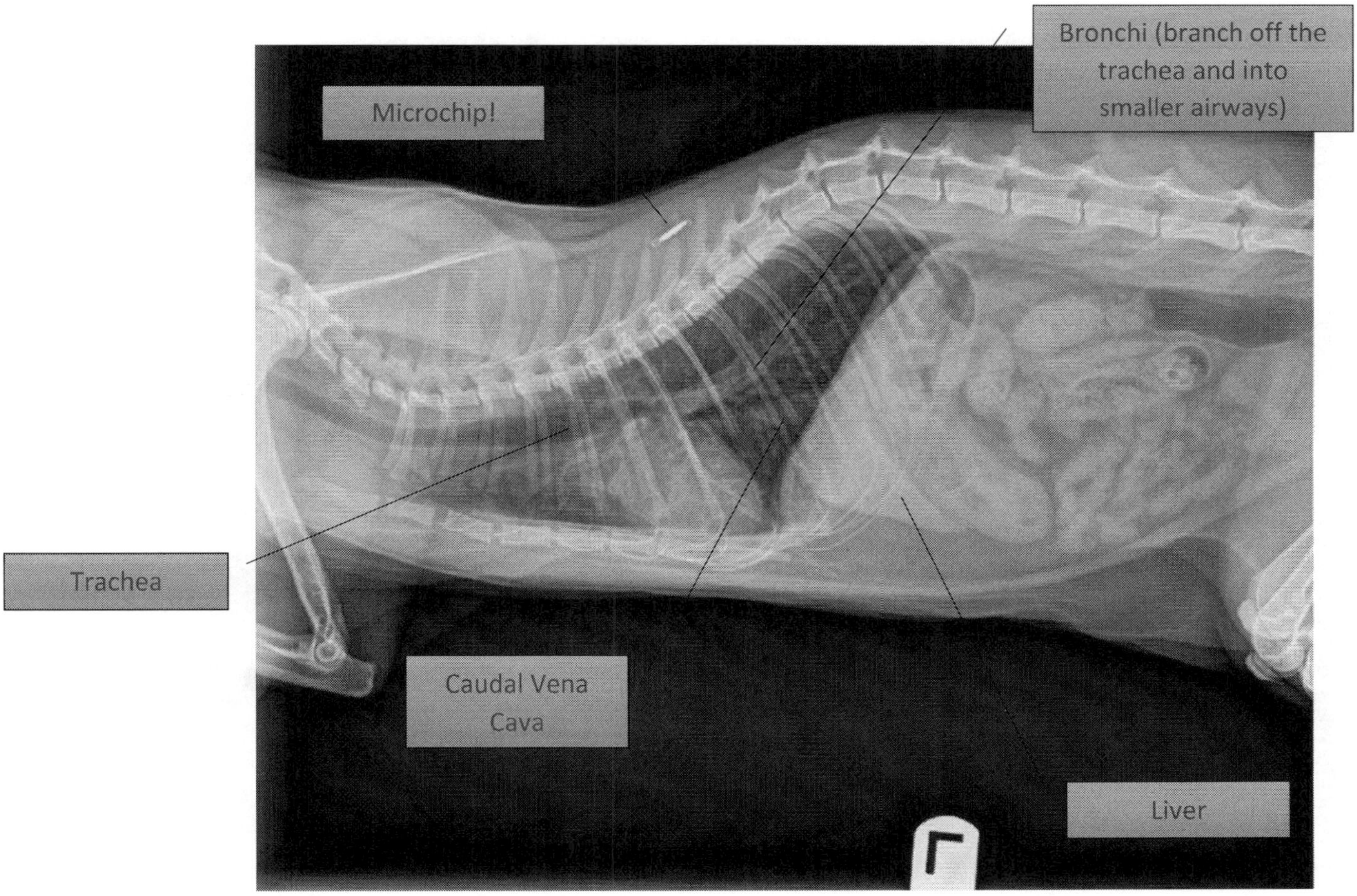
Microchip!
Bronchi (branch off the trachea and into smaller airways)
Trachea
Caudal Vena Cava
Liver

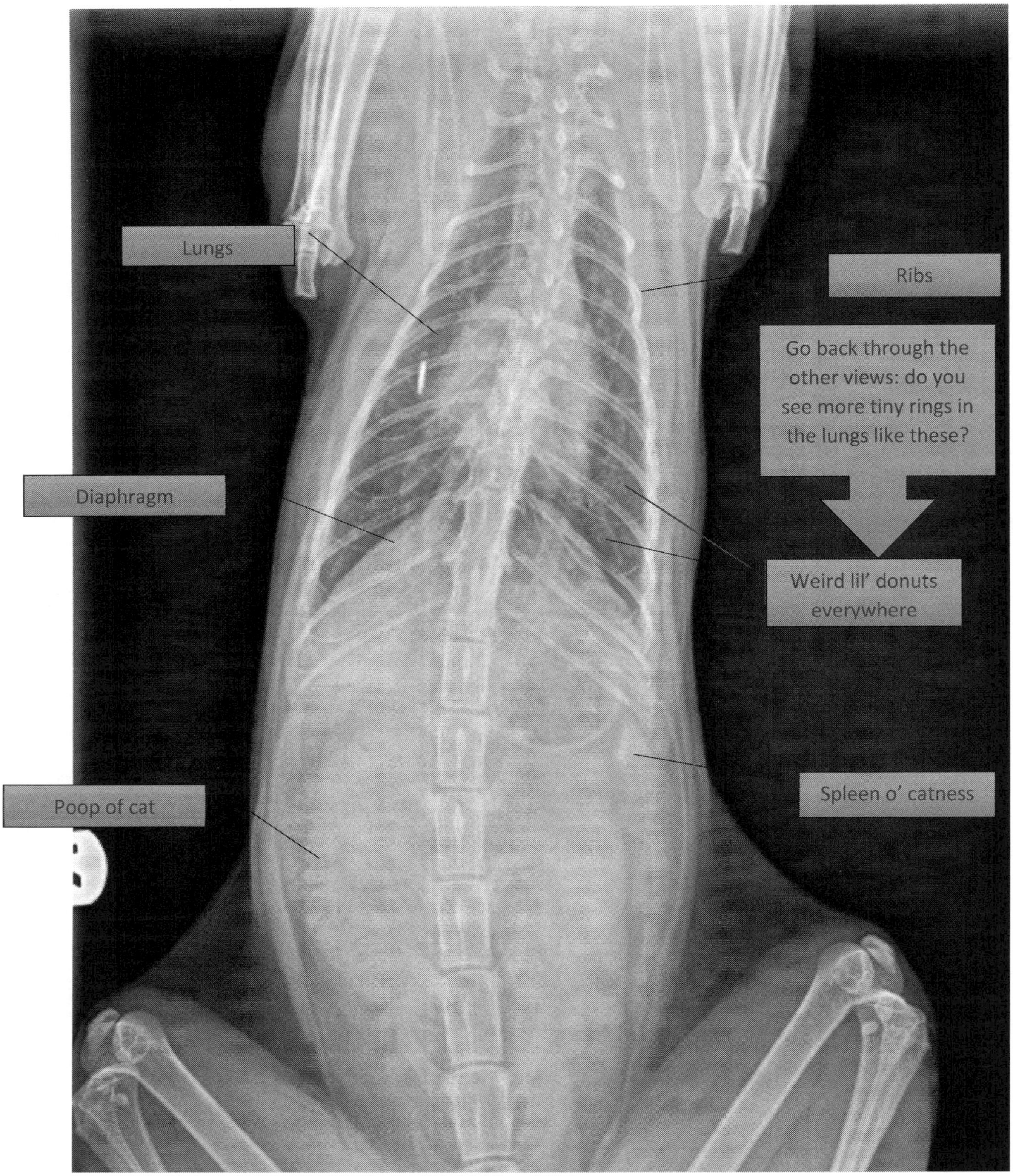
Lungs
Ribs
Go back through the other views: do you see more tiny rings in the lungs like these?
Diaphragm
Weird lil' donuts everywhere
Spleen o' catness
Poop of cat

Alright, that was a boring scan of the lungs. You see good glide sign (an actual glide requires the picture to move in real time, which is very hard to do in this book with today's printing technology: sorry). Radiographs are different. They are a one-time snapshot of the patient's innards.

Sweety Lumpkins calmed down enough to get some radiographs too, I'm sure you noticed. Did you see a pattern on those films? The lungs are tricky for us non-radiologists, who have not been fully trained in the art of the Magical Eye or initiated into the Mystical Vision true radiologists all share. These lungs seem to be inflating OK. Their edges go up against the chest and diaphragm like they should without any air or fluid trapped between.

> Air trapped between the lungs and body wall is pneumothorax. It would look like a black space between the lung edges and the chest wall. Fluid trapped between the lungs and body wall is generally called pleural fluid and more specifically can be named for the type of fluid (like "hemothorax" if it's blood). It looks like white stuff between the lung edges and chest wall on an X-ray.

You also don't see a bunch of fluid in the lung tissue itself (which looks like hazy white splotches in the lungs on a radiograph) or masses in the lungs (which look like round white structures). You do not see an enlarged heart in this patient. "OK already!" You are doubtless shouting. "Enough with what I don't see! There are entire textbooks about what I don't see. Tell me what I do see!" You're very clever with words, by the way.

What you do notice on these radiographs is some thickened small airways, that we often call "peribronchiolar cuffing." That's a fancy radiologist work for "teeny donuts." Look back at those radiographs again and appreciate the teeny donuts. Those are thickened airways deep inside the lungs, and they glom together sometimes to make a sort of hazy, pale pattern across the lung fields that makes them not-quite-as-clear-as-they-should-be. This is what is called a bronchiolar pattern, or bronchoalveolar pattern (depending on how congested the lungs look). Don't be sad if it's hard for you to see. To be honest I often have to stand on my head and squint and make things up to identify a bronchial pattern in a cat (don't tell any of my clients I said that though).

This lung pattern happens with disease processes like bronchitis. Aha!

She was stable enough to get some bloodwork running. Here are the results…

Client: Joe Dertoni	Species: Feline	Sex: FS
Patient: Sweety Lumpkins	Breed: DSH	
Patient ID: 0235579		

CBC

Test	Result	Flag	Reference Range	
WBC	20.6	H	5.5-19.5	$10^3/\mu L$
Neutrophils	11.8		2.5-12.5	$10^3/\mu L$
Monocytes	0.9	H	0-0.85	$10^3/\mu L$
Lymphocytes	2		1.5-7	$10^3/\mu L$
Eosinophils	2.1	H	0-1.5	$10^3/\mu L$
Hematocrit	39		30-45	%
MCV	53		39-55	fL
Platelet Count	357		300-700	$10^3/\mu L$

Client: Joe Dertoni	Species: Feline	Sex: FS
Patient: Sweety Lumpkins	Breed: DSH	
Patient ID: 0235579		

Chemistry Panel

TEST	RESULT	FLAG	REFERENCE RANGE[x]	
ALT	34		8.3-35	IU/L
ALP	52		12-65	IU/L
GGT	4		1.8-12	IU/L
tBili	0.3		0.1-0.5	mg/dL
Glucose	179	H	61-124	mg/dL
Cholesterol	160		71-161	mg/dL
Total Protein	8.5	H	5.7-8.0	g/dL
Albumin	2.9		2.4-3.8	g/dL
Globulin	5.1	H	2.4-4.7	g/dL
Calcium	8		7.9-10.9	mg/dL
BUN	27		15-31	mg/dL
Creatinine	1.5		0.5-1.9	mg/dL
Phosphorus	4.4		4.0-7.3	mg/dL
Sodium	147		146-159	mEq/L
Potassium	4.8		3.8-5.3	mEq/L
Chloride	117		108-130	mEq/L

Also, because he's a great technician and could see this was a respiratory case, Graham went ahead and ran a blood gas with this bloodwork. In some clinics he'd get in trouble because he didn't ask you first. Tonight you don't feel like yelling at him. You feel more like kissing him on the cheek for it. But you don't, of course, because that would be horribly inappropriate. This isn't France after all. Sheesh!

Client: Dertoni, Joe	Species: Feline	Sex: FS
Patient: Sweety Lumpkins	Breed: DSH	
Patient ID: 0235579		

Blood Gas

On a real-life blood gas panel, CO_2 is often listed as PCO_2 (P = partial pressure) and O_2 listed as PO_2.

TEST	RESULT	FLAG	REFERENCE RANGE[xi]	
pH	7.47	H	7.24-7.40	
CO2	22	L	29-42	mmHg
O2	79	L	85-95	mmHg
HCO3-	19		17-24	mEq/L

Oh, by the way, you also got an sPO2 (oxygen saturation) with a little point-of-care reader before putting the patient in the oxygen. It was moving back and forth between 87-90%. Generally, under 92% is a sign of inadequate oxygenation in dogs and cats.

Oooh. Blood gasses… Now you must figure out what those numbers tell you, meaning you have to think about chemistry in the middle of the night while patients are dying and people are crying at you. You don't feel like kissing anyone anymore.

OK kids, let's talk about blood gas panels (we're using a very simplified blood gas panel in this book, by the way).

Oxygen (O2) goes into your lungs when you breathe in, and out into your tissues through the blood. We refer to the oxygen dissolved in your blood "partial pressure of oxygen" (PO2). You get a low O2 in the blood when you can't get enough oxygen because you aren't ventilating (breathing) well, *or* your lungs are messed up and not transferring the oxygen, *or* something's messed up with your hemoglobin levels (the stuff that carries oxygen in your blood).

Carbon dioxide (CO_2) is gasped out when you exhale (after it bubbles back up through the blood, to get it out of tissues, which makes it a waste product).[9] CO_2 can be a good estimate of ventilation (the mechanical act of breathing). You get a low *venous* CO_2 when you hyperventilate, i.e. when you breath really fast and hard (and gasp out that CO_2 waste product as fast as theatergoers chuck garbage). You get high venous CO_2 if you can't breathe well (either through hypoventilation or through something wrong inside your lungs), or when your tissues are making so much of it your breathing can't keep up.

The pH is the measure of your body's acidity (a quality reflecting the amount of hydrogen ions, which has big implications on many chemical reactions important for your functioning). It's a low number when you're acidic, and a high number when you're basic ("OK, boomer?"). The thing is, your body wants to keep the pH in a safe and happy range, and "buffers it" by balancing the base produced by your tissues (metabolic component) with the acid breathed out by your lungs (respiratory component).

Bicarbonate (HCO_3) is a base (think of it as acid's greatest enemy) in solution, produced by your tissues doing their tissue thing.

CO_2 is acidic in blood. HCO_3 is basic in blood. Got all that?

So then… If your tissues are acidic (pH low), you start breathing quickly to get rid of more CO_2 to balance that ("to compensate"). If your tissues are super basic (have a high pH) you start breathing slower to compensate.

When you are looking at a blood gas panel then, you do these things in order:

A. See if the pH is low (acidic) or high (basic).

B. See if the CO_2 is low (respiratory alkalosis) or high (respiratory acidosis).

C. See if the HCO_3 is low (metabolic acidosis) or high (metabolic alkalosis).

D. Decide which one (respiratory or metabolic) is winning, and name the base status to help figure out where the patient is sicker (lungs or tissues).

There are differential patterns for each situation!

pH	CO2	HCO3	Acid-base problem
Low	Normal	Low	Metabolic acidosis
High	Normal	High	Metabolic alkalosis
Low	High	Normal	Respiratory acidosis
High	Low	Normal	Respiratory alkalosis

[9] Which basically means you've got carbonated blood, or soda in your veins…

And if that wasn't confusing enough, in the real world many sick critters have a "mixed acid-base disorder." This means their pH is back to normal, but their CO2 and HCO3 are all over the place, because their body has had time to catch up and balance the pH but not the other numbers yet.

Alright! Now you have the basic information you need to figure out what those few little numbers on the blood gas panel mean to Sweety Lumpkins. Here's what I see:

- The pH is high, so this gal has an alkalosis.
- The CO2 is low in the blood, because she is breathing out really fast. This would cause alkalosis. This is respiratory alkalosis.
- The HCO3 (bicarbonate) is normal, so there hasn't been enough time to make a compensatory metabolic response.

All this mental trauma is telling you that this cat is having trouble breathing. Gee, thanks a lot, blood gases.

But it can help us in two ways. It gives a bit of an idea of how sick the patient is. It also gives us a hint at how long this particular patient has been sick. The pH is barely elevated without metabolic changes catching up to balance it. That *could* mean this cat hasn't been breathing heavily long (which matches what the senator says).

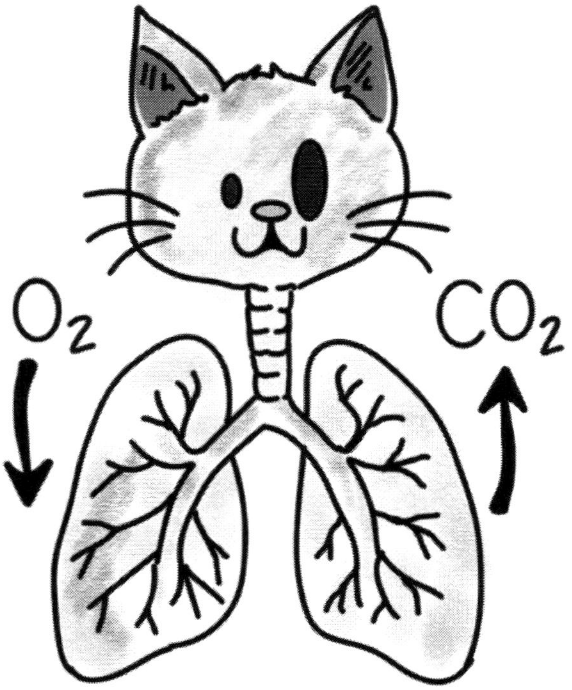

Put all the pieces together and what have we got going on in this cat?

What is your diagnosis?

____

STOP!!!!!!

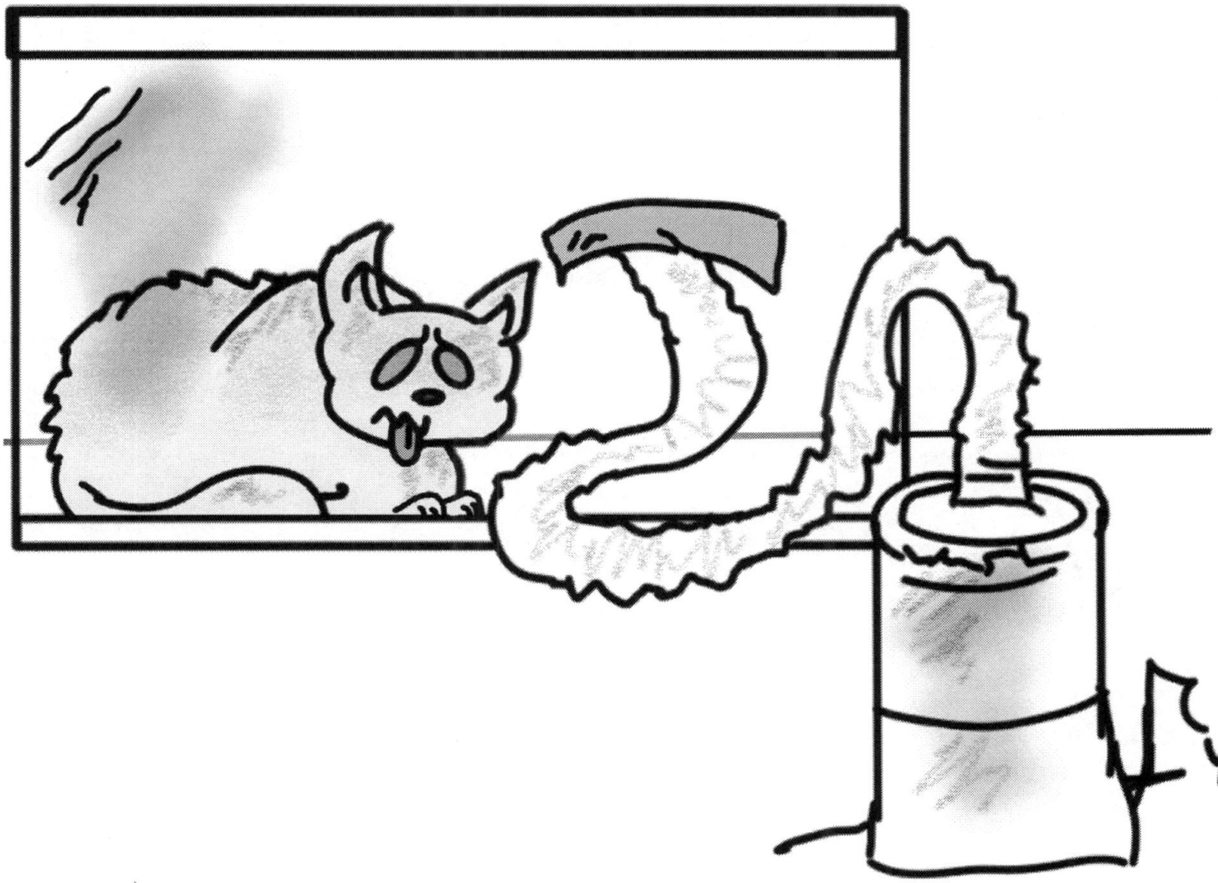

You are absolutely correct! Give that clever kid a prize, Felicia!!

This is **bronchitis**. It is probably an allergic bronchitis, better known **FELINE ASTHMA**. So, if you were all, "Somebody give that cat an inhaler," then you were 100% correct!

Asthma is an allergic reaction in the lungs. This reaction is probably an IgE mediated hypersensitivity reaction (a lot like what's going on inside Superfly too). Instead of the reaction causing histamine and cytokine chemicals to be released throughout the whole body, the effect is more localized to the lungs (which are incidentally the "shock organ," or the more sensitive part of a cat). This causes an eosinophilic inflammation - one in which the eosinophils (a specific white blood cells, which are high on the bloodwork) do much of the freakin' out. There are infections that can cause bronchitis, but this is much rarer than allergic bronchitis in cats. This is a good example of elevated white blood cells meaning inflammation *other than* an infection. The red eyes with a clear discharge probably go along with allergies as well.

Cats in the acute, emergency phase of asthma will breathe out CO2 quickly and have a primary respiratory alkalosis. As time marches on, they develop chronic changes in their lung tissue that blocks exchange of CO2, and develop respiratory acidosis (because CO2 builds up in their blood over time).

The first hint of feline bronchitis is often a cough. Cats with this condition usually have a harsh, hacking type of cough. Sometimes they have a wheezing sound when they breathe. And as the problem progresses (or a more severe reaction occurs acutely) they struggle to breathe at all. Signs of dyspnea in these kitties can be quite severe (even life-threatening). When you listen to their lungs, you often hear harsh crackles everywhere (in up to 82% of cases, according to one study).[xii]

Why is the blood sugar elevated in this patient? I'm glad you asked. It's probably due to stress, which releases hormones that drive glucose up ("stress hyperglycemia"). Not being able to breathe is stressful.

Right! This politician's gasping cat's got asthma… What legal remedy will you apply to this external threat to Sweety Lumpkin's life and pursuit of happiness? How will you pacify this demoralizing force of hyperbole employed by her lungs, and reform a path to health from this toxic last-gasp strategy she seems to be taking?

In other words, Doc, what are you gonna do?

Choose some from this list of treatment options.

What is your treatment plan? (pick several)

a) Aggressive filibustering—talk until *you're* blue in the face

b) Antibiotics

c) Campaign-focused political context analysis by an independent think-tank

d) Coupage

e) Epinephrine

f) Inhaled bronchodilator medications

g) Injectable bronchodilator medications

h) Insulin

i) Oxygen, give her lots and lots of oxygen

j) Pain medications

k) Sedatives

l) Steroids

m) Thoracocentesis—jab a needle into her chest to release the demons

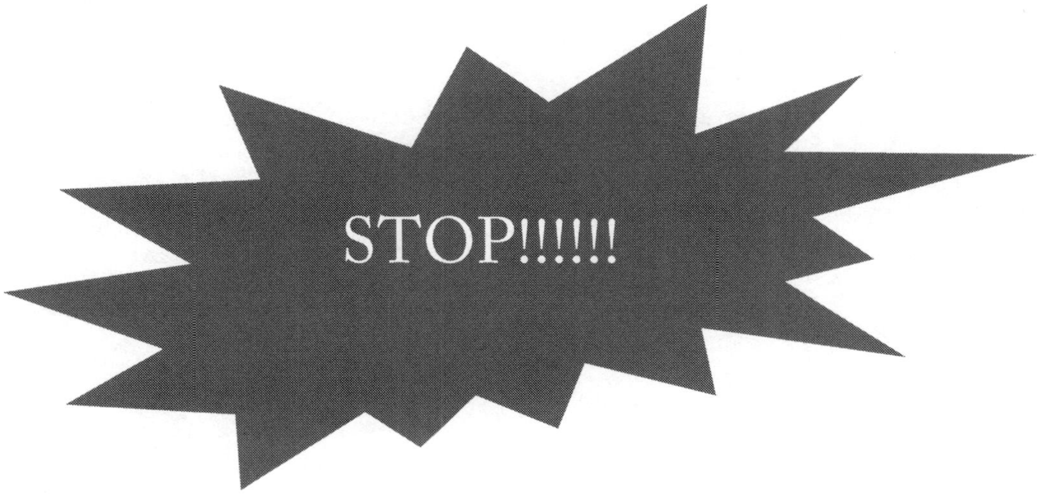

If you answered: **i, k, l, and f OR g** then you are right on track toward a better future for this suffering kitty!

Those are the mainstays of emergency treatment for an asthmatic crisis in a cat. **Get them in oxygen ASAP** (already done) and calm them down. You can use **sedatives** to help get them out of the cycle of panic that makes their breathing worse. You already gave this gal a mild opioid sedative called butorphanol.

Steroids work wonders for the lung inflammation that causes asthma. The word "bronchitis" literally means "inflammation of the bronchi (airways down in the lungs)." And steroids are one of the most potent anti-inflammatory drugs we have. These handy drugs come in many convenient forms. Sadly, they do not come in special collector's edition packaging. And, no, you can't buy them at your local hardware store. But if you are a medical professional (who doesn't care about the packaging) you can give steroids as an injection, an oral medication, or even in an inhaler. In the case of an asthmatic crisis, it's best to start with a short-acting steroid injection (dexamethasone is a common one), then get the patient on oral or inhaled steroids as they become stable. That's because oral and inhaled steroids can take a good 1-2 weeks to really become effective. And it's very inconvenient to be unable to breathe for 1-2 weeks. Also, inhaled drugs won't absorb well when a cat is breathing quick and shallow.

Inhaled or injectable bronchodilator medications are medications that do exactly what their name suggests: they dilate the bronchi and bronchioles. Many vets use an injection called terbutaline for this in asthmatic cats, because it works quickly and can be given as IM (intramuscular) as well as IV (intravenous) injection. It can be repeated within 15 minutes if it doesn't do the job the first time. An inhaled medication like albuterol works too (but shallow, quick breathing makes it challenging to absorb). There are severe cases I've used both together.

Great job! You whip out some doses on your calculating machine of steroid and terbutaline injections and write them on the orders for your technician to give this poor wheezy kitty. Then you make your way through the hallowed halls of this institution to talk to Senator Dertoni about the plan.

"Hey man, can you get the drugs out?" A reedy voice in the darkness interrupts your transit to consult with Dertoni.

You're not exactly sure you heard that right. "Um… Excuse me?"

"Superfly could really use a downer. He seems freakish." You recognize the starry-eyed expression of Dr. Debbie Crimshaw. You'd kinda forgotten about her. You walk over to check on her suffering dog. Superfly looks super better. His vitals have normalized after another fluid bolus and the drugs for anaphylaxis. He does seem agitated though.

"He gets all worked up when we board him," Dr. Crimshaw shrugged. "Especially here. Too many corners that smell of Mel, if you catch what I'm throwin'."

You don't catch it. You have no idea what she is throwing at this point. You suspect she has no idea what she's throwing.

The old doctor nods sagely. "He needs a little sedative. I can give it while you do your thing. I just don't remember the combination to the drug safe."

"Um…" This is not great. This may be a colleague and all, but she does seem exactly trustworthy with control drugs. She also doesn't work here. She's also phishing for access to the drugs, which is super…er…fishy.

'Don't be whack, Youngblood! Give mama some flower power!"

"Um…" It's way too late in the shift for this kind of thing. Where are your technicians?

DING! DONG!

That's the doorbell! Another person is ringing. Oh brother! Not another sick critter. You are beginning to feel very stressed, and probably have mild hyperglycemia. "I have to go check on that…"

You should probably not leave her on her own. But you'll send your staff back as soon as you can. You make your way toward the lobby, glancing at the cat in oxygen as you pass by. She seems to be breathing better. You hear the clap of Exam Room 2, then a familiar wailing from inside it. The voice chills your blood.

"LITTLE BUGS! HAM'S STILL GOT THE LITTLE BUGS!"

Good grief. You really don't have time for this.

Also, why is everyone shouting tonight?!?!??!?!? What's going on!?!?! Who convinced you to sign up for all this misery!?!?!?!?!?

"I'm not absolutely certain of my facts, but I rather fancy it's Shakespeare…who says that it's always just when a chappie is feeling particularly top-hole…with things in general that Fate sneaks up behind him with a bit of lead piping."

— P. G. Wodehouse, Jeeves and the Unbidden Guest[xiii]

Case #3B

"THE LITTLE BUGS ARE BACK!" Harold Wibbly notices you trying to surreptitiously sneak past the exam room and runs to you. "I SAW THEM AGAIN, DOC! THEY'RE BACK AND THEY'RE CRAWLING IN HAM'S HAM-HOCKS AND THEY'RE GOING UP MY ARM AND THEY'RE CRAWLING DOWN MY SHIRT AND THEY'RE PROBABLY IN MY EAR, TOO!"

He shakes you by the lapel while he hollers. You gently remove him, decide not to call the police, and graciously chalk this to the insanity that obviously afflicts people in this city at 3 am.

"Tiny crabs… The tiny crabs…" he continues to mutter.

"Did you go see a human medical professional about this, like we talked about last time?" you sigh. You decide to do a quick once-over of this hairy little Ham dog, just to satisfy his poor, crazed human and then move on (to the patients that have actual problems).

"I did!" Mr. Wibbly replied. "That quack said I was crazy! Said I have something called Morgellan's disease…"

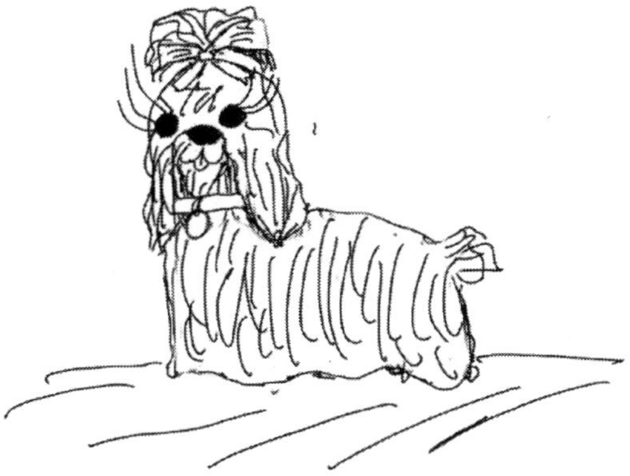

"Aha, well…" you start to say, but he's on a roll.

"I'm not crazy. There are little ant-bugs creeping along Ham. And there are little crab-bugs doing this kind of circle dance around him in my library."

"A circle dance, huh?"

"Yeah. And they stop to wave at the ant-bugs and carry them off with their little crab-hands, and…"

Harold Wibbly's crazed story gets crazier as he drones on. You can't really remember, since his madman voice faded into the background of your consciousness as you do an exam and tune him out. Here's what you see on Ham.

Step 1 – Organize the History

Signalment:

7 years old

Male neutered

Shih Tzu

Presenting Complaints:

Little bugs… Again.

Physical Examination:

Abdominal palpation: No fluid or distension noted, no obvious masses noted. Not painful (not tense or splinting).

Attitude: Bright, alert, responsive. Doesn't seem bothered by little bugs at all.

Cardiac: No heart murmurs or arrhythmias noted. No little bugs hollering "We are here, we are here" into your stethoscope bell.

Ears: Canals appear clear bilaterally.

Eyes: Look clear and super-normal and bug free.

Oronasal: Yep. There's teeth in there. No little bugs hiding behind them though. Gums are pink. Good enough. You're trying to hurry this up.

Respiratory: Lungs sound clear bilaterally on auscultation. Normal respiratory effort.

Integument: No rashes or wounds noted. No little bugs noted and…. Um…. Wait a minute. Was that something moving in the shoulder hair? You part the hair and jump back.

YAAAAH! LITTLE BUG! LITTLE BUG!!!!

A tiny thing that looks very much like a pale crab, or a miniature scorpion without a tail, drops out of Ham's forest of fur and scurries under a cabinet. It's hard to find words. And when the shock fades away, it's replaced by a twinge of guilt for not believing Harold Wibbly. Lemon pops in to check on you after hearing you scream like a toddler frightened by a dark closet.

"Um… I'm OK. Hey! How about you get down there and look under the cabinet. I think a little crab scurried under there…"

The look Lemon gives you is not hard to interpret. But she is a kindhearted person who loves to help, so she looks under the cabinet.

"Oh hey, look at this little guy!" She reaches under and shows you her slim hand. The small, brown thing is scurrying back and forth on her finger, waving its claws like some kind of arachnid protestor. "This is a pseudoscorpion. Don't see too many of these guys around here…"

"A what now?" you ask.

"They're a type of teeny arachnid. Some people call them book scorpions. Completely harmless really, unless you're a louse… I'm double majoring in entomology," Lemon explained. "Bugs are super cool."

Meh. That's debatable…

"THAT'S ONE OF THE DANCING CRABS!!!!!" Harold Wibbly trembles as he points at the tiny thing. This of course reminds you about the reason this little Shih Tzu hitchhiker was important in the first place.

"Do these pseudoscorpion guys usually live on Shih Tzus?"

Lemon laughs. "Not at all. They aren't parasites either, so they won't hurt our little pal." Ham looks at her worshipfully as she rubs his hairy head. "Phoresis, a fancy word for temporarily living on something just for travel purposes, is a common behavior among pseudoscorpions."

"Wait…" Mr. Wibbly wobbles forward, looking with a new expression at the little creature Lemon lets scamper across the floor. "You're saying these little crabs are harmless?"

She nods.

That's when you all notice the pseudoscorpion crush the head off another insect with his tiny claw. Mr. Wibbly jumps up onto the counter.

"LITTLE ANT! LITTLE DECAPITATED ANT!!!!"

"Oho! This is making more sense," Lemon says. "That poor bug was a book louse, Psocopta species, I'm pretty sure. Or it could be a nymph of Lepinotus reticulatus…" she squints at the carcass our murderous neighborhood pseudoscorpion is munching on. "Oh, look! Here's a few more crawling in Ham's fur."

"LITTLE BUGS!"

"It's OK. Book lice are harmless too. They're just catching a ride on Ham's hair. And they also happen to be a favorite food of pseudoscorpions. Mr. Wibbly, do you work around books?"

Harold Wibbly nods. "I'm a librarian."

"You probably need to call a pest control guy out, and maybe clean up the old book section. You've got a book louse infestation."

A light bulb in your noggin' goes blink. "Aha! So it's really got nothing to do with Ham?" Lemon shakes her head. "Mystery of the little bugs solved."

The client blinks and seems calmer. "So they're not ticks or fleas or alien blood-beasts?"

You and Lemon shake your heads in unison.

"Imagine that. Do you know a good pest guy?"

You direct him to the interwebs and Lemon helps him check out. Another mysterious case solved! You write up some discharge notes, then check on Superfly (who's looking every more chill and groovy by the minute) and Sweety Lumpkins (whose symptoms show tendency toward amelioration).

"OK!" you sigh. "It's time to catch up on notes. Glad the rush stopped. Not sure I could handle another case on top of these tough ones coming all at once…"

NEVER say things like that in an ER!

"Help! Help!"

The sound of loud voices echoes after the slam of the front door, chilling your heart like the horrible Banshee-Beast of Phargon-7 froze Corporal Ostinato (in Season 1 of Starship Beethoven). *Now what?*

A few minutes later, Lemon comes jogging back to Treatment with a limp dog in her arms.

Case #7

"We need all hands! The owner said this little guy stopped breathing on the way here. She approved CPR..."

You rush over to the treatment table to find an unresponsive toy poodle. He isn't breathing. His tongue is purple. You can't hear a heartbeat when you slap a stethoscope on him. He looks old...

"What happened to him? Has he been sick? Any vomiting, diarrhea, coughing, sneezing...? How long has it been exactly since he stopped breathing? Is he on any medications?"

"I don't know, and also I don't know," Lemon replies as she starts chest compressions. Graham is already getting an ET tube and pulling up the anesthesia machine to give oxygen. "I'll go talk to them as soon as I can."

Time to assess this guy while your team starts basic CPR. In human medicine, studies have established that the chance of successfully bringing a patient back drops 2.1% with every minute in CPR. Seconds matter! Get moving!!! Go! Go! Go! ACK!!!!!

Step 1 – Organize the History

Signalment:

Pretty old toy poodle

Appears to be a neutered male

Presenting Complaints:

Dead... This guy is apneic and has no heartbeat ("presented with apnea and with no heartbeat on auscultation" is what you write in your notes later). We're hoping to jump-start him with some CPR.

Name: You don't know. We'll just call him Breathless Bill for now.

Step 2 – Gather Clues

Physical Examination: In a situation like this, your exam is a quick assessment while CPR is being performed by your team.

Abdominal Palpation: No obvious distention or fluid wave noted. You don't feel a tumor or organ enlargement.

Apnea: cessation of breathing. Sleep apnea is not very bad. Death apnea is very, very bad.

Attitude: Non-responsive and laterally recumbent.

Cardiac: No heartbeat on auscultation. No palpable femoral pulses.

Ears: You don't have time to look in his ears! You're not gonna find anything in his ears that killed this guy! Keep looking!

Eyes: Yep. He's got eyes. No obvious hyphema or masses on his irises.

Integument: No obvious lacerations or wounds you can see. Skin turgor seems dramatically decreased (estimated 10% dehydration).

Lymph Nodes: No obviously enlarged lymph nodes.

Musculoskeletal: No obvious fractures or luxation that you can palpate.

Neurologic: Non-responsive. Corneal reflex is absent OU.

Oronasal: Slight serosanguinous discharge from his left nostril.

Respiratory: Apneic.

Urogenital: small sized urinary bladder with normal tone.

Differential Diagnoses…

This is a situation where your differential list is going to be growing inside your head as you think through the case, *while your hands are moving*. You need to figure out what disease processes got this patient to the point of shutting down so you have a better chance of targeting treatments that will help him.

But you have two bigger problems at this moment. Those problems are as follows: THIS PATIENT IS NOT BREATHING and THIS PATIENT HAS NO HEARTBEAT!!!!!

So write down your top three differentials here, and you must move on to treatment. What are the three most likely causes of Breathless Bill's symptoms?

____

____

____

Corneal reflex: poking the eyeball with a finger doesn't make him blink. You usually don't want clients to see you do this.
Hyphema: blood inside the eyeball.
Serosanguinous: "kind of bloody;" thin and blood colored, usually because it has serum and blood in it.

Good work! I would probably pick these three differentials:

- Congestive heart failure. Serosanguinous fluid is a common sign at the final stages of heart failure, when soggy lungs full of fluid overflow to drain down the trachea and out the nose and mouth.
- Neoplasia. This is a very common reason for old dogs to die. It could also cause fluid in the lungs that leaks out the nose.
- Renal failure. This dog seems very dehydrated. Kidney disease can happen in older pets and cause serious dehydration.

Alright, say your little, white-coated brain cells, *that's a start. How do we get this guy back into the light long enough to make a real differential list and run some diagnostics?*

Good question, brain cells!

What treatments are you going to do now?

Look over the infographic on the next page, then come back and list some treatments for Breathless Bill before moving on…

PET CPR TIPS

Cardiopulmonary resuscitation (CPR) is indicated when a patient codes (heart and/or breathing stops). Only 5-7% of dogs and 1-19% of cats recover with CPR. Chance of success drops 2.1% with every minute of CPR (humans). The goal with CPR is return to spontaneous circulation (ROSC), meaning trying to restart the heart and get the patient breathing again on their own. CPR consists of BLS (Basic Life Support: compressions and breathing) and ALS (Advanced Life Support: drugs and monitoring).

General Strategy

- BLS in 2-minute cycles
- 10-second pauses to evaluate
- If no ROSC in 10 rounds, consider stopping

1. Chest compressions

Over heart in small dogs and cats, over widest part of chest in big dogs. Aim for 100-120 bpm.

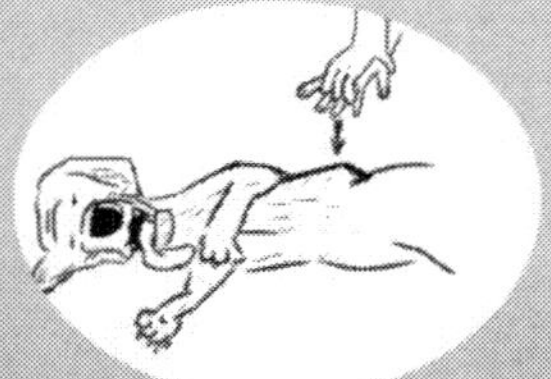

With patient on their side: compress about 1/3-1/2 of chest diameter

Two hands over widest part of chest in big, deep-chest dogs.

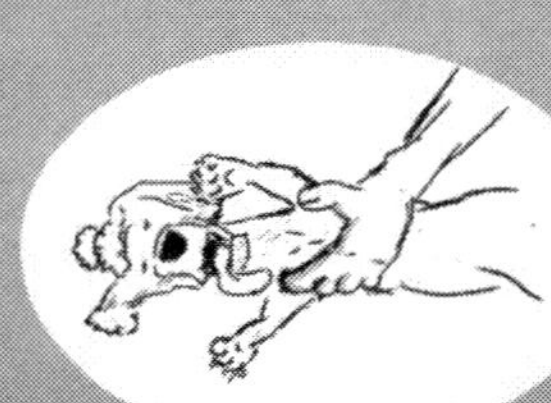

Thumb and fingers around heart in small dogs and cats.

2. Establish an airway

In a clinical setting, this means putting in an endotracheal (ET tube).

3. Breathe for patient

At the clinic this means giving oxygen and hand ventilation (squeezing a breathing bag at 10 bpm).

ROSC Goals

- *Palpable pulse >30 BPM*
- *Systolic BP >60mmHg*
- *Marked increase in ETC02 (>18mmHg)*

4. IV catheter and monitoring

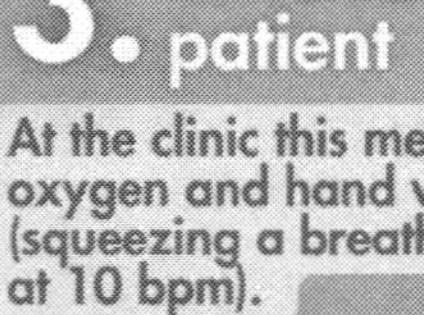

Another rescuer places a catheter and hooks up ECG and capnograph (measures CO2) while others work on breathing and compressions.

5. Give drugs

Such as epinephrine (increase coronary perfusion), atropine (increase heart rate), or lidocaine (treat ventricular tachycardia).

Atropine 0.04 mg/kg once
Epinephrine 0.01 mg/kg (every 3-5 minutes)

Here are some things that should happen in this case:

- **Chest compressions**. In a clinical setting, starting compressions first is recommended, even before checking for an established airway and breathing for the patient. Because you've got several sets of professional hands ready to help, one person can work on the patient's airway while another is doing compressions. If you're the only one present, you might want to make sure the patient's airway is clear before starting compressions. In a little dog like this, the technique used involves one hand compressing right over the heart, by squeezing his chest (about 1/3-1/2 way down) between the thumb and other fingers. If this were a big dog with a narrow ("keel-shaped") chest, Lemon would lay him on his side and use two hands (one atop the other, with fingers interlaced) to compress down the chest right over the heart. If this were a big dog with a barrel-shaped chest, she'd lay him on his side and use two hands to compress over the widest part of his chest. You can find the area around a dog's heart quickly, by the way, by pulling back the front leg and mentally marking where the point of the elbow meets the chest.
    - Your team is going to perform chest compressions in 2-minute cycles, interrupted by 10 second breaks where the person doing the compressions is changed out, and the doctor listens for a heartbeat and feels for a pulse. Lots of clinics have egg timers on hand for CPR. Some use handy phone apps that tick out the heartbeat in 2-minute cycles. You start a log (in this case you rip off a piece of some old bloodwork laying on the counter nearby and scribble a few things with a pen) to keep track of how many CPR cycles have passed, and when you give what meds.
- **Intubation and ventilation.** Graham puts an endotracheal tube into Breathless Bill. He hooks this up to an Ambu bag, which is a portable device you can squeeze to push air into the lung (this is called positive pressure ventilation). Ventilation in this case means moving air in and out, and that's exactly what your technician does for the patient: squeezing the Ambu bag around 10 times per minute. Many clinics use an oxygen delivery system on their anesthesia cart, and squeeze the re-breathing bag instead. If you're not at a clinic, you can provide breaths by holding a pet's mouth closed and blowing into his nose (preferably by making a seal with your hand between your mouth and that germ-coated nose).

Endotracheal tube: a flexible plastic tube that goes down into the windpipe through the mouth, and has a balloon on the tip you blow up with a syringe to make a seal.

  - Chest compressions and breathing for the patient are termed "basic CPR." That's the backbone of your attempts to bring oxygen to this guy's organs while you try to bring him back to life.
- **IV catheter and fluids.** Since there are only three of you, you put in an IV catheter and start some fluids. Fluids will help increase blood pressure (which was 0 mmHg when you started this whole process). Access to his veins allows you to give drugs. There are two drugs you're going to give.
  - Atropine. This potent drug increases the heart rate. It acts within minutes of giving it IV. Current recommendations are to give it once at the start of CPR.
  - Epinephrine. This drug constricts blood vessels around the heart (called the coronary vessels), increasing coronary circulation and helping the heart survive. It also helps treat shock by increasing blood pressure everywhere, and has a "chronotropic effect" (it increases heartbeat). Current recommendations are to give this every 3-5 minutes during CPR, which works out to every other cycle of basic CPR.
- **Monitoring.** You put ECG leads on this patient. This handy doodad lets you see the electrical activity of the heart and if the heart starts beating again. You can see the pulse on a screen this way too, which helps you judge the quality of chest compressions. You also connect a capnograph to the patient, which measures the CO2 coming out of his lungs. If it suddenly spikes and is consistently over 18 mmHg, then Breathless Bill just might not be breathless anymore (he'd just be Bill).

That's the gist of it. Now you know what to do when someone at the vet clinic you work in says, "Do CPR, STAT!" It sounds easy enough, right? Full disclaimer: it's a terrifying, sweat-drenching experience, that moves faster than you expect and usually turns out bad. Exactly *nobody* on their day off says, "What am I gonna do for fun today? Oh, I know, I'll go do some CPR…"

Unfortunately, this patient seems to have read the textbook. Despite all the valiant efforts of your team, he does not show any sign of reviving. Six cycles of CPR go by. No heartbeat, no pulse, no corneal reflex. 10 cycles of CPR and still no response. Evidence in human medicine[10] shows that reviving a patient after 10 cycles (20 minutes) of CPR is very, very unlikely. After 40 minutes chances are extremely, super, uber, mucho unlikely. You may have noticed I didn't say chances are 0%. The only reason for that is that I am not in actual fact (despite what some tribal people on the island of Ucka-matcha-aöloo think) the

[10] There aren't good, controlled studies in dogs and cats for this yet. Sometimes we have to extrapolate evidence from studies in people and hope they hold true in other species.

omnipotent God Almighty. There is no 0% chance of anything in medicine. But CPR beyond 20 minutes is about as close as you can come to it. And after 40 minutes it's even closer.

"Keep suctioning that bloody fluid out of the ET tube, Lemon. There's a lot more coming. That's not good…" You are interrupted from these grim observations by a cheerfully deranged voice.

"Hey groovemiesters! I found this hip chick up in the lobby, just totally freaking out, and figured I'd bring her back…"

Oh, Dr. Crimshaw, what hast thou done?

"This is Jane. She's cool. Say hey to the gang, Jane!"

Jane does not say "hey." What she says is, "AAAAAAAAAAAAAHHHH! WAFFLES! MY WAFFLES! WHAT ARE YOU DOING TO HIM??!?!?! WHAT'S HAPPENING?!?!? WHY IS BLOODY FLUID POURING OUT OF HIS NOSE?!?!?!?! IS HE GOING TO BE OK?!?!?!? AAAAAAAAAAAAAAAAAAAAAAHHHHHHH!!!!"

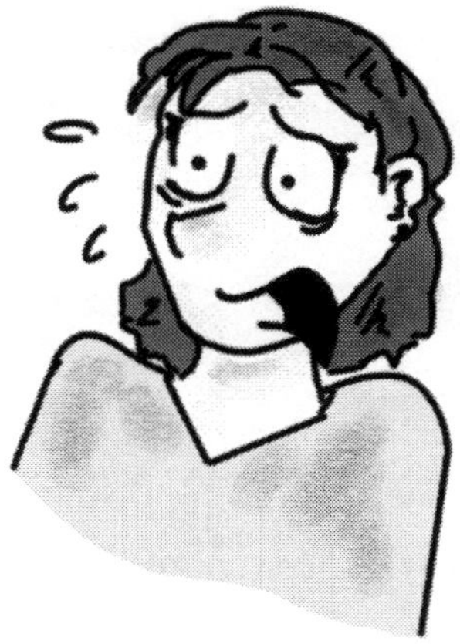

"Little Jane here could use some Mary Jane, if you dig my groove. One of these nice doctor dudes can find you a downer."

"Alright…" You put down the pen and syringe of epinephrine and take charge. "This is not helpful, Miss Crimshaw. Why don't you head back up to the lobby."

"Sure. Wait… Haven't I met you?" She wanders off looking into cabinets. "Is this my clinic? Did I leave something back here? I really need those papers I left in the closet!" Lemon steps over to herd her up front, while you take over the Ambu bag and start talking to Jane (who is pouring tears and babbling at her little poodle).

"I'm so sorry, but Breathless B…um…this little guy is not responding to CPR efforts. It's been 10 (no, 11) cycles of CPR now. Usually if we don't get him back by this time, he isn't going to come back."

She can't answer through her sniffles, and you and Graham silently trudge through more compressions and breaths. More red fluid fills the ET tube, and you have to stop and let it drain into a trash can. You put a stethoscope on the patient's chest. Still no heartbeat. You feel under his hind limb. Still no femoral pulses. You shake your head.

"I'm sorry ma'am, but I think we're not going to get him back."

She nods and sniffles. "H…h…his name is Waffles. He was my first dog. He's 17 years old."

"He sounds like a wonderful little guy. I'm going to stop and call time of death now, OK?"

She agrees, and you and Graham clean Waffles up so she can visit his body. She asks you why he died.

> "It is possible to commit no mistakes and still lose. That is not weakness, that is life."
> —Jean-Luc Picard to Data in *Star Trek: The Next Generation*[xiv]

"I can't be sure at this point, but my best guess would be heart failure, because of the fluid coming out of his mouth and nose." You offer to send him to a local teaching hospital for a necropsy, but she's satisfied with your explanation and would rather not. She thanks you tearfully, as Graham walks her and the dead patient to an exam room for her to say goodbye.

Well, that was awful and heartbreaking. "Whew! Not sure I could take another sad one like that tonight," you breathe to yourself.

NEVER say something like that at an ER!

Two more cases come in over the next hour, both pets presented for euthanasia. Both are in bad shape, and the families are grateful you helped. But it's still emotionally draining. Nobody warned you the ER was such a favorite spot for that horrible specter called Death. You'll put significantly more dogs and cats "to sleep" here than your daytime practice. And you'll watch many more die in front of you despite your best efforts. The ER is a grim place. But it's in the grimmest places that one needs a caring heart and helping hand the most. You genuinely believe you are helping patients and their people with every case: even the sad ones.

The one silver lining to the night is that Graham and Lemon convince Debbie Crimshaw and Joe Dertoni to go home for a few hours while you care for their pets. For a brief hour or two, as the rosy sunlight is just starting to peek over the chilly desert horizon, everything is quiet. You retire to the doctor's office and turn on a rerun of Starship Beethoven for background noise to keep you awake while trying to catch up on your notes.

"Captain Forte, we're heading right into the sun!" the lovely Ensign Dun wails dramatically.

"Carry on, Ensign. Our course has been plotted. We… Will… Come… Through!"

This is one of your favorite episodes, and you turn to watch the crew of the Beethoven link arms and line dance across the deck. You hum along to one of your favorite tunes from the show.

"Carry on, oh Ensign Dun!

Soaring on, we'll pass the sun!

Our starship is brighter,

As our orbit gets tighter,

This will be fun!

Soaring into the light,

Prospects are bright,

Through the endless night of space,

We carry on our flight!

Yeah through the endless night of space,

We carry on our…"

SHHHHHHHPP!

Your happy space-ditty is interrupted by a familiar, yet alien sound. What was that? You've heard it before…when the clinic ghost was walking. Gleep!

You turn the volume down, and your skin crawls at a quiet, but unmistakable clomping sound. Footsteps? It seems to be coming from the room next door, Dr. Short's office. You screw up your courage and open the door to the next room. The sounds stop. You flip on the light. Nothing seems to be moving. No glowing orbs or phantasmic forms greet you.

"Iiiiiiss anyone there?" You're a little embarrassed at the tremble in your squeaky voice. But then, nobody else is back here to hear it… At least, you sure hope not. You open the door to the little backyard of the clinic, a feeling of Déjà vu sweeping over you. The dim rays of an infant sunrise are just starting to penetrate the shadows of the cactus and weeds and piles of junk. But there is no sign of humans, ghostly or otherwise.

As dawn gives way to blazing daylight, your clients pick up their pets, and you crawl out of your cave to blink at the morning like a war-battered troll. You feel fried. You feel sad. Who told you being a veterinarian was a good idea? Tonight you learned that the ER is a particularly rigorous sort of emotional gym, where your willpower and feelings and brain all get stretched to the breaking point…and then a little bit more. Hopefully, like any good gym, exercising your soul will make it stronger.

You return home to doze fitfully all morning (still finding daytime sleep an unnatural and difficult task). The next week, your latest paycheck comes and you feel glowing satisfaction as you order Samuel his Squishwidget in time to arrive for Christmas. He'll love squishing it, twisting it, and coloring it with crayons. Your smile fades just a little as you step out into the chilly winter atmosphere to journey toward your next ER adventure. You're scheduled for several nights in a row.

Are you really up for this?

One drive later, you pause as you stand up outside your car and stare into the middle distance, while your hair is whipped epically in the icy breeze like some intrepid explorer in Antarctica. The clinic stares back at you as if challenging you to another night. You have a metaphorical mountain to climb. You were trained for this mission, and you can do it.

"You OK?" You jump (and your squeak of surprise kinda negates your epic pose). Doug, the unhoused guy who periodically haunts the parking lot, is leaning against the cinder-block wall of the clinic shivering in a layer of tattered jackets. "You just sorta stared for a bit, and I thought you might be havin' a stroke or somethin'."

"Oh, um… Nope. Just thinking," you stammer.

"Thanks for letting me sit in the lobby the other night. You're a good person."

You mutter something, but your words fade as he stares at you with puppy dog eyes. "Why don't you come on in and warm up a little now?" You sigh, wondering how you're going to explain this to whatever tech is on shift tonight. It's generally a bad idea to let random people into your clinic, especially at nighttime and in bad parts of town. But Graham did vouch for Doug, and you don't get any dangerous vibes. He seems chatty as he comes in from the cold, and his praises make you blush.

"I can always tell when a person has a kind heart! You ain't at all like the ol' lady that used ta run this place. I been comin' round here for a long time. And back in those days, she was mean!"

Fred Kawalkovitch waves at you from behind the desk in the lobby. "Good morning," he hollers cheerfully. You're relieved that he seems to know Doug too. "Good to see you, Doug. Sit a bit, but you know the rules. You've gotta leave when the customers roll in. Hey Doc, have you met Harlow?"

A short girl with auburn hair and intense eyes pokes her head up from the counter (where she'd been counting the opening balance to get ready for tonight's shift). She nods and grins.

"Good to meet you. Are you one of the regular techs, or is this your first shift?"

"A little of both, actually," she laughs. "I was a tech here a few years back, then took a break. I missed it though. This job kinda gets in your blood, doesn't it?"

"Word," you answer, feeling like one of the cool kids.

That's when the door opens and a blustery breeze blows about the knees of a guy who looks like William Wallace. All he seems to be missing is a set of bagpipes. Instead, he holds a wiry looking terrier beast in his arms.

"Crivvens! Kin ye help ma wee pup?"

CASE #8

A wee 20-pound Scottish Terrier soon sits panting on an exam table.

His owner is a big man with a red beard and a sleeveless shirt on which is emblazoned a blue Scottish flag. He is also wearing a Utilikilt, a man-skirt made of leather with multiple pockets, which you didn't know was a real thing until now. It fits into the wide category of Things you'd be quite happy not knowing about: but it's too late now.

"Ach mon! Ma pal MacWoof here seems pure done in!" Your ruddy client barks as his owner tries to hide the tear glinting in his left eye. Despite the skull and crossbones tattoo on his shoulder, Stewart Abernathy is evidently a big softie. "I tried rousin' him with a tune on me pipes, but even that didn't help."

You start your exam and ask questions as you go. "What symptoms are you seeing at home?"

"Two days ago, young MacWoof here started actin' like a deflated set o' pipes. Dinnae even ett his meat, ye ken? On Tuesday he vomited. Today he started in ta coughing. An' I noticed a totesy, wee trickle o' blood from his nose."

Fred seems to know a highland term or two, and translates for you. Fred seems to know a lot about lots of things and you often wonder what he does on his time off to gather such a cornucopia of factoids.

Step 1 – Organize the History

Signalment:

Scottish Terrier dog

5 years old

Male neutered

Presenting Complaints:

Lethargy

Vomiting (resolved)

Inappetence

Coughing

Epistaxis (bloody nose)

Step 2 – Gather Clues

Physical Examination:

Abdominal palpation: No splinting or pain noted. You suspect a possible fluid wave, with very slight distension. No obvious masses or foreign material palpated.

Attitude: Quiet, lethargic, but responsive.

Cardiac: Tackycardia with a steady rhythm. Grade 2/6 murmur noted. Adequate femoral pulses.

Ears: Canals appear clear with no debris noted.

Eyes: Appear clear OU.

Integument: Decreased skin tenting (~7% dehydrated). No wounds or draining tracts. No obvious hives or rashes or other problems noted. There is a bruise on the underside of his belly (right ventral abdomen).

Lymph Nodes: Mild enlargement of submandibular lymph nodes (under the neck) suspected.

Musculoskeletal: NSF. Weight bearing on all four limbs. No obvious fracture or luxation.

Neurologic: Quiet and responsive patient, but does seem generally lethargic. Normal menace reflex and palpebral response.

Oronasal: Slight bloody discharge noted from the left nares. Petechiation suspected.

Respiratory: Tachypnea with a few slight crackles noted on the left. Minimal increase in expiratory effort. No cyanosis noted.

Urogenital: NSF. Urinary bladder palpates soft and moderate in size.

Vitals: Mucous membranes are pale pink, tacky, CRT<2s.

Right, mon! Ye've looked the wee beastie over. Now show yer heid's nae mince, and come up with a brilliant list o' differentials to guide ye!

> "Every solution to every problem is simple. It's the distance between the two where the mystery lies."
>
> -Derek Landy, *Skulduggery Pleasant*[xv]

Think of some differentials before turning the page.

STOP!!!!!!

Ye're pure dead brilliant! Oh aye, ye are! Check my list on the next page. See how we compare.

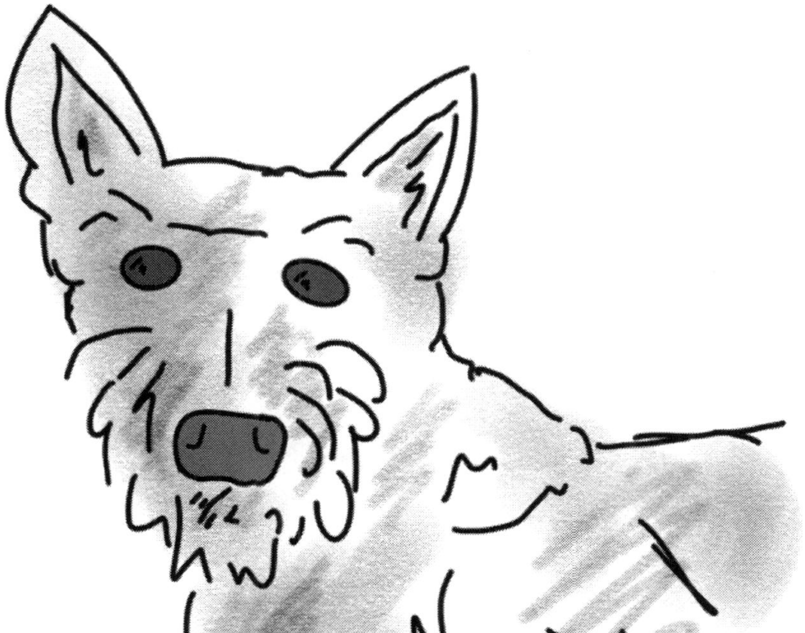

Differential Diagnoses for MacWoof:

Allergic reaction

Anemia — Differentials like blood loss, bone marrow cancer, blood infections.

Clotting disorder (leading to internal bleeding)

Congestive heart failure

GI foreign body

GI parasitism — Like roundworms or giardia.

Hypovolemic shock with DIC or blood loss

Infection — Like canine distemper.

Nasal foreign body

Neoplasia — Nasal tumor, splenic tumor, etc.

Pancreatitis

Pneumonia — Such as GI disease with secondary aspiration pneumonia.

Toxicity

Trauma

Some of these (like GI parasitism) would cause a few of the presenting complaints but not all of them (i.e. vomiting and inappetence, but not cough or bleeding or lethargy). It's less likely, but certainly possible, that this wee laddie has several conditions causing his list of symptoms. All of this is why it's sometimes helpful to organize your differentials into sets of signs. If you find one that explains everything, put it on the top!

- *DDx (vomiting, inappetence, lethargy, coughing, epistaxis, bruising)*-> toxin (anticoagulant toxins like rodenticide), DIC and shock (potentially from differentials like neoplasia or allergic reaction).
- *DDx (vomiting, inappetence, lethargy, coughing)* -> infection (distemper), neoplasia, GI disease with aspiration pneumonia, allergies/reaction.
- *DDx (Vomiting, inappetence, lethargy)*-> GI parasitism, GI foreign body, pancreatitis, neoplasia, toxin (plants like English Holly or American Mandrake, chemicals like soap, etc.).
- *DDx (coughing, epistaxis)*-> nasal and/or pharyngeal foreign body, neoplasia.

Do you see something interesting on these lists?

Woop! Woop! Woop!

DDx: shorthand for differential diagnoses.

Rodenticide: rat poison.

Alerts go off in your head like the strobing red lights on the Command Deck of the Beethoven during a Category 14 asteroid shower. One differential is not like the others. One differential stands out, because it keeps showing up on your lists.

You wisely ask Mr. Abernathy about toxin exposure.

“Och, aye! There are a couple o’ wee bait boxes fer the barn mice me bairn boy barks aboot.”

You turn to Fred for help. “There’s some rat poison in the barn,” he translates for you.

“Ah!” you exclaim, feeling a rush of adrenaline at your detective training, at the same time you feel a growing sense of dread.

Stewart Abernathy feels chatty. “Scottie dogs were bred to hunt vermin, ye know, but not MacWoof. Wee fella’s a bone idle slaodair. He just sleeps in the shafts o’ light slantin’ through the barn doors…”

You tune him out as you consider what to do next. What tests wheest ye ta run, laddie (or lassie)-buck?

Decision time!

What tests do you want to run first?

Here’s what you can do in your clinic:

- ✓ Basic bloodwork (a chemistry panel and CBC)
- ✓ Benchtop Ethylene glycol test
- ✓ Blood gas analysis
- ✓ Clotting times
- ✓ Cytology
- ✓ Fecal floatation and direct saline exam
- ✓ FeLV/FIV test
- ✓ Giardia test
- ✓ Heartworm test (with rickettsial diseases)
- ✓ Leptospirosis test
- ✓ Pancreatic lipase
- ✓ Parvo test
- ✓ Pregnancy test
- ✓ Radiographs (X-rays)
- ✓ Skin scraping
- ✓ Thyroid hormone level (T4)
- ✓ Ultrasound
- ✓ Urinalysis

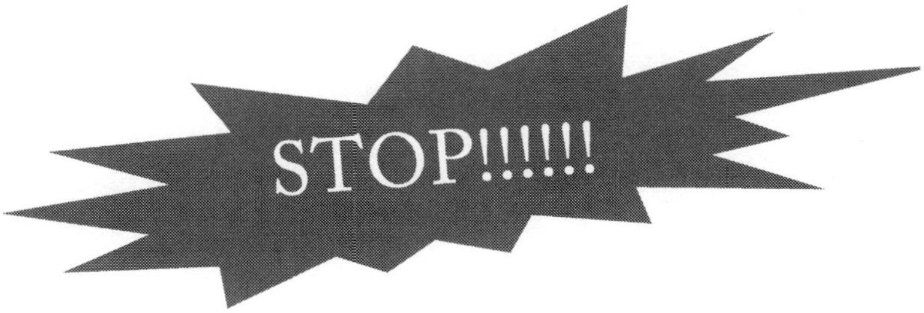

The tests I picked were as follows, and I quote: **bloodwork** (a chemistry panel with electrolytes, and a CBC), **clotting times, a pancreatitis test, ultrasound** (or radiographs if your ultrasound machine is full of gremlins, or you suddenly forgot how to use it).

Why? Good question! At this point toxicity is increasingly suspicious, and these wee tests will hone in on the diagnosis of rodenticide toxicity, and help rule out a lot of other items on the list of differentials.

Why am I more suspicious about toxins? Good question. Because they fit the history findings of a previously healthy young dog, they fit the symptoms of vomiting and acute lethargy and bleeding (and explain signs on more than one of your lists), and because Stewart Abernathy told you there was poison around for this patient to munch.

Do bear in mind that these reasons (as brilliant as they are) do not a diagnosis make. Other diseases could still cause these signs as well. Let's run some test then and see how this all shakes out…

"Facts are stubborn things; and whatever may be our wishes, our inclinations, or the dictates of our passion, they cannot alter the state of facts and evidence.

—John Adams, 1770[xv]

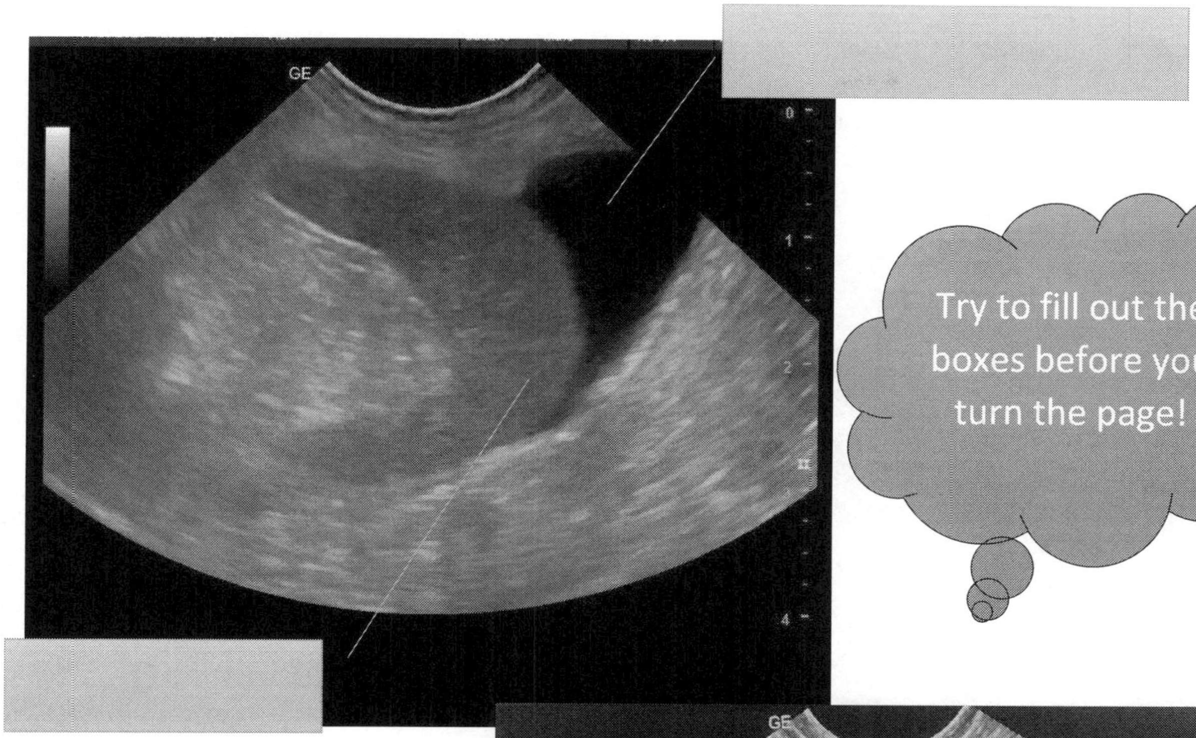

Try to fill out the boxes before you turn the page!

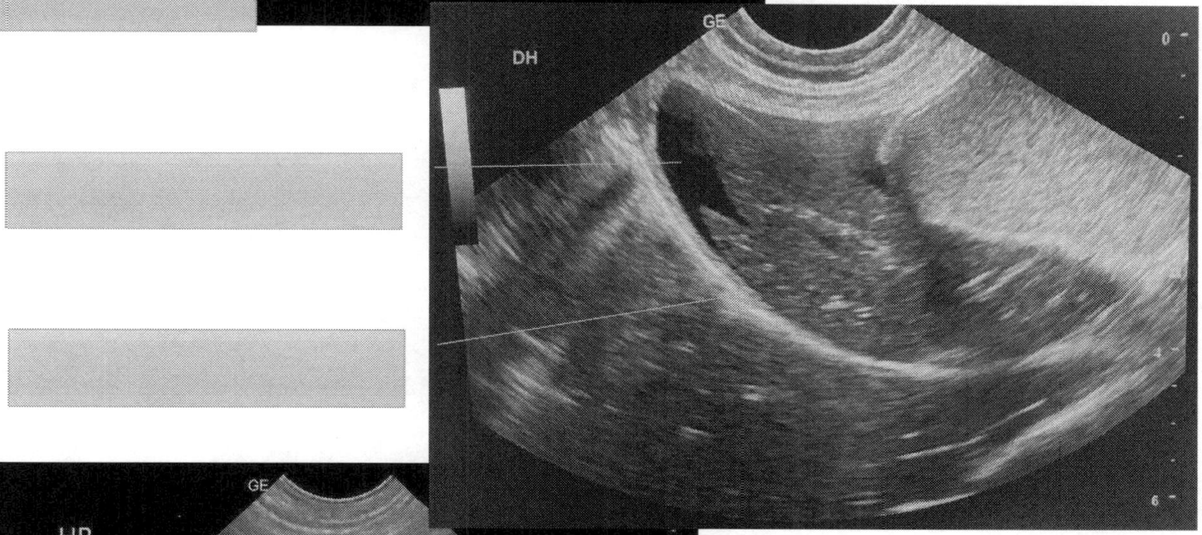

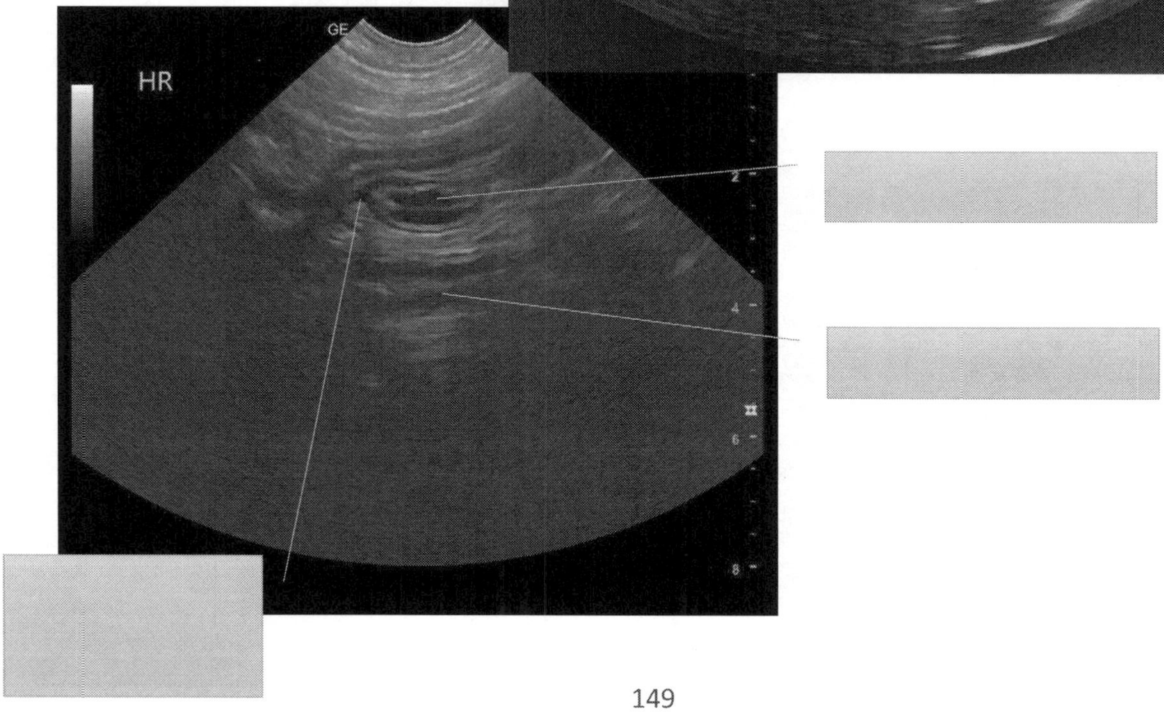

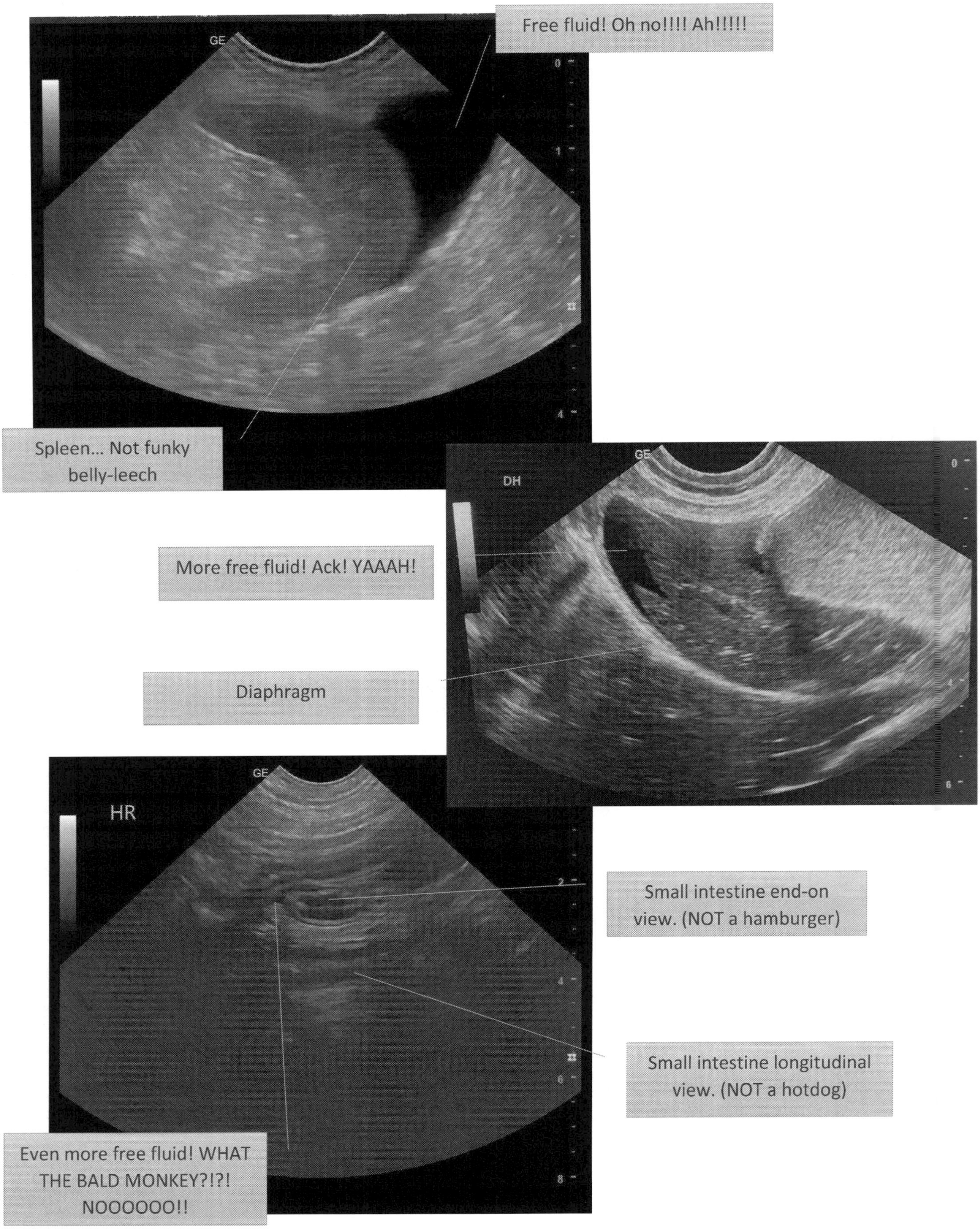
Free fluid! Oh no!!!! Ah!!!!!
Spleen... Not funky belly-leech
DH
More free fluid! Ack! YAAAH!
Diaphragm
HR
Small intestine end-on view. (NOT a hamburger)
Small intestine longitudinal view. (NOT a hotdog)
Even more free fluid! WHAT THE BALD MONKEY?!?! NOOOOOO!!

The important thing to note here is free fluid in the abdomen. Remember that fluid on an ultrasound looks like black patches. Free fluid (floating about the abdomen where it shouldn't be) usually has some shape to it: you see square or triangular edges. I see free fluid in this wee beastie near his spleen, near his urinary bladder, and just a hint near some of his small bowel.

What kind of fluid is it, you may ask?

You go ahead and sample some with a needle (abdominocentesis) and it looks like blood. Then you cringe as you see a bruise where you poked this guy, and realize you might have caused increased bleeding by sampling the fluid (if there is a problem with blood clotting). You have Harlow put pressure on the area for a while and move on to check bloodwork.

Client: Abernathy, Stewart	Species: Canine	Sex: MC
Patient: MacWoof	Breed: Scottish Terrier	
Patient ID: 0321668		

CBC

TEST	RESULT	FLAG	REFERENCE RANGE	
WBC	12		6.0-17.0	$10^3/\mu L$
Neutrophils	10		3-11.4	$10^3/\mu L$
Monocytes	1.1		0.15-1.35	$10^3/\mu L$
Lymphocytes	2		1-4.8	$10^3/\mu L$
Eosinophils	0.6		0.1-0.75	$10^3/\mu L$
Hematocrit	21	L	37-55	%
MCV	77		60-77	fL
Platelet Count	302		200-900	$10^3/\mu L$

Client: Abernathy, Stewart	Species: Canine	Sex: MC
Patient: MacWoof	Breed: Scottish Terrier	
Patient ID: 0321668		

Chemistry Panel

Test	Result	Flag	Reference Range
ALT	55		8.2-57 IU/L
ALP	98		10.6-101 IU/L
GGT	9		1.0-9.7 IU/L
tBili	0.2		0.1-0.6 mg/dL
Glucose	84		62-108 mg/dL
Cholesterol	123		116-254 mg/dL
Total Protein	4.0	L	5.5-7.5 g/dL
Albumin	2.5	L	2.6-4.0 g/dL
Globulin	1.9	L	2.1-3.7 g/dL
Calcium	9.2		8.7-11.8 mg/dL
BUN	30	H	8.8-26 mg/dL
Creatinine	3.1	H	0.5-1.6 mg/dL
Phosphorus	5		2.9-6.2 mg/dL
Sodium	142		140-154 mEq/L
Potassium	3.0	L	3.8-5.6 mEq/L
Chloride	102		102-117 mEq/L

Client: Abernathy, Stewart	Species: Canine	Sex: MN
Patient: MacWoof	Breed: Scottish Terrier	
Patient ID: 0321668		

Clotting Times

TEST	RESULT	FLAG	REFERENCE RANGE
APTT	>300	H	84-72 seconds
PT	39	H	11-17 seconds

This means "too high to read a number."

There is evidence of anemia and decreased clotting factors (increase in clotting times). Protein is low (both globulin and albumin). There is azotemia (a fancy word for BUN and creatinine being elevated together) and a slightly low potassium. What's going on here?!?!?

What is your diagnosis, Doctor?

____

One line to fill.

One diagnosis.

Eliminate each differential,

Ye cannae use hypnosis...

I'll tell you what I think is going on here (and you should listen closely, because I wrote this book)...

The most likely diagnosis here is **rodenticide toxicity**—I think little MacWoof got into rat poison!

We have signs of anemia (low blood cells) that are likely from blood loss. Low protein along with anemia is a clue blood cells are leaking out, rather than being destroyed inside the veins or not being produced in the bone marrow. That's because proteins leak out with the blood. You found blood pooling into the abdomen, and blood under the skin (bruises) already, which tracks.

Why is there blood loss? Probably because the blood is not clotting (since you have severely elevated clotting times). PT and aPTT measure clotting factors in the plasma, and prolonged PT and aPTT mean low numbers of clotting factors.

What makes low clotting factors? Common options are:

- Rat poison
- Severe liver disease
- DIC (disseminated intravascular coagulation).

There's no evidence of liver disease on your ultrasound or bloodwork. DIC is a horrible complication of severe disease (it's secondary to something else) and involves microclots forming all over the body (which uses up clotting factors fast). DIC is usually going to make a dog sicker and cause other bloodwork changes you don't see in this case - such as low platelet counts, elevated or low white cell counts, and more evidence of organ failure. You do have mild elevation in BUN and creatinine, which could be early renal injury consistent with DIC. You can also get renal injury from anticoagulant poisons too, though. If you had it available, you could check another blood test called D-dimer assay or FDP (fibrin degradation products) measurement to help diagnose DIC. But you don't have those here.

What you do have is a little terrier bred to hunt rats, who spends a lot of time in a barn with anticoagulant poisons, and has signs of bleeding and elevated clotting times. If it squawks like the dread chicken-beast of Coda-5 (S3E7 of Starship Beethoven), it probably is the dread chicken-beast of Coda-5.

You have a most likely diagnosis at this point! What are you going to do about it? Look over the beautiful infographic on the next page and formulate a plan.

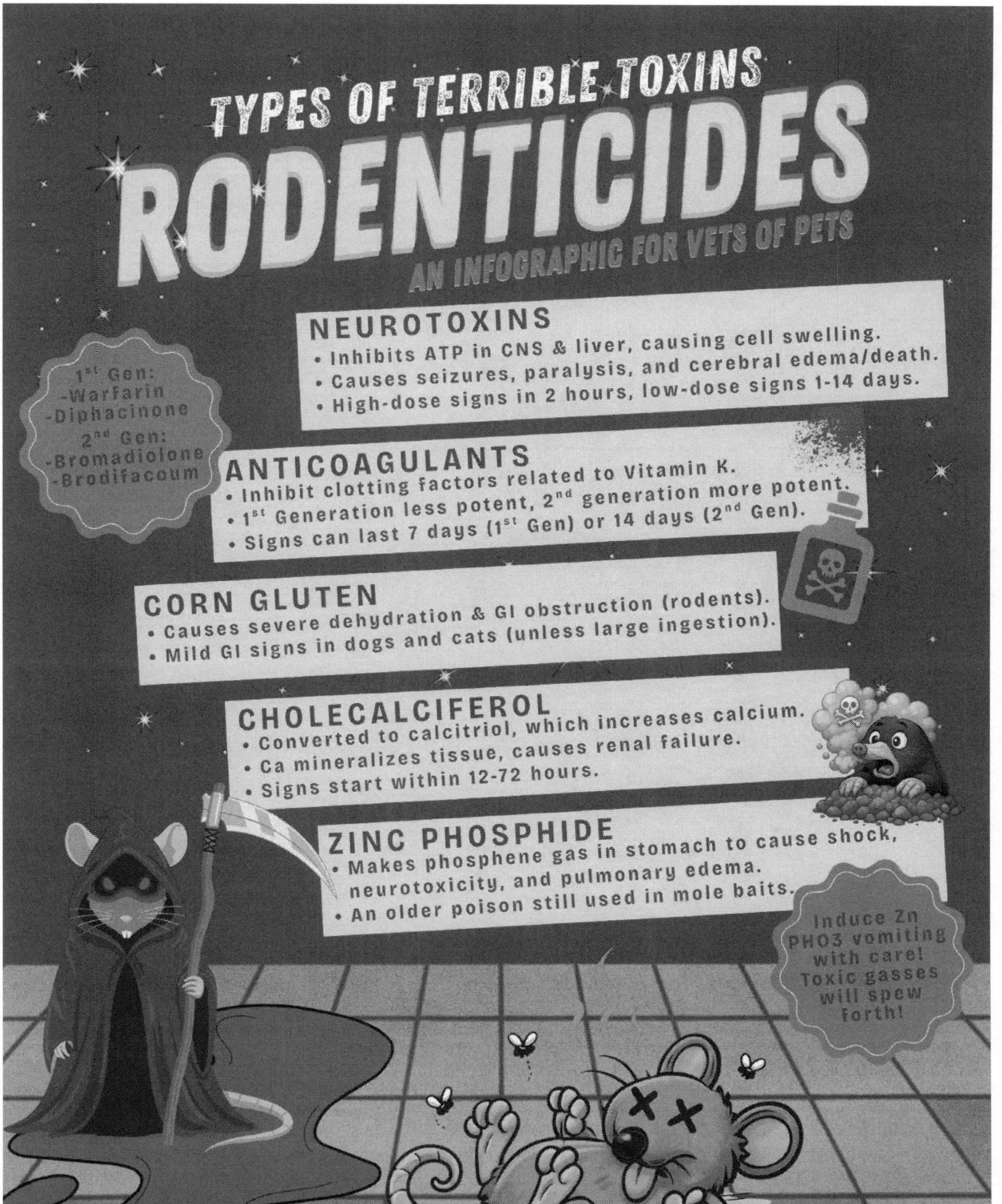
TYPES OF TERRIBLE TOXINS
RODENTICIDES
AN INFOGRAPHIC FOR VETS OF PETS
NEUROTOXINS
• Inhibits ATP in CNS & liver, causing cell swelling.
• Causes seizures, paralysis, and cerebral edema/death.
• High-dose signs in 2 hours, low-dose signs 1-14 days.
1st Gen: -Warfarin -Diphacinone
2nd Gen: -Bromadiolone -Brodifacoum
ANTICOAGULANTS
• Inhibit clotting factors related to Vitamin K.
• 1st Generation less potent, 2nd generation more potent.
• Signs can last 7 days (1st Gen) or 14 days (2nd Gen).
CORN GLUTEN
• Causes severe dehydration & GI obstruction (rodents).
• Mild GI signs in dogs and cats (unless large ingestion).
CHOLECALCIFEROL
• Converted to calcitriol, which increases calcium.
• Ca mineralizes tissue, causes renal failure.
• Signs start within 12-72 hours.
ZINC PHOSPHIDE
• Makes phosphene gas in stomach to cause shock, neurotoxicity, and pulmonary edema.
• An older poison still used in mole baits.
Induce Zn PHO3 vomiting with care! Toxic gasses will spew forth!
© J. Aaron Gruben

What is your treatment plan? (pick several)

a) Antibiotics
b) Anti-emetics (drugs to prevent vomiting)
c) IV fluids
d) Give activated charcoal
e) Give a blood transfusion
f) Give clotting factors
g) Give vitamin K
h) Induce emesis (make him puke)
i) Oxygen therapy
j) Smear the blood of a rat slain under a waning moon across the patient's nose and forehead
k) Splenectomy (surgically remove the spleen)
l) Write a letter to your congressperson

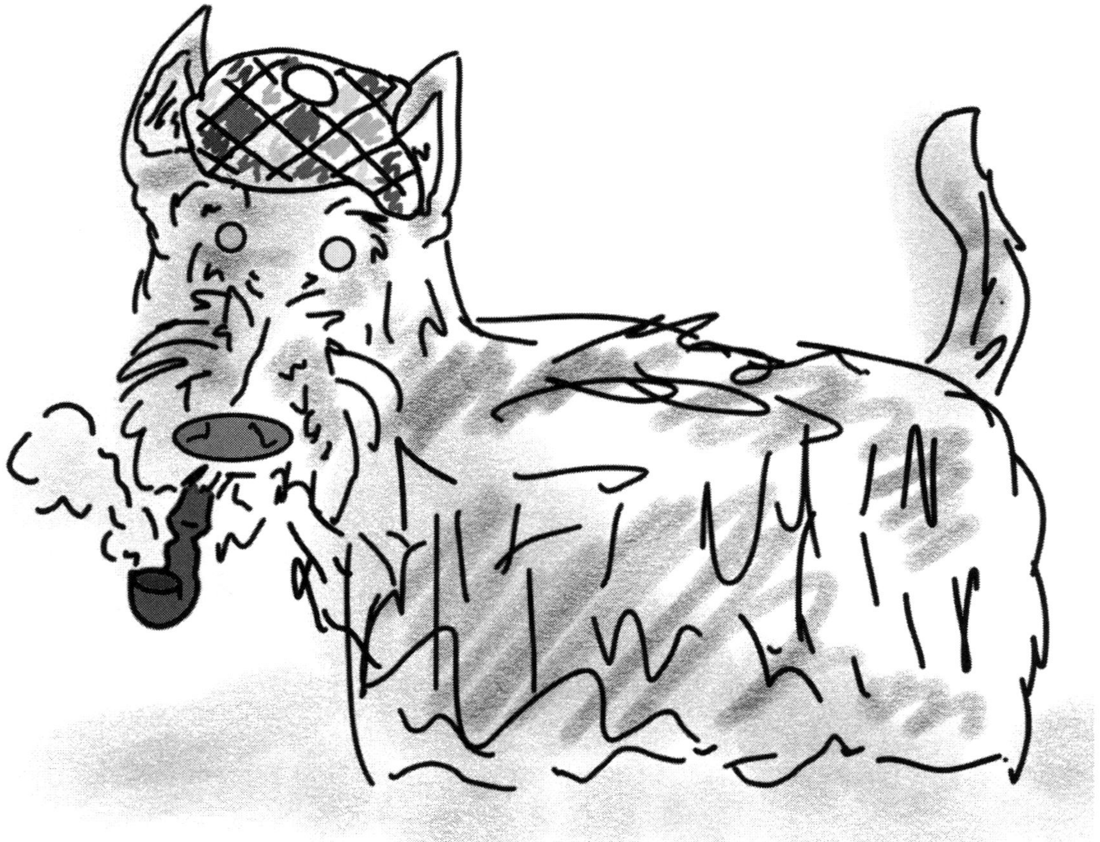

What is your treatment plan for this poor guy?

STOP!!!!!!

"Make your choice, adventurous Stranger,

Strike the bell and bide the danger,

Or wonder, till it drives you mad,

What would have followed if you had."

-C. S. Lewis, The Magician's Nephew[xvii]

So many options! I'm excited to see your treatment plan. Does it look somewhat like this one?

I'd probably pick: **b, c, f, and g**. Let's go over the whys, and possibly also the wherefores…

- **Give anti-emetic**: This pup's been vomiting and is not eating. Drugs for vomiting and to help with nausea might help him recover quickly.
- **IV fluids**: This guy is a little dehydrated. Also, his kidneys are questionable (BUN and Cr elevated). Not every rodenticide toxicity case needs IV fluids, but this dude seems to be asking for them.
- **Give clotting factors**: Lack of clotting factors is this guy's most immediate problem. It's what's making him leaky inside and bruisy outside. The fastest way to correct that is by giving clotting factors right into his veins. And the best way to do that is by giving plasma! Plasma is the fluid part of the blood that contains clotting factors (it becomes "serum" when the clotting factors are all used up). A transfusion of a special product called fresh frozen plasma (FFP) would give him an emergency supply of clotting factors to help stop the short-term bleeding. You'll want to monitor clotting times periodically (probably every 6-8 hours after giving plasma until it looks better).
- **Give vitamin K**: This is the antidote to rodenticide toxicity. Anticoagulant rodenticides block an enzyme (hepatic vitamin K epoxide reductase, if you must know) that helps keep up the body's supply of vitamin K. And vitamin K is required to make clotting factors II, VII, IX, X (numbers your more sadistic professors at vet school made you memorize). You'll start with a vitamin K injection but also put this guy on oral vitamin K for around three weeks. You'll also want to monitor clotting times during this treatment.

You might also have answered: d, e, h, or i. Let me tell you why these would not be best in this case.

- **Give activated charcoal.** We do often give activated charcoal to help absorb many toxins. But it's way too late for this to help in MacWoof's particular case. Also, charcoal can inhibit absorption of the oral vitamin K you want to give this guy, and has potentially serious side effects like hypernatremia (really high sodium) or aspiration pneumonia.
- **Give a blood transfusion.** This is not wrong, and there are cases of rat poisoning that do need to fix anemia from blood loss. MacWoof's HCT of 21% is probably not low enough to kill him, and will come up when you make the bleeding stop.
- **Induce emesis.** This is a great idea soon after a patient eats the poison (within around 4-8 hours post ingestion). Like the charcoal, in MacWoof's case, way too much time has already

gone by, and the poison is already absorbed into his little dog-bod.

- **Supplement oxygen.** This is sometimes needed in anticoagulant toxicity cases, *if* there's signs of bleeding in the lungs and dyspnea (trouble breathing).

Whew! That's a lot to think about. Your brain feels a bit tired, doesn't it? You tell your good buddy Stewart all about your tests and the treatments you want to do. Then you build a treatment plan and Fred goes over it with the client.

Fred returned with remarkable quickness. "He said 'there's nae so wheen o spoondoolies in me sporran! Awa' an bile yer heid!'"

You raise an eyebrow in what you hope is a questioning look. "Is that good?"

Fred shakes his head. "It means he can't afford it, Doc. Please try again."

You take a long breath. This is one of your least favorite part of emergency medicine: building a plan B (and C, and D, and E, and F…) to fit the quality medicine you learned to practice (which nobody at school told you was so very, very expensive) into a real world filled with people who have budgets. It turns out your clients need to pay for things like food and shelter and transportation, and don't always approve expensive things like plasma transfusions or hospitalization. As you gain experience working in this muddled mess of the real world, you'll learn to go into a case with a plan B, C, and D in mind already.

In veterinary medicine we often refer to this idea of tailoring a treatment plan to a family's resources as "spectrum of care." The term "contextualized care" is similar but includes practical considerations other than money (like ability of an owner to give medications or living arrangements of the patient) that could affect the treatment plan. In the end, these considerations are very important, even though it makes you feel like you're haggling over your patient's well-being. Always offer the best care but be willing to pivot if the situation needs it: because the reality is that the situation will probably need it in 8 cases out of 10.

You make a plan for MacWoof without a plasma transfusion that's about $1000 less than the first one. McWoof's human declines that one, too. Turns out he spent all his money on the tests and is declined for the medical credit lines your clinic has to offer. What Steward can do is pay for an injection of vitamin K and a couple of weeks of oral vitamin K tabs. That's a start. You warn him there's a chance this patient (who is teetering on the edge of instability) might crash and burn. You review a list of serious signs that mean he should bring MacWoof back right away. You also tell him to rest this wee fella: bumping into things will make him bleed more.

Then you try (mostly in vain) not to worry about it.

As time drags on and no more clients appear, you grab a coffee and a Fred to chat outside.

A chilly, high-desert breeze blows across the dingy backyard of Owlhoot Veterinary Emergency Clinic as you stare up at a winter sky, brilliant with astral pinpricks. It's one of those magical midnight moments that occur on night shifts, when time seems to slow its rushing stream and the world is blanketed in a silence that's sylvan and almost sacred.

"So what do you think about this clinic ghost, Fred? Is this place really haunted?"

Fred sips his coffee, the stars twinkling in his always cheerful eyes. "Well now, that's a big question, Doc. I haven't worked yet in an ER that didn't have a few ghost stories. If you're asking if I really believe them all, then…probably not. Still, I have heard some weird sounds, seen a shadow once or twice that I couldn't explain…"

"Yeah, but I've only worked here a week, and heard the ghost shuffling around this place several times. Why's he…she…it…so busy right now?"

"Maybe because it's Christmastime. The Victorians always claimed Christmas was ghostly prime time. English folks still save up their ghost stories for this time of year."

You shrug. That could be one explanation. Or… Perhaps you could say it was one differential. Could that ever-helpful differential thinking help puzzle through this ghostly phenomenon?

"OK then, let's think through all the possible identities of this ghost," your tone becomes very matter-of-fact, and the crow's feet beside Fred's eyes deepen just a little. "Let's make a differential list…"

What do you think? What could the weird noises and flickering shadows be?

Write out some possible differential diagnoses for the clinic ghost's identity before you turn the page…

STOP!!!

"You know my methods. Apply them."

—Arthur Conan Doyle, *The Sign of Four*[xviii]

So, to be honest, this is not a differential list I've made in my career (though I, like other characters in this book, have indeed found tales of ghosts to be ubiquitous to every ER I've worked in).

Here's what I'd put down. The strangeness could be…

- An actual ghost, as in a spirit in limbo, mysteriously tied to the place of their death and doomed to haunt it.
- Some other kind of spiritual entity.
- A natural phenomena (like plumbing problems, flickering fluorescent lights that need to be changed, rodents scampering around in the walls, etc.).
- A flesh and blood human being, tromping around and making weird sounds at strange hours of the shift.
- The product of overstimulated brains, hopped on caffeine, with nothing to do all night but wait around for emergencies to happen and make up ghost stories…

"Well, I guess that about covers all the possibilities," Fred nods. "But a few of your differentials could use some clarification. What do you mean by 'some other spiritual entity' first off?"

"Like a demon… or something? Darn it, Fred! I'm a doctor, not a theologian!"

Fred grins, then stares silently at the empty yard for a minute. "But now I'm actually scared."

"It's just one of several differentials," you remind him in your best professionally reassuring tone.

"What about a flesh and blood human being? What kind of person would be tromping around a clinic at night? And why do we never actually see them?"

"Well, there are a couple of possibilities. It could be a prankster. It could be a thief. It could be a staff member sneaking in for something they left behind. Maybe it's an unhoused person like Doug, who's coming inside to warm up while we aren't looking."

Fred rubs his chin in thought. "Doc, we keep the doors locked from midnight to 6 am…"

"Most of the time."

He shrugs in silent acknowledgment that a policy does not always equal adherence. "Also, why would any of these classes of humans keep coming back frequently enough to make a rumor of it?"

"Maybe they don't. Maybe they just come in occasionally, or even just recently, and our imaginations have filled in the rest of the rumor from things like rats in the walls."

"Huh. Could be, Doc, could be." He takes another sip at his coffee and stares up into the pristine sky. "Or it could be that it's still just a good old-fashioned ghost. You do know I named him 'Marvin' don't you?"

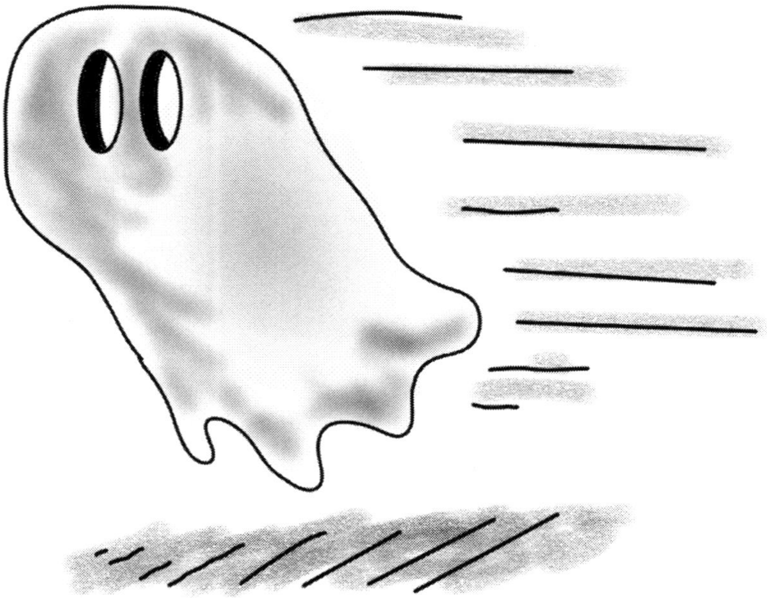

“Wait, what? Don’t name him, or you’ll have to keep him…”

“I figure he’s not a human ghost at all, but a big Labrador that died here years ago, whose spirit roams the clinic chasing spectral rubber balls and squeaky toys.”

You laugh, despite not being entirely sure he’s joking.

But at that moment, you hear, through the open back door, a chorus of cat screams blaring from the lobby…

Case #9

YOWL! MEOW! WOH! WOH-RORRR!

Yeah, that is one distressed cat: a sound you've come to recognize and dread in your short tenure at the ER. Frederick goes to triage this new patient, and returns shortly with a cat carrier full of furry fury.

"This appears to be some kind of mini-tiger?" Fred laughs. You're prone to agree, as you stare in the cage at a hissing, yowling, orange furball of spit and fury. "This is Edgar Allen Paw. Owner says he's lethargic and has been trying to pee all over the house for the past 36 hours."

"*That's* lethargic?" you ask.

"Heh! Evidently. I'll get more history, while you do your assessment. Owner said a pain injection and something to calm this guy is OK."

A few minutes later, you've got a syringe full of methadone and acepromazine in hand. You glance at Harlow, and then at the carrier (which rattles and bounces over the exam table as hissing and growling echoes from inside it). "You first," you politely offer.

"Gee, thanks…" Harlow gives you a dirty look, and suggests she tips up the carrier so you can poke the patient's backside through it (an IM, or intramuscular injection is sometimes possible this way). Miraculously it works, and you wait for the patient to calm down and get drowsy. By the time Edgar Allen Paw is in a workable mood (still growling but drunk), Fred returns with a history.

"Edgar Allen Paw is a 4-year-old, MC domestic shorthair, who presents today for straining to urinate." His professional presentation of the signalment and presenting complaint shows the experience this technician has! "Mrs. Bagsby (his owner) noticed him acting a bit less energetic yesterday, and hiding a lot. When she did see him, he was always trying to urinate in unusual places. Today she noticed him doing it again, and noticed he isn't leaving urine behind. He's also vomited twice today, and refused to eat his dinner. He's vaccinated and is not on any medications currently. No known toxin exposure."

Harlow gingerly restrains this guy, as he growls low and angry. He's just drunk enough with his injections to perform a physical exam.

Step 1 – Organize the History

Signalment:

4 years old

Male neutered

Domestic shorthair cat

Presenting Complaints:

Dysuria (abnormal urination)

Vomiting and inappetence

Lethargy

Step 2 – Gather Clues

Physical Examination:

Abdominal palpation: Very large, hard, rounded something in the caudal abdomen. Patient acts painful (and tries to murder everyone) when palpated.

Attitude: Quiet, sedate (you did that!), and responsive.

Cardiac: Bradycardia (slow heart rate, at about 100 bpm), but steady rhythm with no murmur noted.

Ears: Appear clear AU with no debris or swelling in the canals.

Eyes: Appear clear OU.

Integument: Skin turgor is mildly decreased (~5% dehydrated).

Lymph Nodes: All palpate WNL.

Musculoskeletal: WNL.

Neurologic: Sedate but otherwise WNL.

Oronasal: You're not gonna look in his mouth! There are fangs in this beast, and he's still growling!

Respiratory: Normal rate and effort noted. No cyanosis noted. Lungs sound clear.

Urogenital: Large rounded something structure in caudal abdomen. This patient resists your attempt to lift his tail and examine his perineal region.

Vitals: You are able to lift his cat-lip with a tongue depressor and see that he has pink gums and a CRT<2 seconds.

Can you think of any differentials before you look at the page?

Differential Diagnoses:

Behavioral change

Congenital disease (like a urethral stricture he was born with)

Constipation or obstipation

Feline Idiopathic Cystitis (FIC)

Neoplasia

Renal failure

Toxicity

Urethral obstruction

Urinary tract infection

Urolithiasis

One thing to be clear about is the anatomy involved in peeing. A cat's urinary tract consists of the upper urinary tract (the kidneys and the tubes that flow from them, called the ureters) and the lower urinary tract (the bladder and the urethra that flows from it). Urine (i.e. pee) is produced in the kidneys and flows into the bladder where it's stored up until the cat pees (when it flows out of his urethra and hopefully into his litter box). Technically the act of voiding urine from the body is called micturition, just in case you wanted to impress your friends (without getting yelled at by your parents for talking about gross stuff).

Now admire my world-class artwork…

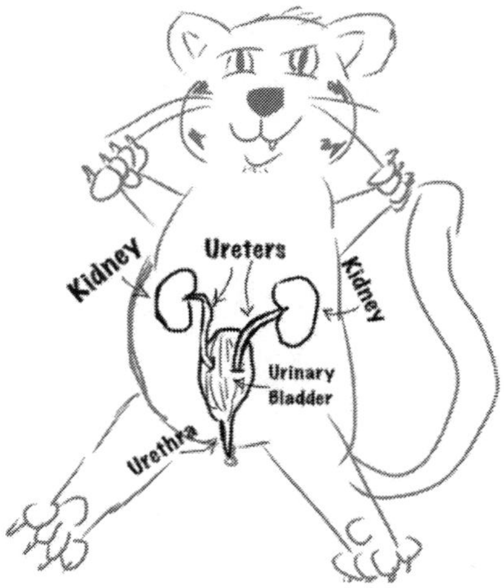

Feline Idiopathic Cystitis (FIC): a condition causing inflammation in the bladder (and often urethra) without an infection. It's related to stress in cats, neurologic and hormonal abnormalities, and has genetic predispositions.
Obstipation: really bad constipation.
Urolithiasis: a fancy word for urinary stones. Often, in cats, this manifests as sandy, crystalline substance, but can be actual little rocks.

You'll notice that the opening from the urethra is very teeny in this drawing. That's going to be important. Is there a test you want to run? Maybe one that costs the clinic next to nothing, and rules out major differentials?

Ooh! Good idea! Let's do a quick **ultrasound** of this cat's caudal abdomen. After all, you feel something big and hard and painful (which is probably not a baseball). Also, he is currently sedate enough to let you look. Harlow bravely holds down this grumbly patient full of teeth and venom (cats have tons of bacteria on their sharp teeth). You put an ultrasound probe on him. This is what you see.

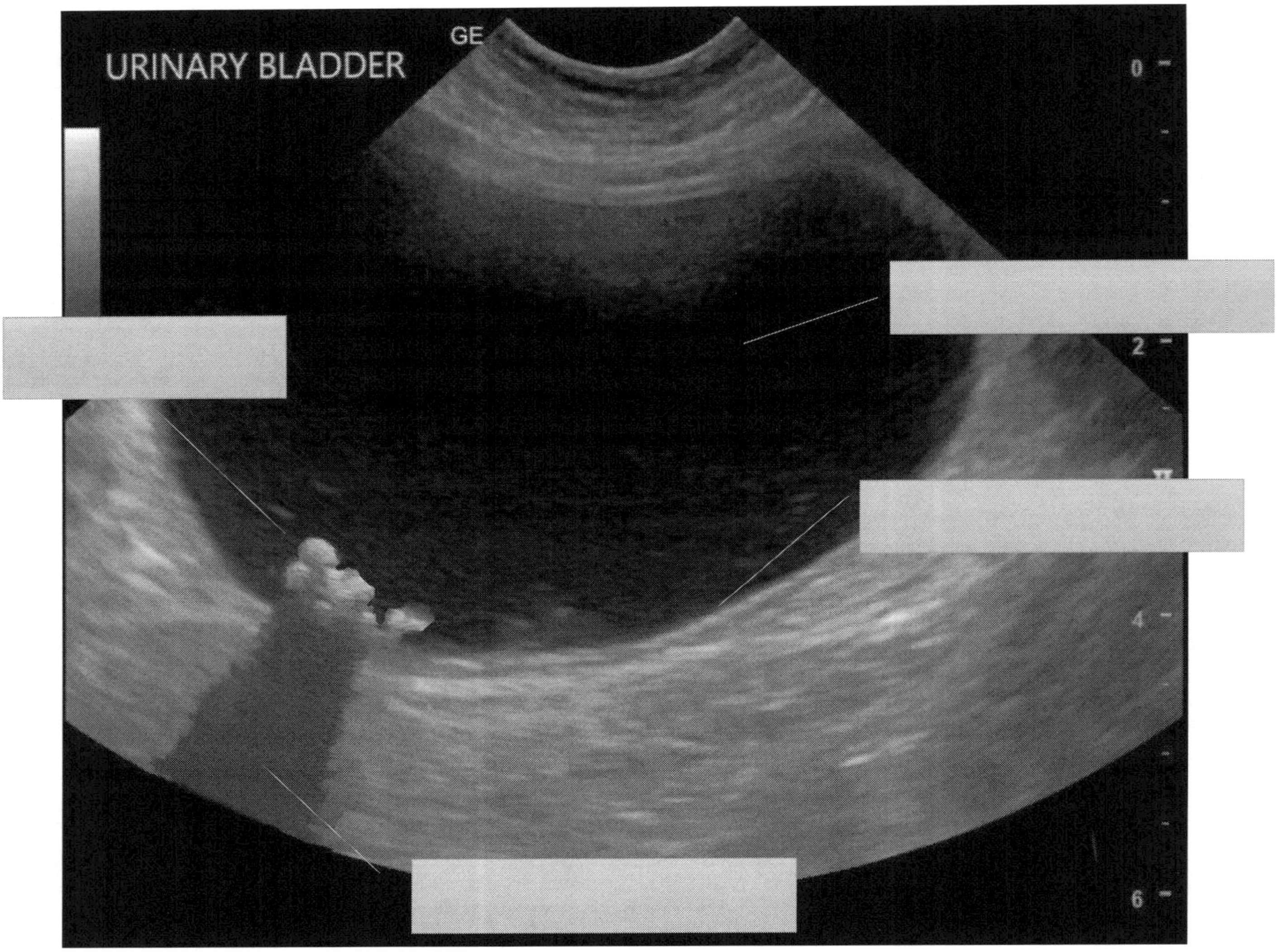

"Aha! It's not a baseball after all!" you holler. Harlow and Fred cast odd looks at you but graciously refrain from snide comments.

What exactly do you see here? Fill in the blank labels…

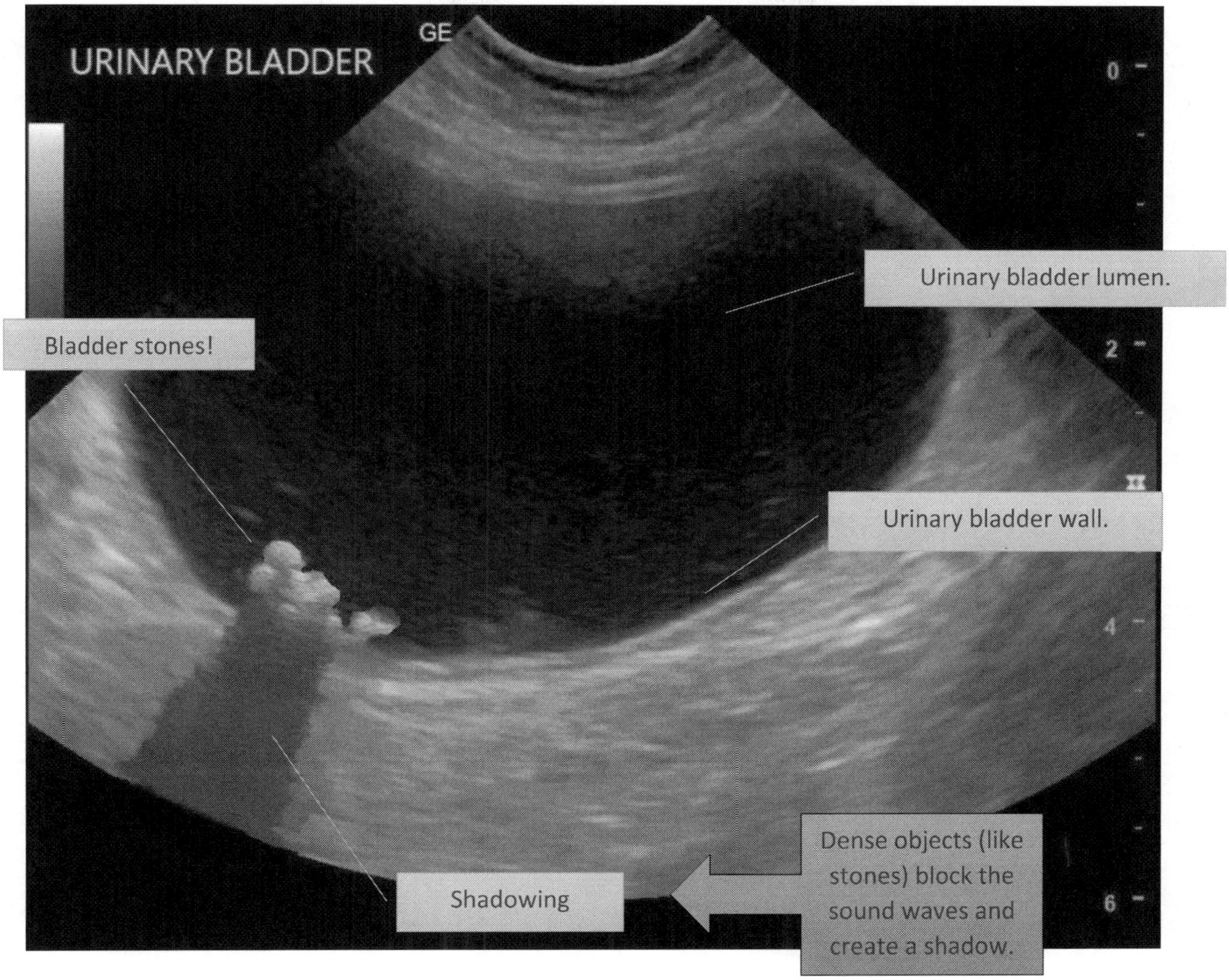

Wowsers! You might just have a diagnosis already with one quick ultrasound! This cat has a really big urinary bladder. That must be the hard thing you feel in his abdomen. Those little white ("hyperechoic") guys against the bladder wall seem to be blocking sound waves and causing shadowing on the screen beyond them. Those look an awful lot like bladder stones. You try to follow the urethra from the bladder but lose it partway down (this is not abnormal: it's very hard for many of us to trace the urethra with an ultrasound). However, stones in a really big, painful bladder make you think of a urethral obstruction. Even if the urethra is not blocked by a stone itself, the inflammation caused by uroliths can clog a urethra and keep a cat from normal micturition. This here's a blocked tomcat!

We sometimes call this a "triage diagnosis": a case where we figured out the basic problem right away without doing lots of tests.

You march into Exam Room 1, armed with information. You half expect to find an elderly lady draped in diamonds with a servant in the corner. But the Mrs. Bagsby that you find is a millennial 30-something, wearing a flannel shirt, thick-framed glasses (which just might be recording you), and skinny jeans. When you walk in, she lowers a biodegradable cup she's been sipping (emblazoned with the logo of a local coffee shop) and looks at you expectantly through intense brown eyes.

"Violet Bagsby," she replies, after you shake her hand and introduce yourself. "Nice to meet you. Were you humming 'The Astrasian Carol' from Starship Beethoven just now?"

"You're a fan too?"

She holds up a hand-made purse with a crocheted picture of The Beethoven on it and smiles. "My cats and I listen to Season 1 soundtrack on vinyl almost every day."

"Nice!" You grin. You like this human-of-Edgar-Allen-Paw.

"How's my boy doing?" she asks.

"Better. We've given him a pain injection with a sedative, and he calmed down enough to do an exam. I noticed a big, turgid urinary bladder during my exam that seemed painful when I palpated him. That's usually something you'll feel on a blocked cat."

You chat about the history a little bit and confirm the things Fred already told you. This is a smart move you've learned over the years, since clients will often tell you a different story than they tell your technicians. You move on to describe your findings in your brief ultrasound.

"Poor Edgar Allen Paw!" she exclaims. "He sounds really bad. What should we do about it?"

This is a very good question. What should you do?

First off, are there any more tests you want to recommend? You've found out already that the patient has urinary stones, and probably a urethral obstruction, but there are several potential differentials/causes that can go along with those problems. Think about the consequences of not being able to pee, and having stones rubbing around inside the bladder…

Turgid: a fancy word for "hard and tense."

What are a couple other tests to run?

Here's what you can do in your clinic:

- ✓ Basic bloodwork (a chemistry panel and CBC)
- ✓ Benchtop Ethylene glycol test
- ✓ Blood gas analysis
- ✓ Clotting times
- ✓ Cytology
- ✓ Fecal floatation and direct saline exam
- ✓ FeLV/FIV test
- ✓ Giardia test
- ✓ Heartworm test (with rickettsial diseases)
- ✓ Leptospirosis test
- ✓ Pancreatic lipase
- ✓ Parvo test
- ✓ Pregnancy test
- ✓ Radiographs (X-rays)
- ✓ Skin scraping
- ✓ Thyroid hormone level (T4)
- ✓ Ultrasound
- ✓ Urinalysis

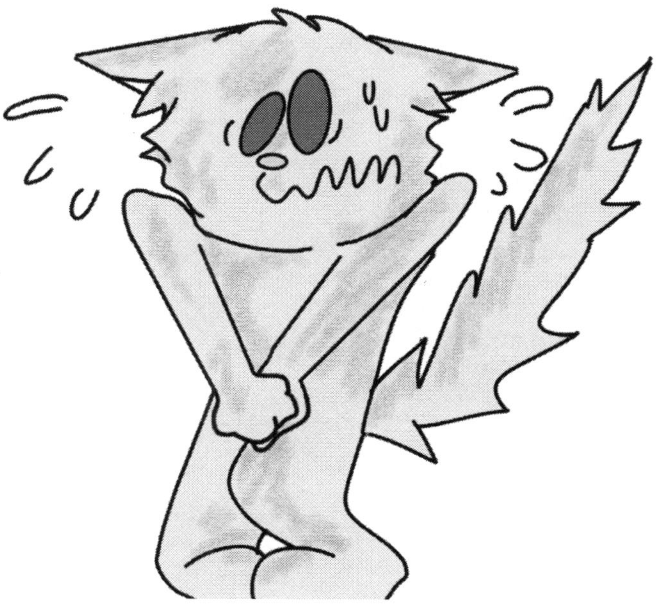

What tests do you want to run?

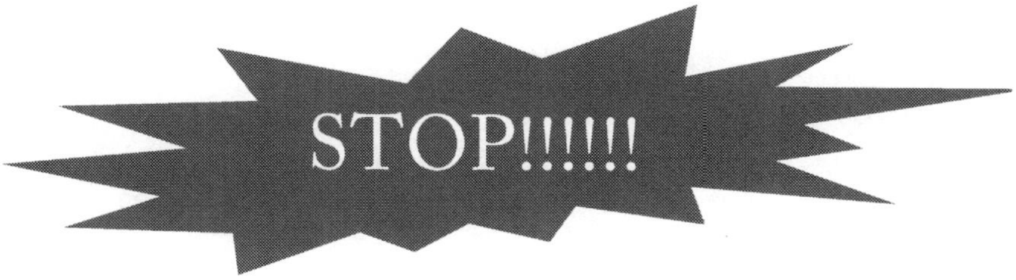

Word, man. You're good at this. Pretty sure we picked the same tests, but let's compare them just in case. I'd additionally recommend: **bloodwork** (a chemistry panel, electrolytes, and CBC), **ECG** (because this patient has a low heart rate, and you know a factoid about potassium in blocked cats), **urinalysis** (once we can get urine safely), **radiographs** (to look for more stones in the upper or lower urinary tract).

"Sure," Violet says. "Those sound like good ideas. But how much will that all cost?"

Much, you almost say. Instead, you say you'll make her an estimate. She approves bloodwork and an ECG, but wants to wait on radiographs. You've got to wait for a urinalysis since you're worried about poking that big bladder under pressure with a needle.

Here's the bloodwork and ECG…

Client: Bagsby, Violet	Species: Feline	Sex: MC
Patient: Edgar Allen Paw	Breed: DSH	
Patient ID: 03783		

CBC

TEST	RESULT	FLAG	REFERENCE RANGE	
WBC	29	H	5.5-19.5	$10^3/\mu L$
Neutrophils	18	H	2.5-12.5	$10^3/\mu L$
Monocytes	0.98	H	0-0.85	$10^3/\mu L$
Lymphocytes	8	H	1.5-7	$10^3/\mu L$
Eosinophils	0.1		0-1.5	$10^3/\mu L$
Hematocrit	33		30-45	%
MCV	46		39-55	fL
Platelet Count	357		300-700	$10^3/\mu L$

Client: Bagsby, Violet	Species: Feline	Sex: MC
Patient: Edgar Allen Paw	Breed: DSH	
Patient ID: 03783		

Chemistry Panel

Test	Result	Flag	Reference Range[xix]
ALT	26		8.3-35 IU/L
ALP	56		12-65 IU/L
GGT	4		1.8-12 IU/L
tBili	0.4		0.1-0.5 mg/dL
Glucose	194	H	61-124 mg/dL
Cholesterol	201		71-161 mg/dL
Total Protein	7.4		5.7-8.0 g/dL
Albumin	2.1	L	2.4-3.8 g/dL
Globulin	3.5		2.4-4.7 g/dL
Calcium	1.9	L	2.0-2.7 mg/dL
BUN	87	H	15-31 mg/dL
Creatinine	5.7	H	0.5-1.9 mg/dL
Phosphorus	8	H	4.0-7.3 mg/dL
Sodium	137	L	146-159 mEq/L
Potassium	8.7	H	3.8-5.3 mEq/L
Chloride	110		108-130 mEq/L

What have you got here? Remember, when looking over bloodwork it helps to "zoom out" and look at the abnormal numbers in terms of body systems. What are the kidneys doing? What is the liver doing? What is the immune system doing? Here's what I see…

- **There is inflammation.** This guy has a high white blood cell count (leukocytosis) with elevated neutrophils, monocytes, and lymphocytes (different types of white blood cells).
- **There is kidney dysfunction.** This guy has severely elevated BUN and creatinine (called "azotemia" when they go up together). He also has a really high phosphorus, which is one of the values that goes up in the blood when the kidneys aren't working (since they usually filter out phosphorus). Now, does this mean his kidneys are diseased and failing? Maybe. Maybe not. He has something blocking his urethra, backing up pressure to his whole urinary tract, which makes the kidneys temporarily unable to do their jobs (even if the kidney tissue is healthy). Of course, as time goes by and more pressure builds up, they may become permanently damaged.
- **There are serious electrolyte changes.** Kidneys filter electrolytes and waste them in the urine. Now this guy's urine is pooling inside him, and his kidneys aren't working like they should, so electrolytes are all over the place. In particular, his potassium is scary high…
- **Blood glucose is high.** This goes up with stress. Not being able to pee is generally stressful.

Right. Those trends in the bloodwork fit the picture of a cat whose body is in some major distress because he cannot let out any urine. This whole discussion is starting to distress me and cause sympathetic discomfort. Excuse me a moment while I visit the bathroom…

*** Friendly jazz rendition of The Astrasian Carol from Starship Beethoven played here***

OK. Sorry about that. Now where were we? Oh yes! The ***dreaded ECG***.

It looks a bit like this:

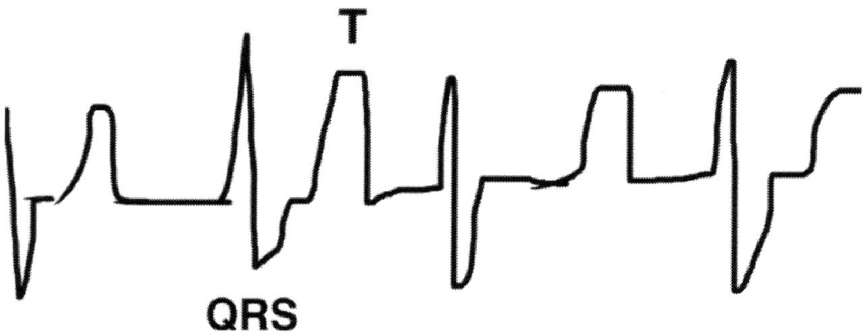

"Yaaaarg! Look at all those squiggles!! What does it all mean?!?! Make it stop! Make it stop!" This, of course, you do not say out loud but keep firmly inside your head…

Look over the infographic on the next page to learn about what exactly an ECG measures. Then you can better appreciate Edgar Allen Paw's ECG.

BASIC ANATOMY OF AN

ECG TRACING

ECG (sometimes written EKG) stands for electrocardiograph, and is a tracing of electrical activity of the heart made in real time. Electric leads are placed in specific locations on a patient, and record the waves of electrons that move toward and away from them through the heart muscle.

BIOELECTRIC!

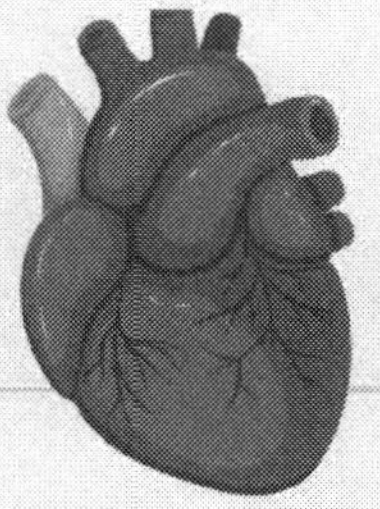

The heart is a complex organ made of specialized muscles that physically contract in response to an electrical signal (depolarization) and relax when that signal is over (repolarization).

The action potential (AP) is a rapid change in electrical potential created by cardiac cells (which normally maintain a polarized gradient of charge across their membrane). The AP has a voltage peak, which plateaus then drops back down. Action potentials are created by movement of charged sodium, potassium, and calcium ion flowing across the cell membranes.

DYNAMIC SYSTEM!

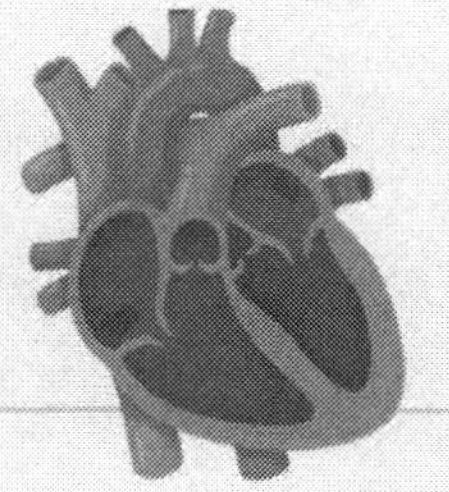

The electric signal is started at a specific area (SA node) and conducted through a pathway designed exactly to stimulate the right chambers to contract and relax in the proper sequence needed to move blood.

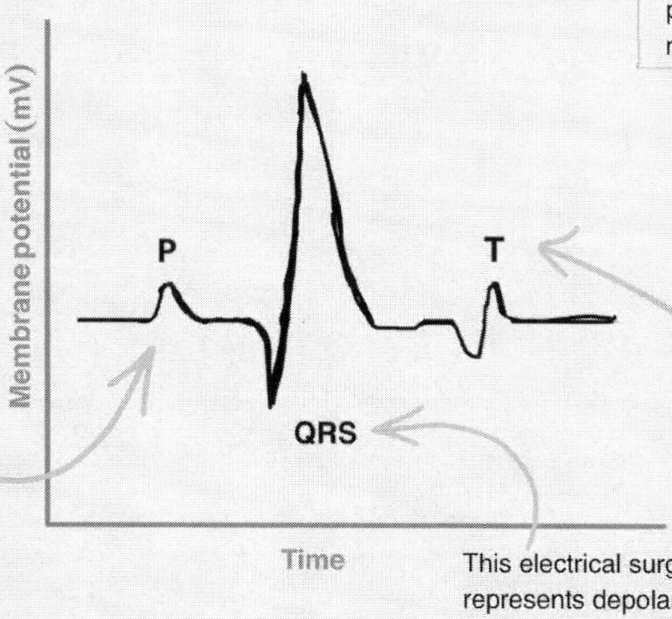

This electrical surge represents depolarization of (and precedes contraction of) the atria, the small heart chambers.

This represents the repolarization of the ventricles.

This electrical surge represents depolarization of (and precedes contraction of) the ventricles, the largest heart chambers.

Now that you see what a normal ECG tracing should look like, you can appreciate how abnormal our patient's is right now. Here's a quick snapshot of the lines blipping across your machine again.

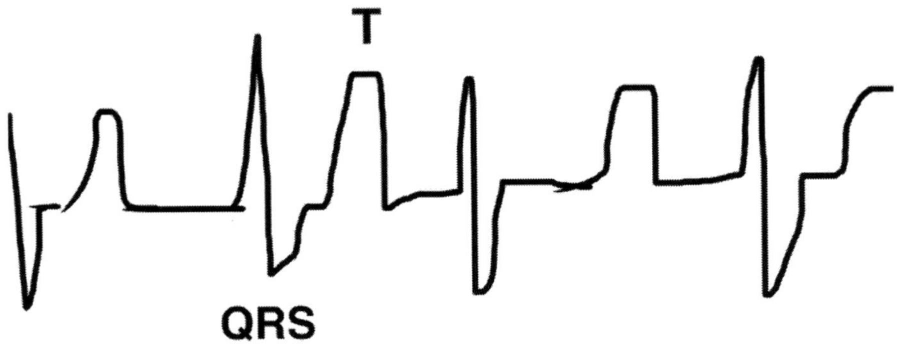

Hmm… Somethin' ain't right, Cletus! The QRS complex seems short and wide. The T-wave seems tall and weird looking. You can't see any consistent P waves at all.

Your brain is ruminating in response to these squiggles, trying to dredge up something you learned in school. *Something can create all those abnormalities, and cause bradycardia. Now what was it…?*

Then your brain screams out loud a sudden revelation (which is super annoying and almost gives you a headache: brains should never scream). *That's right! Hyperkalemia!*

Potassium ions (K+) play a huge part in maintaining the right balance of charge across the cell membrane of the heart muscle. When the blood is flooded with too much potassium (as might happen when the bladder can't empty and pee out used potassium like it normally would), that electric charge across the heart goes haywire! At K levels of 5.5-6.5 mEq/L you can see tall T waves. At K levels of 6.6-7 mEq/L you can see shortened QRS complexes (the R part in particular) and longer spaces between the P wave and the QRS. At K levels of over 7 mEq/L you can see decreased P wave height and AV block (when some beats don't have a P wave). When K levels are over 8.5 mEq/L you lose all the P waves entirely.

You should be starting to worry…

Your patient has serious pressure on the kidneys, limiting their function. That much pressure could potentially tear the bladder. Your patient also has so much potassium building up in his blood that his heart is not beating right. A bit more potassium (over 10.1 mEq/L specifically, if you really want to know, you nerd, you) will cause ventricular fibrillation: a REALLY bad arrhythmia where the nice "lub-dup" heartbeat changes to a frantic jiggle just before the heart gives out entirely and stops. And just in case you fell asleep during that part of vet school, a stopped heart is bad.

"Uh oh!" you say. "Someone really ought to do something about this."

Fred and Harlow blink. Oh yeah. You're the doctor. *You* ought to do something about this. But what?

Choose some from this list of treatment options.

What is your treatment plan? (pick several)

a) Antibiotics

b) Apply 4 leeches to the base of the ears to release the phlegmatic humors

c) CPR

d) Give anti-inflammatory medication

e) Give a cardioprotectant drug (one that protects the heart)

f) Give drugs to prevent a seizure

g) Give drugs to relax the urethra

h) Give insulin

i) Give terbutaline (which opens the small airways) or albuterol

j) Give up. This patient can't be saved

k) Hand the patient a litter box

l) IV fluids

m) Nausea medications

n) Pain medications

o) Pass a catheter up that cat's urethra and unblock him

p) Poke a needle in that bladder and relieve all the pressure!

q) Surgery to remove the stones in the bladder (cystotomy)

STOP!!!!!!

> "Oh, I don't know, you know, don't you know!"
>
> —P.G. Wodehouse, *The Inimitable Jeeves*[xx]

Whew! That's a lot of possibilities. Is it even legal to make multiple choice questions that long? Here's what I'd recommend in this patient: **e, i, l, and o**. Already done: **g and n**.

Give cardioprotectant drugs. This guy's heart is about to go kablooey. And in case you fell asleep during that part of school... Never mind. We did that joke already. The specific drug you'll use is called calcium gluconate, and it protects the heart temporarily against the effects of the high potassium.

Give terbutaline or albuterol. Haha! Fooled you, didn't I? Those are drugs we usually give for dilation of airways, but have a handy side effect of reducing potassium levels in the blood quickly. A puff of albuterol in an inhaler, or an injection of terbutaline, is a common way to treat dangerously high levels of potassium in cats. Another way to treat dangerously high levels of potassium is to give some insulin, which drives K into cells. The problem is, it will also drive glucose down to dangerously low levels, so if you do it, you're gonna have to give dextrose (an injectable form of glucose) all night long and monitor the blood sugar.

Give IV fluids. Fluids help rehydrate the patient and improve his kidney function. You can choose fluids that help drop potassium too, which is sometimes enough by itself (with special drugs like terbutaline) in cases where the potassium isn't as high as it is in this guy.

You already gave **pain medications** and **a drug that relaxes the urethra**. Good job. Acepromazine (which you used to sedate this guy a few pages back) has the handy side effect of relaxing the muscles in the urethra. I have had cases of urethral obstruction that "magically" started peeing after an acepromazine dose before I could move on to unblock them.

Oh yeah. **Unclogging the urethra** is the treatment that will ultimately make this guy better. The other treatments are aimed at stabilizing him and getting him ready to unblock. Why? Because he must be sedated (usually anesthetized completely) for this procedure. What you do is, you take this little slippery urethral catheter and put it up the urethra through this kitty's tiny penis. It is *not* easy, especially in cases like this where there are uroliths clogging up the urethra. In this case you're probably gonna have to do a little something we veterinarians like to call URETHRAL RETROGRADE UROHYDROPROPULSION. This is one of the best terms ever, because it's a *huge* word for a simple process. Retrograde urohydropropulsion is flushing the blockage (stones or sand) down the urethra and back into the bladder.

What did you think of p) poke a needle in that bladder and relieve all the pressure? It sounds risky and brutal. Years ago, it was a big "no no." But there have been studies that show that the risk of cystocetesis (poking the bladder with a needle) to suction out urine and relieve the pressure is low and a viable option to help stabilize a patient—especially in cases where putting in a urethral catheter isn't possible. Obviously, this isn't fixing the problem of blockage, but can help keep the patient comfortable and alive while you figure out Plan B.

Well, you go in and explain all these things to Violet Bagsby, who promptly begins to panic. Then you have Fred show her an expensive estimate to do all these treatments and hospitalize Edgar Allen Paw, because that'll surely help her stop panicking…

You contemplate what to do if Violet declines treatment.

What would be Plan B?

That's a tough one! There are several options you could consider, but you're going to have to prioritize the most important treatment goals.

- The potassium is going to have to be lowered, or this guy will die.
- The pressure in the bladder will need to be relieved.

You could maybe give some drugs for the potassium, then either perform a cystocentesis or go ahead and unblock him but remove the urethral catheter. Usually you would leave it in for hospitalization overnight, but if the patient doesn't stay, you risk causing bad infections if you don't remove it. Colorado State University[11] did a study specifically describing an outpatient treatment plan for financially restricted cases of urethral obstruction in cats, which many veterinarians have found useful.

Fortunately, Mrs. Bagsby does approve your very expensive treatment Plan A. This leaves you glad for your patient and wondering if you can change careers to do whatever Mrs. Bagsby is doing. But you can't wonder long. Gotta get busy. This is the sort of case that can keep you occupied for a while.

You give calcium gluconate while monitoring the ECG. Then you give some terbutaline and start IV fluids. Blood pressure is OK. ECG looks a little better. Everything is set up to unblock this guy. You give more sedatives and get him to sleep completely. Harlow shaves and preps the area, then you take your 3.5 Fr catheter and try to slip it in. It's a lot like trying to feed a thread to a floppy earthworm that keeps trying to go back into his hole. There's this stiff bit inside the catheter called a stylet you use to help, but it's still very tough. You manage to get it past the opening but find the catheter tip is clunking up against something. Time to pull out the old retrograde urohydropropulsion! Harlow gets a saline syringe and flushes it into the catheter in little pulses while you try to push it in further. No dice!

Then you remember a trick the hospital manager here told you about. You have atricurium in the fridge here! This is a potent muscle relaxer that can loosen the urethral muscles and give you a better chance at

[11] My own Alma Mater. Go Rams!

flushing this blockage back into the bladder. It is also, coincidently, a cousin of the toxin in poison dart frogs (epibatidine). You slop a bit through the urethral catheter (OK… What you actually do is carefully inject a specific amount through the catheter). Then you get back at it. About half an hour later, you holler and do a happy dance, because the blockage flushed through finally, and you got that catheter into the bladder! Bloody urine flows out of the catheter like oil gushing from a Texas oil rig!

"Excelsior!" you holler.

You take a sample for testing later, then flush the catheter and bladder with saline to help dilute out grit and mucous plugs and hopefully reduce inflammation. Then you take a radiograph to make sure the catheter is where it should be. It looks like this…

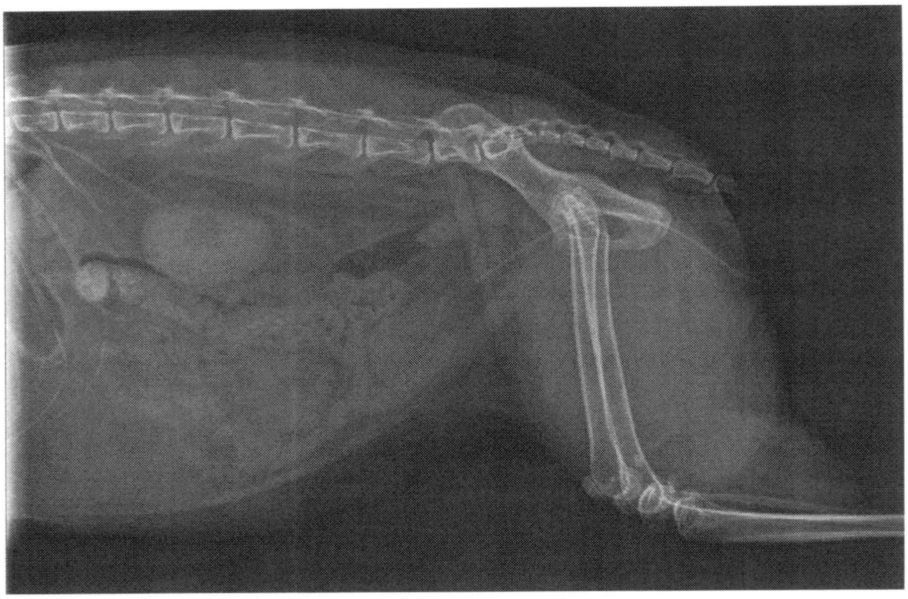

Could be just a little further in, but that should work fine. You visually confirm there is flow of urine through the catheter into the collection system, then send him with Harlow to get his accommodation for the night set up. Your radiograph confirmed something else.

What are these?

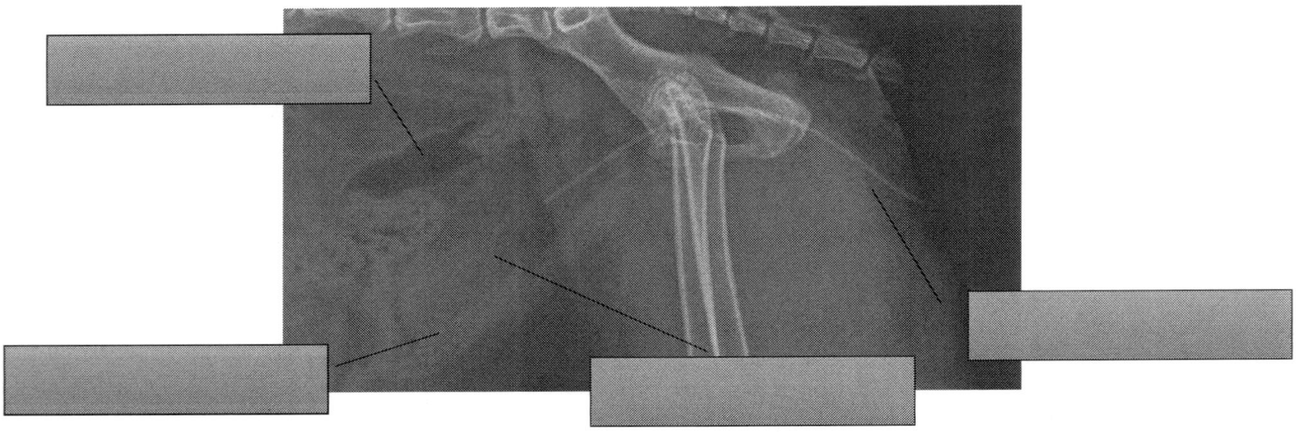

Did your labels look like this?

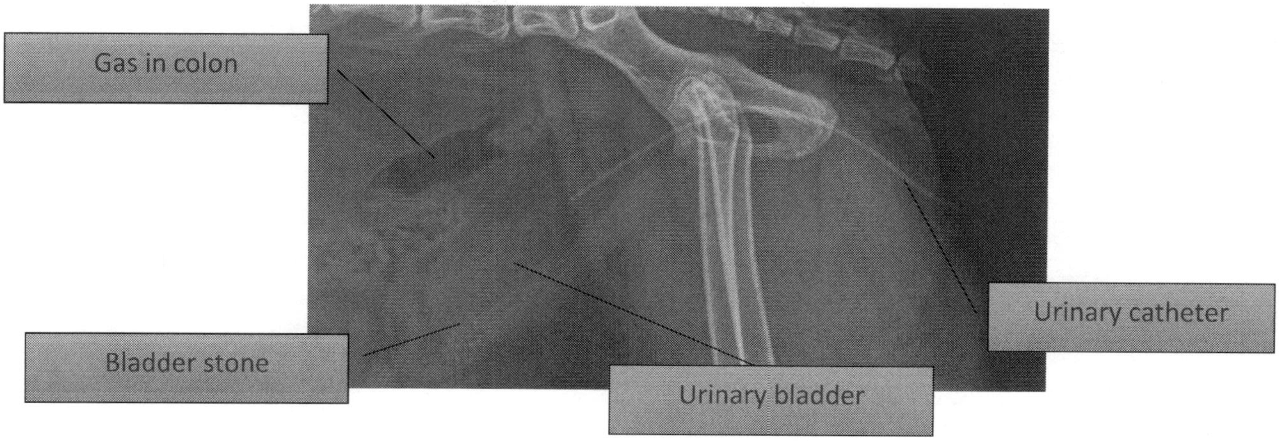

That's right! Those are **bladder stones**. And there are a lot of them. It may be an entire shoal, flock, or pack. With these many stones it seems likely that this cat is going to need a cystotomy (surgical removal of the stone) when he is more stable. This intra-abdominal surgery involves an incision into the urinary bladder to physically scoop out those little rocks. The alternative is attempting medical dissolution. This means putting the patient on a special diet that might dissolve the stone away. Some types of stones will not dissolve well, and there is a high chance of the patient blocking again while trying to pass smaller stones.

Did you know there are different types of bladder stones a cat or dog can get? The chemicals that make them up will change how bright they show up on X-rays and how easily they dissolve at different degrees of urine acidity or alkalinity. How are we gonna know what type of urolith this is? Well, we could send a stone off to a lab to analyze, but that would mean we have to surgically get them. We can also do a urinalysis which will usually tell us the type of microscopic crystals these uroliths are shedding. A urinalysis will also look for clues to other problems like urinary tract infections (which sometimes go along with stones in the bladder) or diabetes or kidney injury. Fortunately, you have collected lots of urine in this patient. You also collected a sterile sample (one not contaminated by bacteria from the table or the patient's skin or your hands) when you first got in the urethral catheter. That's important because having signs of inflammation on a urinalysis (like white blood cells and proteins) doesn't necessarily mean there's an infection. You'll have to send a sterile sample to a lab to culture for bacteria if you really want to be sure about an infection.

You can check a urinalysis "in house" (we usually say to sound all cool and suave and hip and stuff). This usually involves a special paper strip that changes colors when dipped in urine, and is often slipped into a little machine that reads the color change. Frustratingly, that means results are a little more nebulous, and don't usually come with clear-cut reference values. A tiny amount of urine is spun down in a centrifuge to get a sediment (i.e. a bunch of gunk pushed down to the bottom of the tube by gravity) you can look at under a microscope.

Here's your in-house urinalysis…

Client: Bagsby, Violet	Species: Feline	Sex: MC
Patient: Edgar Allen Paw	Breed: DSH	
Patient ID: 03783		

Urinalysis

TEST	RESULT	FLAG	REFERENCE RANGE
Color	YELLOW		
Clarity	CLOUDY		
Specific Gravity	>1.040		1.020-1.040
pH	7.0		6.0-7.5
Urine Protein	1+		
Glucose	NEGATIVE		
Ketones	NEGATIVE		
Hemoglobin	NEGATIVE		
Bilirubin	NEGATIVE		
White Blood Cells	1-2/ HPF		
Red Blood cells	2-3/ HPF		
Bacteria	COCCI 3+		
Epithelial Cells	1+		
Casts	NONE SEEN		
Crystals	STRUVITE 3-4/HPF		

And here's what you see in the sediment under the microscope…

What is all this stuff?

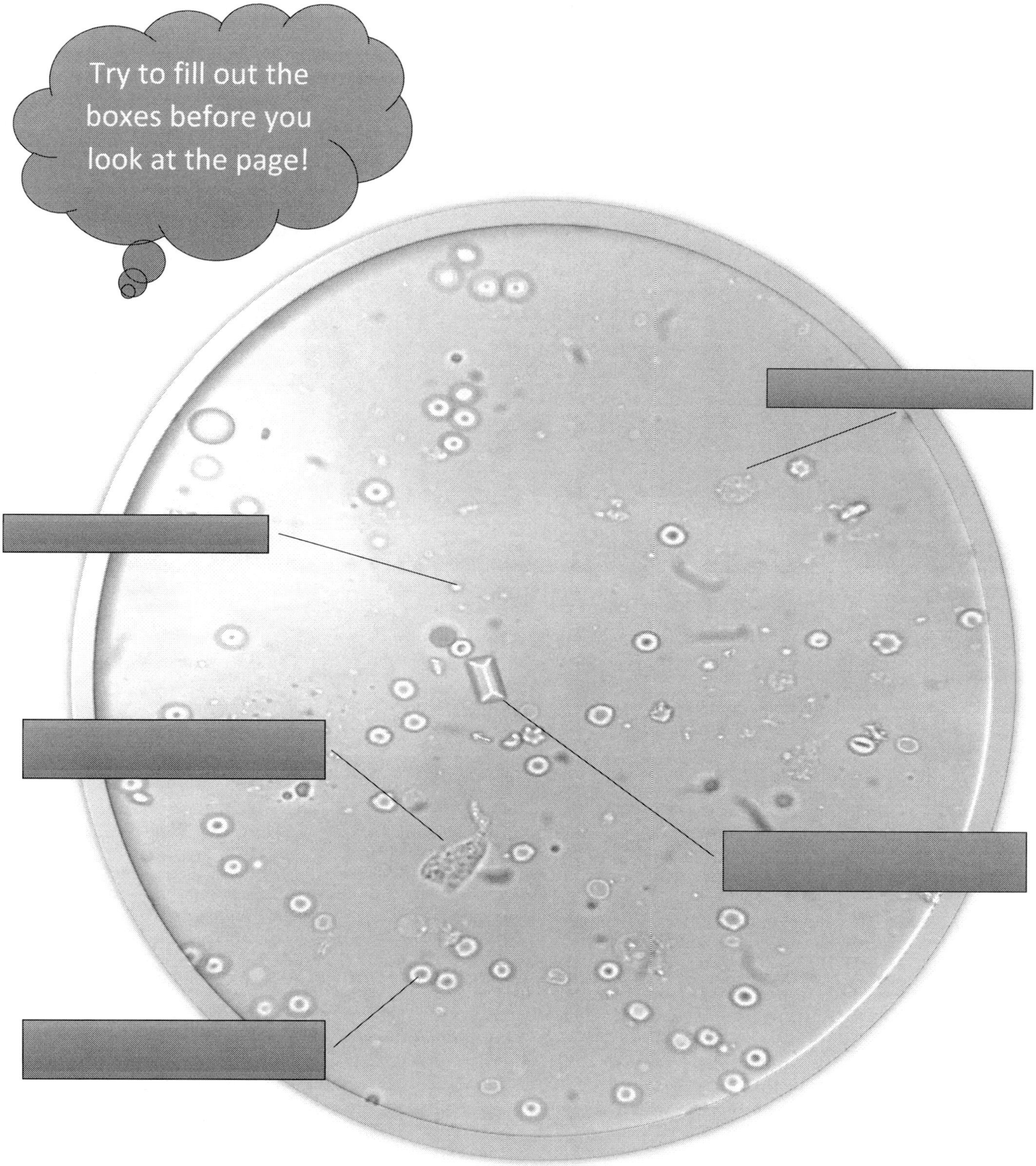

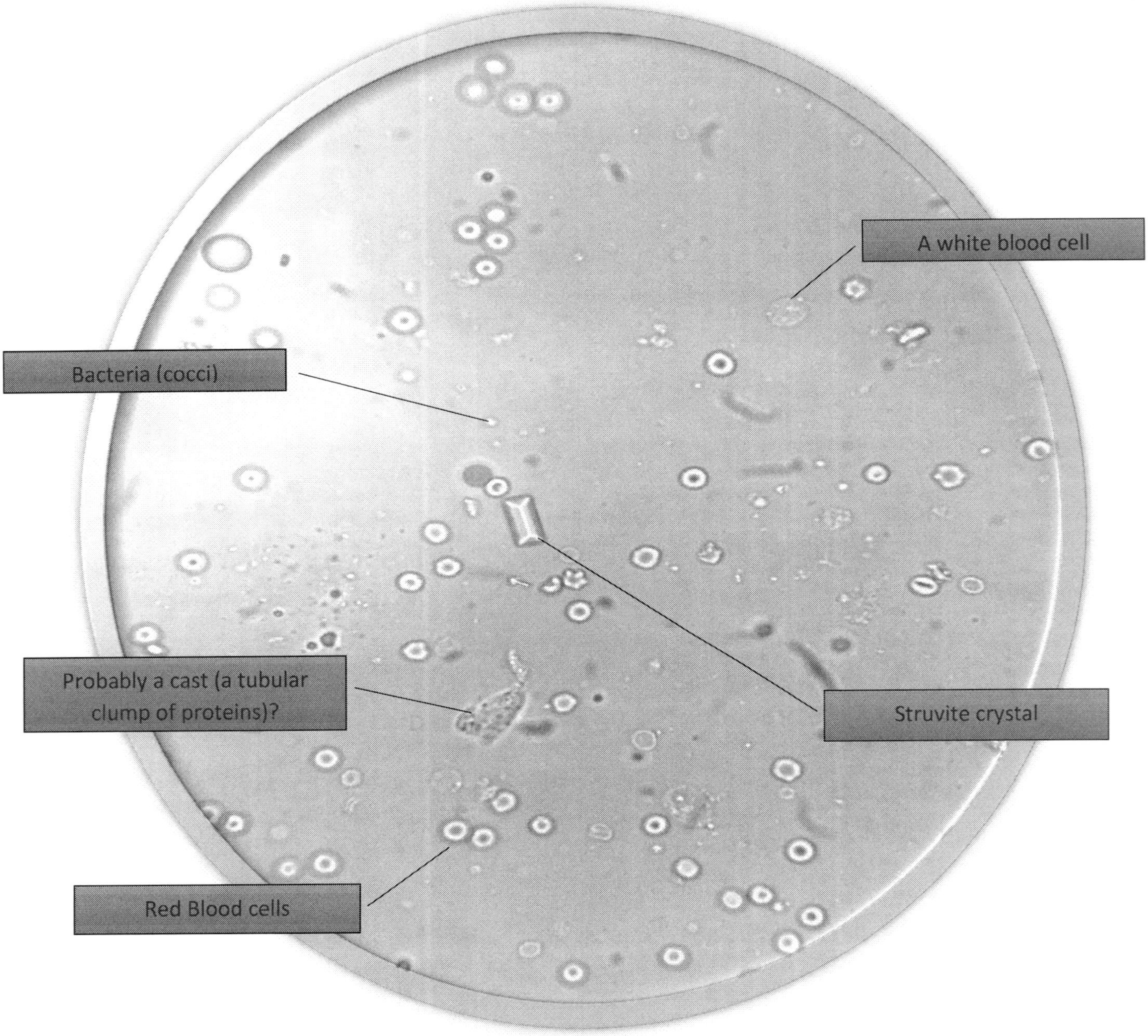
A white blood cell
Bacteria (cocci)
Probably a cast (a tubular clump of proteins)?
Struvite crystal
Red Blood cells

"What does it all mean???"

You ask the question famously sung in minor key by Lieutenant Quarternote on the Quasideck during the Battle of Kashioto-hamburi (Starship Beethoven S3E14). Then you take a step backward, and a shape emerges. Yes…yes! It's all becoming clear!

There's an increased specific gravity. That's just a measurement of the concentration of the urine, meaning there's more stuff than normal in the urine. There are increased white blood cells and blood and proteins, all things you might find with inflammation. But wait! There's also a large amount of bacteria - cocci (which are round bacteria in particular). On the sediment exam under the microscope, you can confirm all these: cocci bacteria, red blood cells, white blood cells.

But there is also another…thing. It's shaped like a tiny coffin. It's crystalline and alien to the bladder of a normal cat (though there can be a miniscule amount of struvite crystals in a healthy cat). It's a struvite crystal! You find more of them with every field you scan under the microscope. This proves there are a lot more than a miniscule amount of struvite crystals in this guy. Aha!

It's a tale as old as time. Struvite stones are a great place to grow bacteria. And bacteria lead to an infection. Both of those together cause big amount of inflammation, bloody urine, and a feeling of urgency and straining when voiding urine. And all of that can cause urethral obstruction.

"Case closed," you whisper (out loud…embarrassing yourself). You try to drop the magnifying glass you imagine yourself holding in your right hand, before you forget it's not there.

Fred laughs. Harlow just looks confused.

Alrighty. So you've got Edgar Allen Paw unblocked and catheterized, you have his potassium under control, IV fluids are helping to flush out his kidneys, and he's had some good pain medications. What's another treatment you could consider starting, with the new information you've got now?

Pick another treatment from the previous list…

____

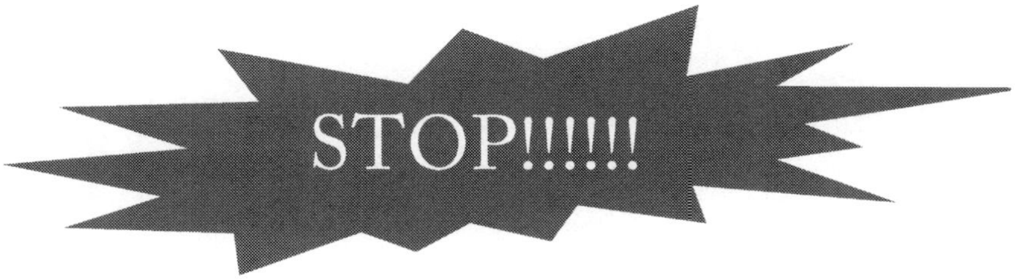

If you picked **antibiotics**, give yourself a high five!

An antibiotic would not be bad to start now that you've seen evidence of a lower urinary tract infection (like white blood cells *and* bacteria). A urine culture will confirm infection, and tell you what antibiotics these bugs might be resistant to. You don't want to start antibiotics before you collect urine to culture, since they could mess up the results of the test. But now that you have some "pre-antibiotic" sterile urine off to the lab you could start a broad-spectrum antibiotic with the plan to stop it if culture comes back negative. This is what we often call "empiric antibiotic therapy," fancy words to mean we're trying out an antibiotic, by guessing what bugs are probably there.

If you picked **give an anti-inflammatory**, give yourself a medium five. You've seen plenty of evidence of inflammation in this poor guy's urinary tract, and it would not be wrong to give anti-inflammatory medication. The one most vets pick for cats is robenacoxib, a type of NSAID anti-inflammatory. The problem is it can be hard on the kidneys (which are already straining like Trebble Snifflet, when he lifted the Stone of Doom from the volcanic shaft on Vorbon-6 while singing "Let it out, let it all rush out!"). So NSAIDS this early could potentially be risky. Steroids also have some risky side effects. But they might help. We often must balance the risks with the benefits of a treatment in a complicated case like this. Being the one to make those tough choices is one of the biggest challenges of being a doctor.

You go talk to Violet Bagsby. You go over the case so far, and she's grateful to hear her little guy is unblocked and stable. You're grateful you talked to her about NSAIDs and antibiotics before starting them, since she does not want to risk harming the kidneys and seems anxious about starting antibiotics.

"I don't like giving any more medication to him than we have to, Doctor," she says, the careful tone in her voice signaling that she's probably been ridiculed for those words before.

She seems relieved when you agree with her. "Yeah, I understand. Every drug has side effects. It's probably OK to wait on both of those until he's been on fluids and we have results from the lab. If the inflammation isn't getting better tomorrow or the next day, we can always decide to start them then."

"Good! I try to be environmentally conscious and worry about contributing to antibiotic overuse."

This is an interesting statement to hear from a client. She thanks you and leaves her cat for the night, and you find yourself contemplating her words. Do you think she's right? Have you ever thought about potential risk antibiotic use in your patients could have on everyone else around you?

Look over the infographic on the next page…

Antibiotic Stewardship

Veterinary decisions make a difference in preserving antibiotic success!

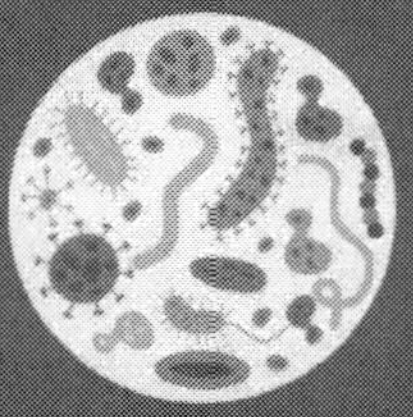

Impact of Antibiotic Resistance

1.27M

Deaths in people worldwide directly related to antibiotic resistant organisms in 2019

2.8M

Antibiotic resistant infections in humans in USA every year

$4.6B

Spent in US yearly to treat antibiotic resistant infections

Methods of Antibiotic (AB) Resistance

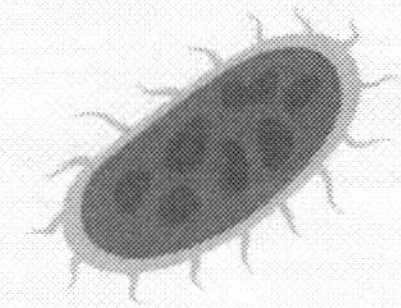

Microorganisms use 4 basic stategies to develop resistance to antibiotics...

- Inactivation of AB inside the cell
- Decreased AB penetration (block it from entering)
- Expulsion of AB through pumps in membrane
- Modification of the antibiotic's target in the cell

Definitions

Multidrug Resistant (MDR)
Resistance in 3 or more antibiotic classes

Extensive Resistant (XDR)
Resistance in all but 1 or 2 antibiotic categories

Resist the Resistance

Test Running culture and sensitivity panels more often helps to target antibiotics where they'll work

Timeout Pausing to evaluate response in 48-72 hours can prompt de-escalation of AB if needed

Treatment Pick the propper drug, dose, and duration ("3 D's of antibiotic use")

Animal Impact

Statistical data on the impact of veterinarians in AB resistance is lacking, but it is almost certainly underestimated.

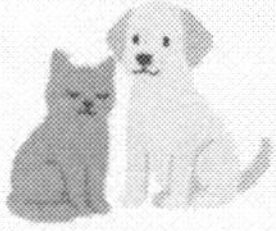

Increased contact between humans and small animals, and inappropriate antibiotic use creates resistance. Up to 47% of veterinary cases had resistant E. coli in one study!

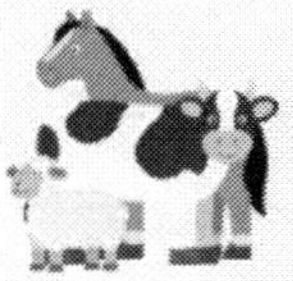

Use of antibiotics prophylactically and to treat diseases in large animals spreads resistance to pathogens like Moraxella and E. coli.

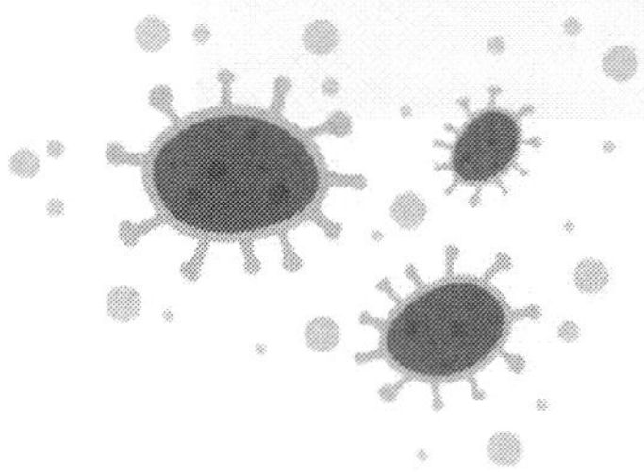

Sources:

Antimicrobial Resistance Facts and Stats. CDC 2025

Menard, Julie. *Antimicrobial Stewardship and Antimicrobial Resistance.* EVECC2020

Antimicrobial-Resistant Pathogens Affecting Animal Health in the United States. AVMA 2020

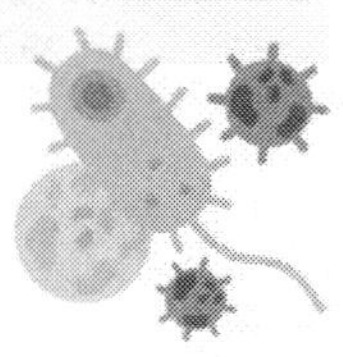

J. Aaron Gruben

"So how's your week?" you ask Fred during one of the many awkwardly long commas of silent boredom which often punctuate ER shifts. The ER is sometimes a place where friends and acquaintances sit and stare at each other while wondering what Thing will happen next.

"Oh, you know," he yawned, "just another week of battling terrorists to keep space-time from unraveling and exploding the universe…"

You and Harlow stare before laughing at his odd sense of humor. "Sounds like someone's spent too much time on the AI-deck this week!" you comment.

"Ha! I couldn't stay there long with Sonja's Theme running in the background like it always does."

Your eyes light up. You've met another fellow Starship Beethoven nerd! You and Fred sing Sonja's Theme, which plays on the show every time a character uses the AI-deck. True fans will, of course, know that the AI that runs this special room with simulated adventures is called Sonja.

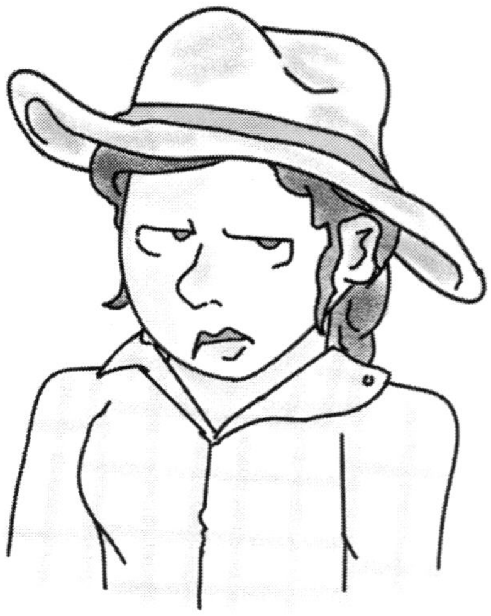

"*Imagine it! Imagine it!*
Take a ride, side by side
On a flying carpet!
On the AI deck, anything is possible
It will fool your brain
And possibly your nost-i-ril…"

Harlow groans. "Who writes this stuff?"

"Not a fan of Starship Beethoven?" you laugh.

"Never heard of it. I pretty much only watch crime shows, if I watch anything. I spend most of my time with barrel racing, and don't have much left."

You feel genuinely puzzled. "How fast can a barrel really go?"

Fred bursts out laughing. He generally seems ready to do that.

This time Harlow joins in. "No, no, Doc," Harlow pulls out her phone to show you a picture of her hobby. "Barrel racing is western riding sport. I ride my quarter horse around a pattern of barrels in competitions. Guess you're a city slicker after all, huh?"

That makes more sense. Santa Fe (like a lot of New Mexico) has a significant cowboy culture. That's what comes from vast amounts of open spaces for ranching, and generations of cowboy history. Because of its rich Hispanic influence, there's a unique mingling of vaquero traditions around the capital. You ask Harlow about her quarter horse, and a broad smile crosses her friendly face. It's always nice to find a topic someone likes to talk about.

"His name's Jack. Well, it's officially Jack of All Trade HD24 on his papers. Been training with him since I was 12!" She swipes on her phone to show you a picture of Jack. "He's a big guy. Bit over 15 hands!"

You decide against saying, "Looks like a horse to me," and instead go with, "He's handsome!"

She nods. "I have two more horses, but he's my favorite."

"Harlow's our farm girl," Fred smiles. "If you're nice to her, she might bring you eggs from her chickens."

"I just pretend to be a farm girl. Only have a few acres out by Chalupa Drive."

That street name sounds familiar. "Didn't I see that somewhere recently? Oh yeah! Dr. Crimshaw put it down as her address. I remember, because I looked over her paperwork after she checked in, to make sure it was coherent."

Fred and Harlow chuckle, obviously understanding. Then Harlow's brow darkens a bit. "Yeah. Old Doc Crimshaw's place butts up against my property. Used to work with her, back when she owned this place."

"Wait a minute… You're not the neighbor she thinks has been poisoning Superfly are you?"

This time Harlow's chuckle sounds wry. "She said that? That old so-and-so is getting as mean as she is forgetful. Er… Sorry. Hope you're not friends or anything."

You can't stop the grin from breaking out over your face at the goofiness of this small, small world. "Not at all. I just met her, and she is a character."

At this point the doorbell rings, and a gust of cold air with snowflakes accompanies a limping dog into the clinic. It's a friendly and very energetic Australian shepherd mix of some kind. A middle-aged couple follow him into the clinic.

Case #10

"Our dog Spot broke his leg!" the lady he gasps out, wide-eyed and panicked.

"We just got back from the gym," the man pants, flushing with obvious anxiety and talking quickly. "Spot was in the backyard when we left, and seemed fine then."

"Now he can't walk on his right back leg!" she interrupts.

"Won't put any weight at all!" he adds.

"He yelped when I tried to move it," she says.

"Bark!" Spot says.

"I think it could be broken! Is it broken? How do we tell if it's broken?" he says.

"Can you fix a broken leg?"

"Does it need a cast?"

"Arf! Arf!" Spot adds cheerfully.

"Does it need surgery? I don't think we can afford surgery, can we, Linda?"

"Does it need an amputation? He's only five years old! Oh, Gary, I don't think we can take care of a three-legged dog!"

At this point you wisely intervene to stop this unhealthy, spiraling cycle of panic. The ER is sometimes a billboard to display how unchecked panic can lead to disastrous drama, but a cool head can calm any fire. "Hang on a minute. Let's get you guys checked in. We don't know if this fella's leg is broken yet, but there are certainly things we can do to find out and help fix it."

"But he's not putting any weight on it!" Linda nearly screams, having worked herself into a frenzy.

"Lots of things can cause that. Harlow and I will take him to the exam room and look him over. Can we give him a pain injection while you're filling out your paperwork?"

They nod approval, and you take Spot to do an exam. You've brought the situation to a more peaceful Spot, you might say. Here's what you find.

Step 1 – Organize the History

Signalment:

5 years old

Male neutered

Mixed breed

Presenting Complaints:

Left hind limb lameness

Step 2 – Gather Clues

Physical Examination:

Abdominal palpation: Palpates normally. Pliable with no splinting. No distension or fluid wave noted. No obvious organomegally or mass noted.

Attitude: BAR, calm and friendly.

Oronasal: Mild dental calculus noted, with minimal inflammation of the gingiva (gums).

Cardiac: Thoracic auscultation is unremarkable (no murmur or arrhythmia noted). Strong femoral pulses noted.

Ears: Appear clear AU.

Eyes: Appear clear OU.

Integument: No lacerations or wounds noted. Normal skin turgor.

Lymph Nodes: Palpate normally.

Musculoskeletal: Toe-touching lame on the right hind limb. Flexion of the hock and digits is unremarkable, but the patient seems uncomfortable when flexing his stifle (knee) and coxofemoral joint (hip). No pain on spinal palpation noted. Positive cranial drawer motion[12] suspected in the right stifle.

Neurologic: No significant findings. Normal menace response and palpebral reflex. Normal conscious proprioception on all four paws.

Respiratory: The patient is panting, but no increased respiratory effort is noted. Pulmonary auscultation is clear (no crackles or wheezes noted in the chest, etc.).

Urogenital: No significant findings. Urinary bladder palpates normally.

Vitals: MM are pink and moist, CRT<2 seconds.

[12] This is a special type of movement you can produce in a loose knee joint if there's a problem with the big ligament called the "cruciate ligament" in the knee.

Right! You have some information.

Make a differential list before you turn the page…

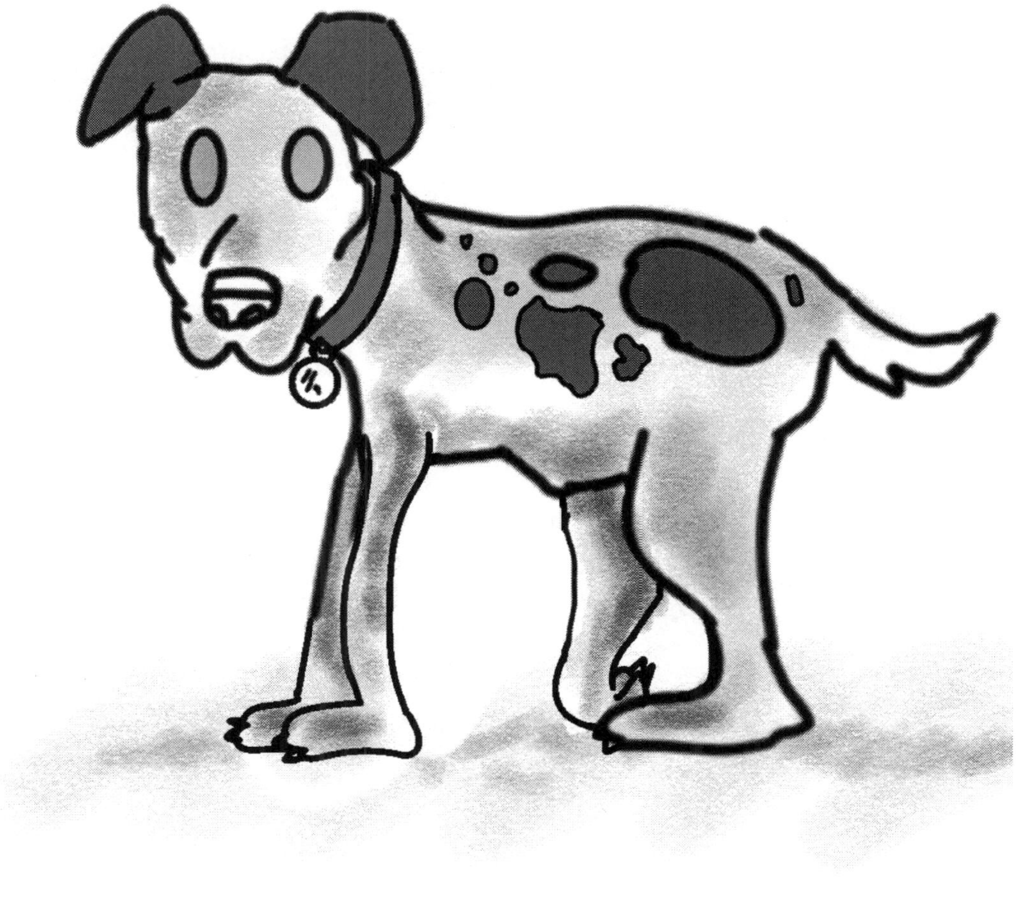

"There is nothing like looking, if you want to find something. You certainly usually find something, if you look, but it is not always quite the something you were after."

—J. R. R. Tolkien, *The Hobbit*[xxi]

Differential Diagnoses that limped out of my mind:

Infection

Fracture

Luxation — A joint popped out of place.

Neoplasia

Neurologic — Such as: central nerve disorder (like a slipped disc pushing on a spinal cord) or peripheral nerve injury.

Soft tissue injury — Such as: muscle tear, sprain, or strain.

As you can see, there are quite a few possibilities even with something that seems simple. Some of those (like fungal infection or neoplasia) are far-fetched. Spot wouldn't be able to fetch them right now…

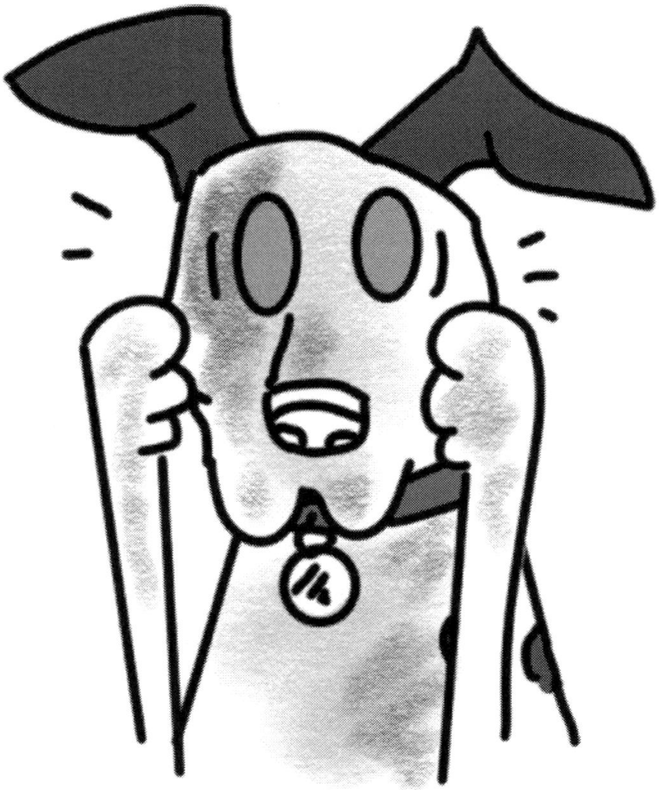

Considering these possibilities, what's the best test to recommend?

Here's what you can do in your clinic:

- ✓ Basic bloodwork (a chemistry panel and CBC)
- ✓ Benchtop Ethylene glycol test
- ✓ Blood gas analysis
- ✓ Clotting times
- ✓ Cytology
- ✓ Fecal floatation and direct saline exam
- ✓ FeLV/FIV test
- ✓ Giardia test
- ✓ Heartworm test (with rickettsial diseases)
- ✓ Leptospirosis test
- ✓ Pancreatic lipase
- ✓ Parvo test
- ✓ Pregnancy test
- ✓ Radiographs (X-rays)
- ✓ Skin scraping
- ✓ Thyroid hormone level (T4)
- ✓ Ultrasound
- ✓ Urinalysis

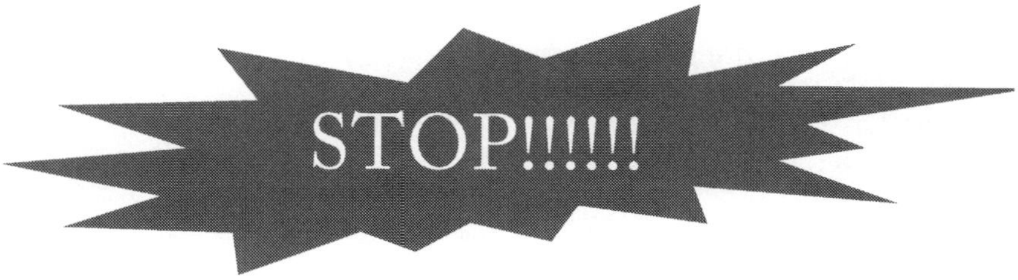

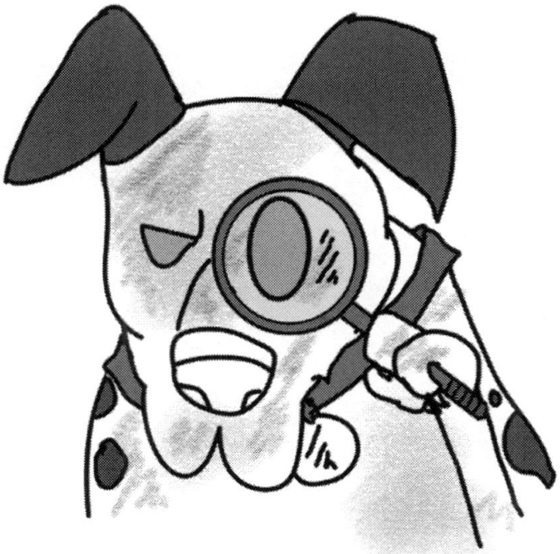

If you picked **radiographs**, you're Spot-on! Give yourself a million dollars![13]

The most likely differentials at this point are musculoskeletal problems. X-rays will be the best way to investigate. They show bones really well in particular. If this is a soft tissue injury (like a sprain or strain) then a CT scan would really be the best way to image that. But Owlhoot Veterinary Clinic has no CT scanner.

You are probably wondering why musculoskeletal differentials are more likely. Good question, you!

There are several clues you can pick up on in the physical exam and signalment to tell you this (if you pay close attention like the brilliant veterinary detective I know you're becoming).

- Neoplasia: This is a young, healthy dog and bone cancer, though possible, tends to affect older dogs.
- Neurological: There is pain in the knee and hip of this patient. That probably means this is not neurologic (though there are some *really* rare cases of peripheral nerve pain).
- Spinal problems: The reflexes were normal, and he wasn't painful in his back. That makes spinal problems (central neurologic) less likely.
- Infection: There is not a fever in this patient, which you'd expect from infectious causes of lameness.
- Fungal or tick-born infection: There is no vomiting or inappetence, or other signs of systemic (whole body) diseases like you'd expect from fungal or tick-born infections.

So those things are all on the list of possibilities, but are less likely than some kind of bone, muscle, or tendon injury based on your exam.

Harlow helps you give this guy some methadone, which is a strong pain injection that has the really nice side effect of sedating him a little. Now he's a still Spot, and you can take some radiographs of his leg and hips.

Can you identify anything on these radiographs?

[13] Toss me a few hundred thousand while you're at it, huh? I did teach you all this stuff, after all...

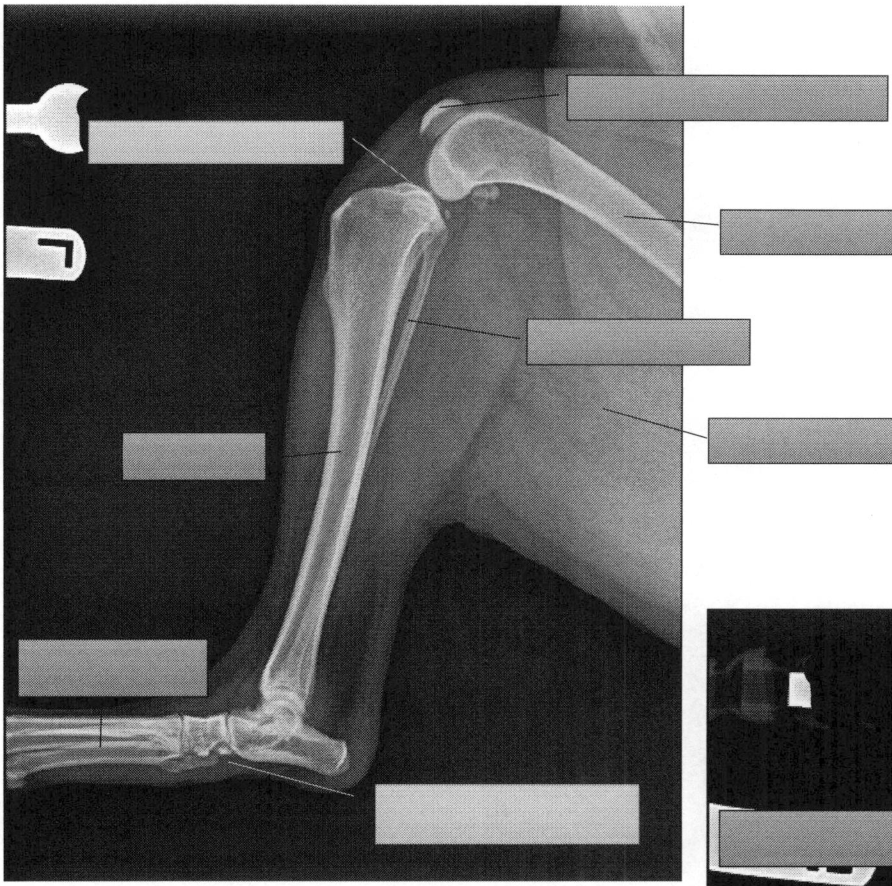

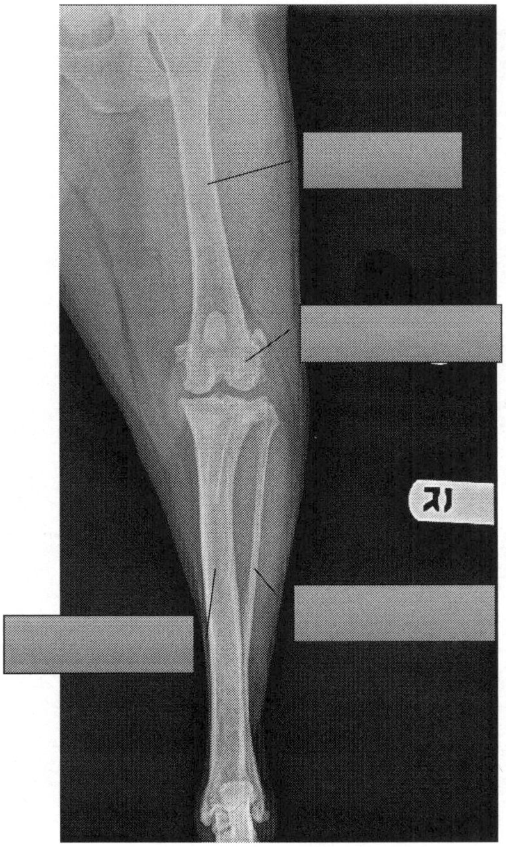

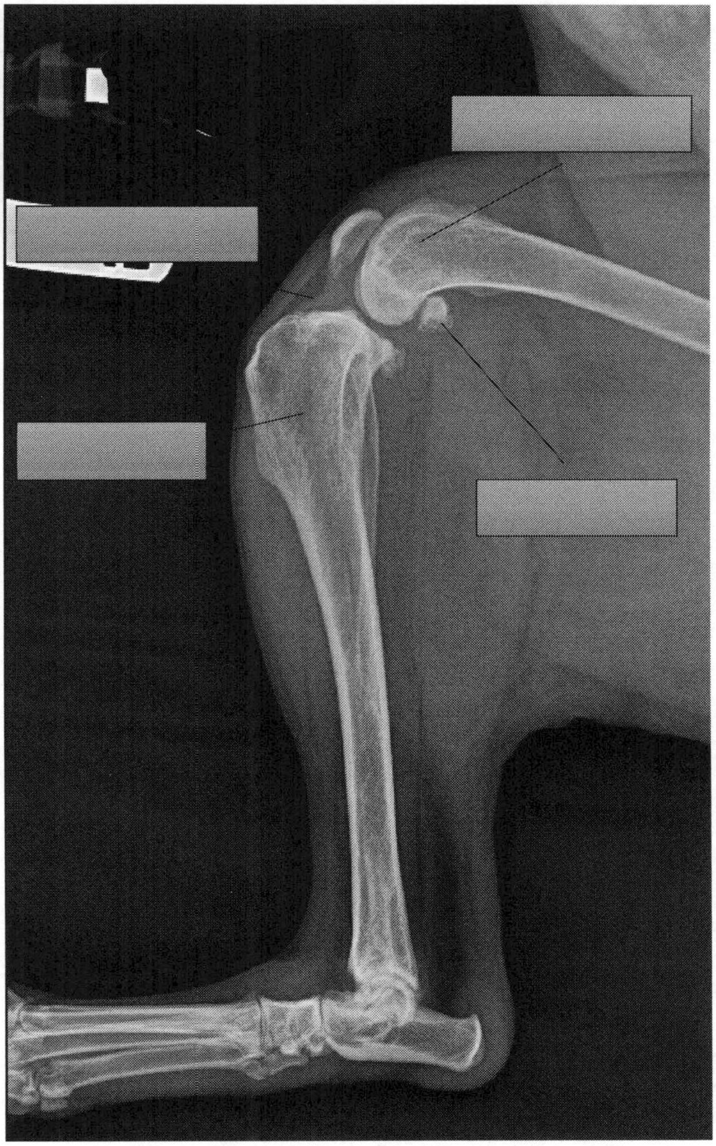

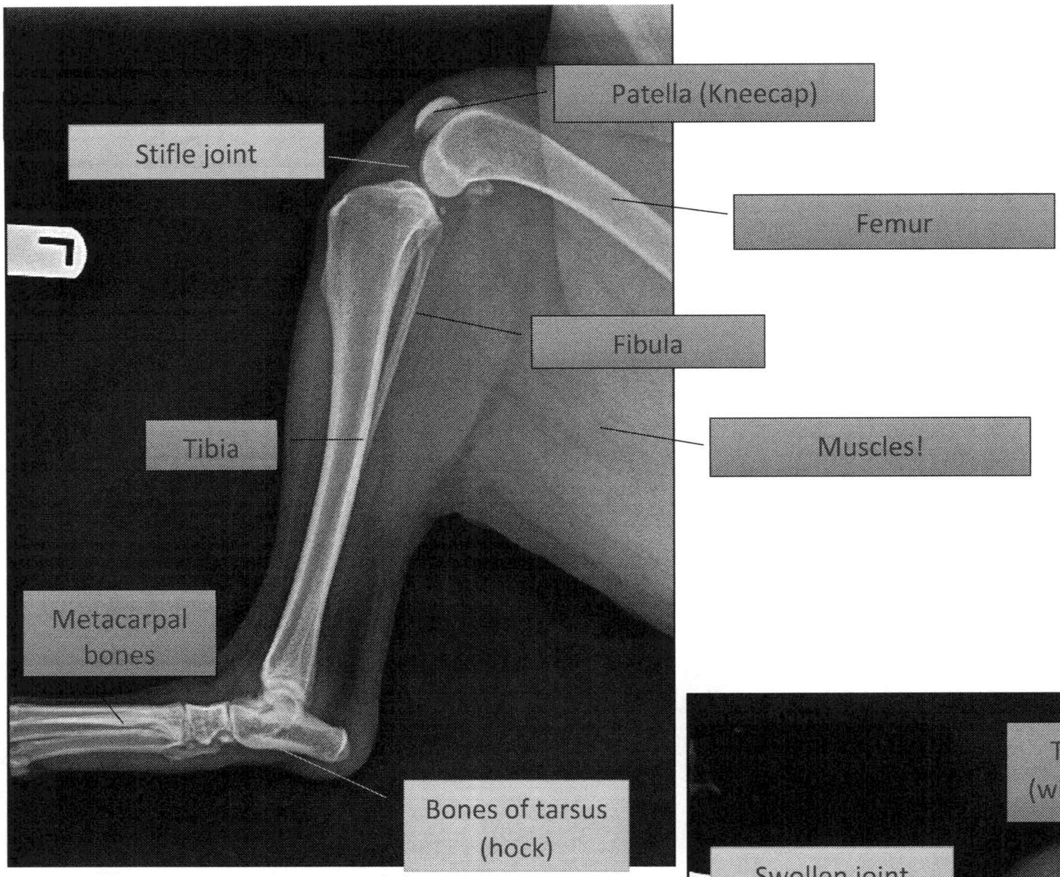
Patella (Kneecap)
Stifle joint
Femur
Fibula
Tibia
Muscles!
Metacarpal bones
Bones of tarsus (hock)

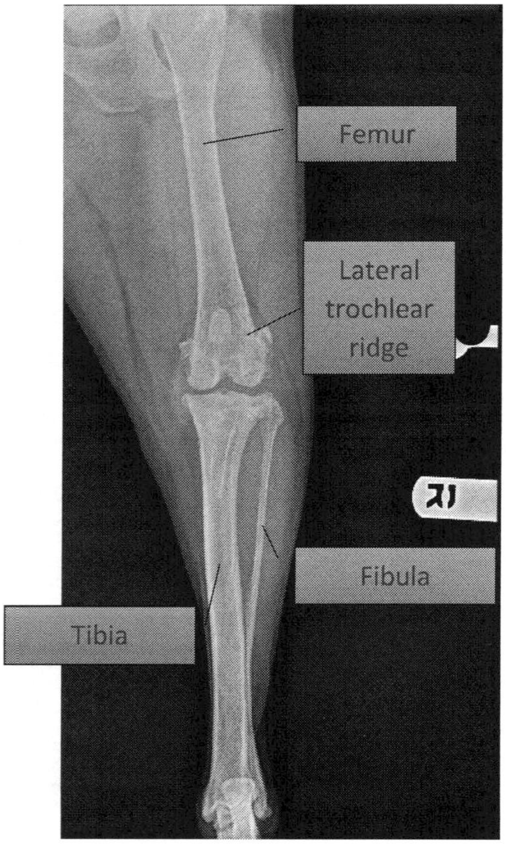
Femur
Lateral trochlear ridge
Fibula
Tibia

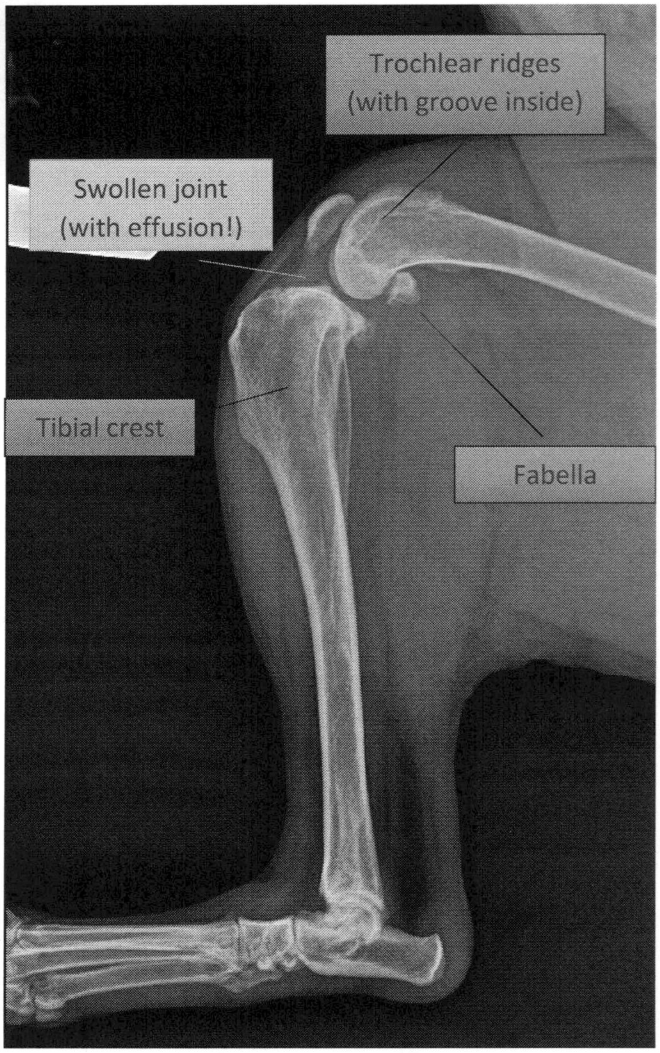
Trochlear ridges (with groove inside)
Swollen joint (with effusion!)
Tibial crest
Fabella

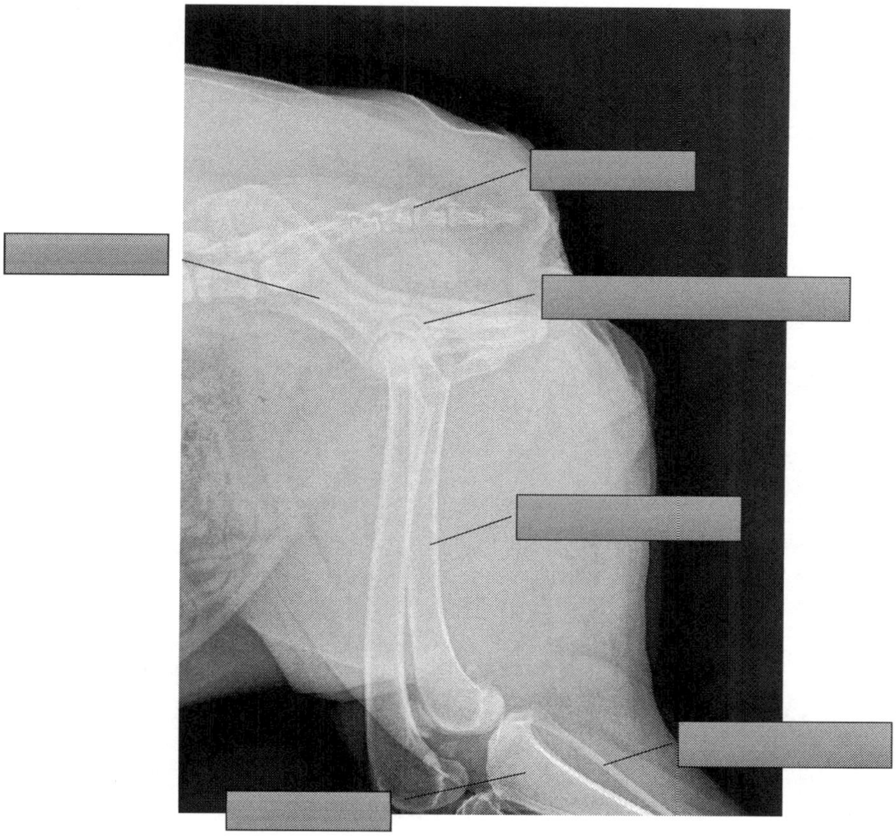

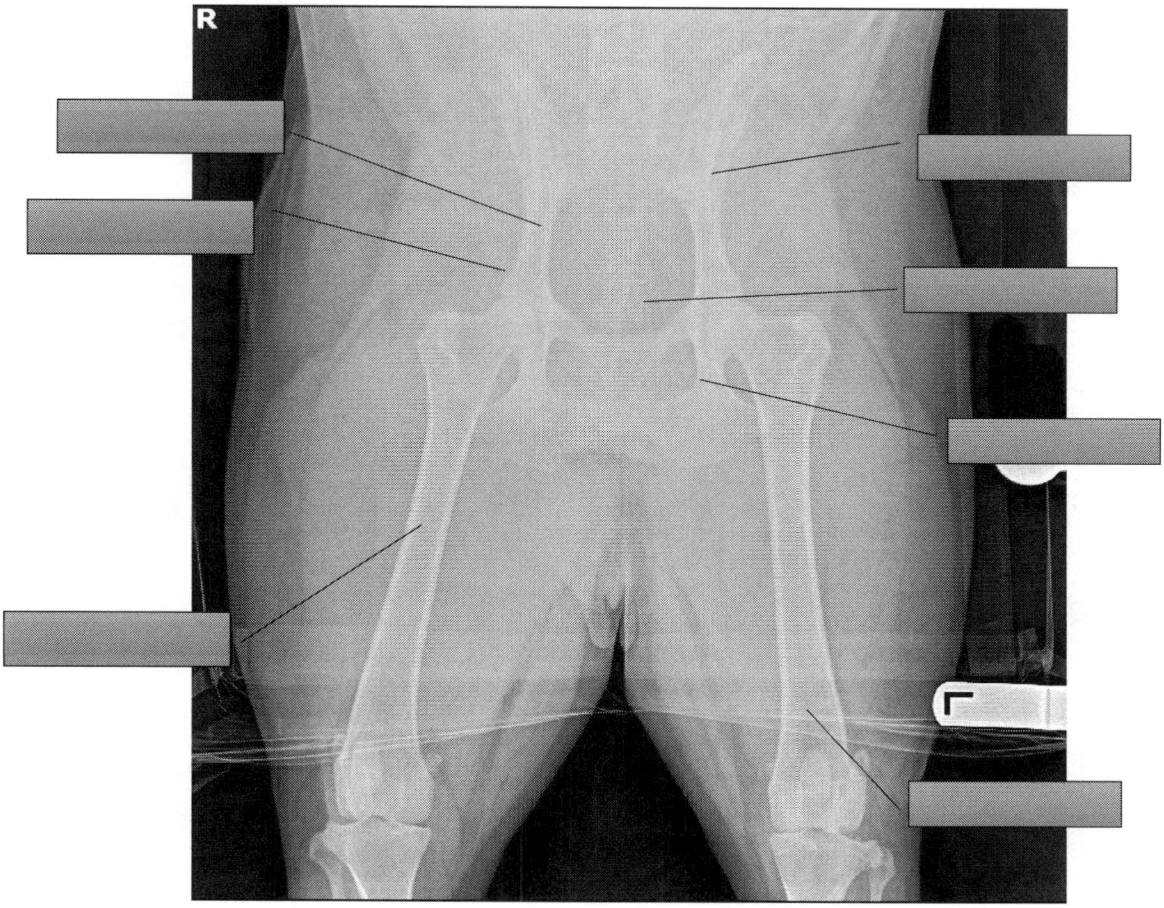
R

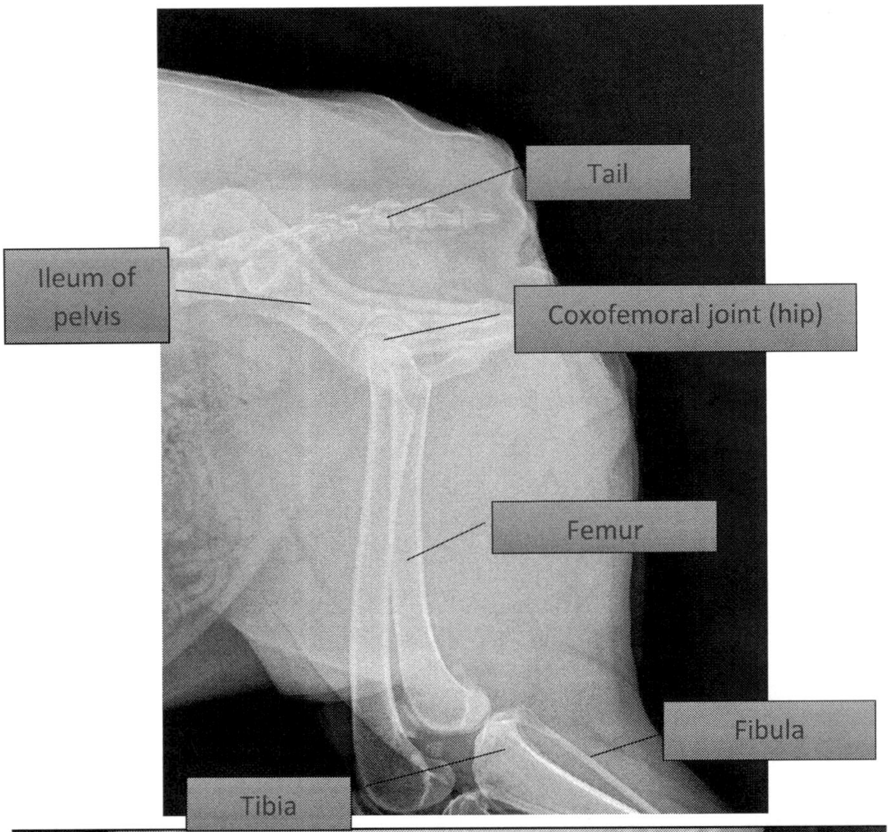
Tail
Ileum of pelvis
Coxofemoral joint (hip)
Femur
Fibula
Tibia

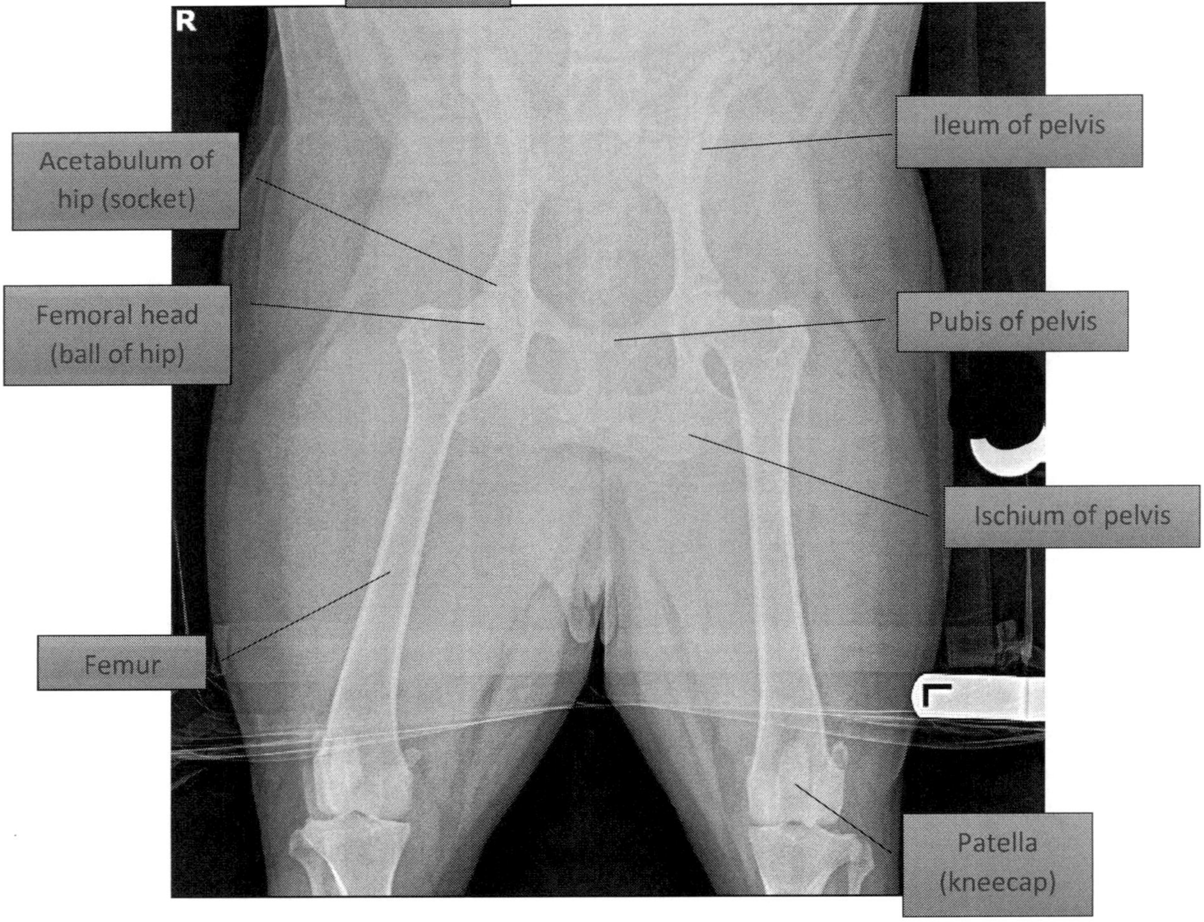
R
Ileum of pelvis
Acetabulum of hip (socket)
Femoral head (ball of hip)
Pubis of pelvis
Ischium of pelvis
Femur
Patella (kneecap)

Wonderful! You've identified lots of spots on Spot's anatomy. Pay close attention to the stifles (the joint between the femur and tibia) and hips (the joint between the femoral head and pelvis), since that's where he was painful during your exam. Did you see any fractures or luxation (a popped joint)?

I did see one thing that was abnormal, among that forest of text boxes.

Did you catch it? What's your diagnosis here?

What is your diagnosis?

____

STOP!!!!!

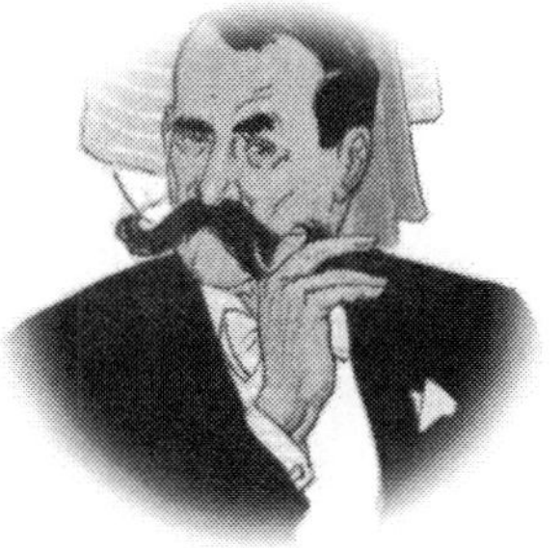

"You should employ your little grey cells."

—Hercule Poirot in *The Murder of Roger Ackroyd*[xxii]

That's right! This dog has a **soft tissue injury** (a sprain).

You figured this out mostly by ruling out fractures and luxation (there aren't any on the radiographs), by clues on your physical exam, and by one more thing: joint effusion! In this patient's right knee (stifle) you can see increased amounts of fluid in the joint compared to the left knee (most easily seen on the right lateral view). That's what effusion is: more fluid than there should be.

And what might cause more fluid inside a joint? Several things could. But the most common is an injury to a ligament (a little something we call a sprain). You start to do a happy dance, then remember that Spot's people are freaking out and convinced he has a broken leg. They might not find a happy dance appropriate. At least not yet…

"Well guys," you beam a smile you hope is disarming, "you can now do a happy dance, becauuuuuse there is no fracture! Spot does not have a broken leg."

Linda casts a skeptical look toward Gary. Somehow it infects his face, and they both turn skeptical looks toward you. Fortunately, you've come armed with a tablet to show them Spot's X-rays. You explain everything, and their skepticism gives way to belief so quickly it probably made Santa envious.

"We believe now!" Linda gasps.

"We do!" Gary chortles (while doing a happy dance). "We believe the doctor!"

Well, maybe it wasn't quite like that… But it was close. Good work! You've diagnosed the problem, and convinced the owners you are smart. Specifically, you suspect this to be a **cranial cruciate ligament injury**. There are two cruciate ligaments that hold the knee together like little crisscrossing ropes in the center. In dogs the knee joint is at an angle, and strain over years can cause chronic microtears in the ligament (especially the cranial cruciate ligament) which makes it prone to snapping or (more commonly) partially snapping. This makes the knee joint all loose (which we feel as cranial drawer motion during an exam). You stop to confirm cranial drawer motion when this guy's sedate too (it's easier to feel then). And joint laxity (looseness) can damage the meniscus (a flat ligament over the surface of the knee joint) and hurt the dog even more.

Now how do you treat it?

Chose from the options below:

a) Amputation
b) Anti-inflammatory medication
c) Cast
d) Lidocaine to slow the heart rate
e) Nausea medication
f) Pain medication
g) Physical therapy
h) Rest
i) Rub some dirt on it
j) Surgery

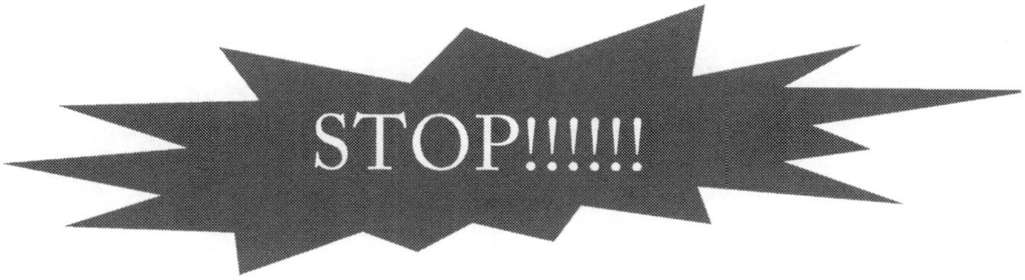

Pick some treatments before you turn the page...

"Look here, if it's all the same to you
I'll continue the melodrama!"
— Margery Allingham's detective Albert Campion[xxiii]

I would pick: **b, f, and h** and see if the owners would consider **j**.

This is not a fracture, so we don't need to cast it or repair it with a plate or wires or anything. There is a lot of inflammation inside the joint around the torn tendon, so **an anti-inflammatory** (usually an NSAID) is helpful. **Pain medication** will help as well. **Strict rest** is important to prevent injuring the knee further now that it's all loosey-goosey.

I wouldn't give lidocaine to this patient. (Trick question! Trick question!) The fast heart rate you noticed was due to pain, so pain medication and rest are the main ways to help.

There are surgeries that can help fix this. In fact, it is considered by most vets to be primarily a surgical problem, so **surgery** is important to consider. There have been several types of surgeries developed to help stabilize the knee. A TPLO (tibial plateau leveling osteotomy) is the most common today. Usually this will be performed by a special board-certified surgeon (not a general practice vet like you). You recommend surgery, and Spot's humans are interested enough to send in a referral form to a local surgeon. Spot goes home on some medications, and you finish up your notes.

Next you suture up a few lacerations on a critter that got into a fight at the dog park (or as we ER vets call it, "Canine Fight Club"). A cat with an ear infection comes in afterward. You always find it surprising when people bring you simple things like ear infections at 2 am. But it's easy enough to treat, and you quote them your motto "Happy to help!" with exhausted cheeriness.[14] Then you slink into the office for a couple of hours rest. Dawn pokes up her rosy cheeks upon a sprinkling of snow.

Fred pulls you aside just after Harlow leaves. The look of concern on his face brings a weary frown to yours. "How much methadone did we use on Spot?" he asks. You tell him the amount and he nods, staring at the log book in his hands. "That's what the computer said. Doesn't quite match the log, though. If you see Dr. Short before I do, let her know, will ya?"

You promise to do so, wondering how much you should be worried. But right now, you're too tired to worry, and bid farewell with an overall feeling of pride in a job well done. You've helped save a blocked tom-cat, calmed some panic, relieved some pain, fixed some wounds, and treated an infection. You're not such a bad doctor after all! Sometimes the ER is a lighthouse mirror that makes your healer's skill shine.

"I want to be a healer, and love all things that grow..."

—J. R. R. Tolkien, *The Return of the King*[xxiii]

[14] You don't quote your other motto: "Meh, it's good enough for the ER!" Clients don't seem to appreciate that one.

Drab blankets of clouds cover the normally clear New Mexico skies when you wake up from a dead sleep in the afternoon. You stumble around for a few minutes, wondering what year it is and who exactly you are, before your befuddled brain rights itself enough to remember you need to get ready for another ER shift. A chilly breeze meets you as you walk to the car, and you ponder how very unnatural the weather looks in the normally cheery setting of the high desert.

Doug waves at you in the parking lot as you pull into the ramshackle overnight clinic. You nod briefly but try to rush past without engaging him. Fred and Lemon greet you with a smile and chit-chat ensues until the first case of the night walks into the door.

Three grown men carry a 50-pound dog. You notice something odd about this dog: his head is stuck through the rim of a tire. Not the rubber bit, mind you, but the big heavy, metal rim that goes inside. Two of the guys are carrying the rim, while one carries the hound.[15]

"Um..." is all you can think to say.

"How can we help you?" Fred says, managing not to raise his eyebrows.

"Our dog was chasing a cat and got his head stuck in this tire rim. We can't get him out."

"Um..." is still all you can think to say.

A little while later, you've sedated the dog and applied about three bottles of sterile lube to his neck. This was Fred's suggestion, and it sounded like the best course of action. Never be too proud to accept good suggestions from your staff!

You gently push, while Fred and Lemon roughly tug, and the three other guys hold the tire rim. At one point you put pressure on the eyeballs of this patient, which start to bulge forward terrifyingly with the pressure. But fortunately, both eyes stay in place, and the shaggy head finally pops through the hole in the tire rim. A careful exam of the hound's skin doesn't reveal any laceration, and he recovers fine from sedation and walks out the clinic.

The three dudes wave happily as they roll their tire rim out the door.

"Well, that's something they never told me about in vet school!" you comment. Lemon and Fred laugh. "I nearly threw up when I had to hold his eyes in place!" you say. Even vets have a right to feel grossed out. "Eyes are useful, but they feel disgusting. Guess that's why ophtho cases are my least favorite..."

---

[15] Just so you know, this is a real case I once saw at an ER! And just to prove that real life is often stranger than fiction, the next week another case came in with a dog whose paw was stuck in a bathtub drain. The fire department had been called, and a couple of burly firemen accompanied the patient (who still had a piece of pipe and drain attached to him which they'd cut off with a blow torch). Whatever else it may be, the ER is certainly a house of surprises.

Uh oh! You said it.

The Universe took it as a challenge…

Ding dong! The bell rings and Fred opens the door.

Case #11

A cat stares at you from the threshold in his owner's arms. It stares with its right eye, because the left eye is hanging out of the socket.

"My cat's got something wrong with his eye," the man comments dryly.

"Urp!" you tell Fred and Lemon you'll just be in the back looking a few things up while they check this patient in.

A few minutes later you've settled your stomach and steeled your nerves, and Fred comes in to give you the history on your new patient.

"Mr. Tafoya is an elder in one of the local Pueblo tribes. He got back from a tribal function today and found his cat Náshdóitsoh outside with her eye popped out. He doesn't know what happened to her. She was inside the living room in the morning, so he thinks it couldn't have been more than a few hours ago that she got hurt. She's a fancy Persian kitty that they originally meant to keep inside (on a pile of silk cushions, eating imported tuna from a gold bowl… You know the type). But she had other ideas and runs out the door a few times a week. She's fully vaccinated and not on any medications. They haven't noted any coughing, sneezing, vomiting, or diarrhea. And that's pretty much all I've got. Passing the ball do you, Doc. Run it across the, er…yard line!" He looks a bit embarrassed and shakes his head. "It that right? I don't know football really."

"Sounds right to me," you shrug and march off to the exam room.

"Miguel Tafoya," your new client introduces politely as you enter the room. His hand trembles slightly as you shake it, and he seems unnerved: probably because his cat's eye is hanging out.

You look at the pancake-snouted, mutant felid snuffling in his arms and resist the urge to say, "Who smashed your cat's face?" or "Your cat's noseless! Does the breeder do partial refunds?" Instead, you just mutter "Poor kitty!" and pat her on the back (trying not to look at the bloody eye bulging out of her left socket.)

"I saw Náshdóitsoh's eye and rushed her right in." He confirms the story Fred told, and doesn't really have any more details. You ask what her name means, trying to make conversation as Lemon takes the patient and you start your exam.

"It means mountain lion," Miguel grins, obviously aware of the humor in naming a fluffy, posh, smashed-nosed purebred such a fierce name. It lightens the mood as you continue with your exam.

Step 1 – Organize the History

Signalment:

9 years old

Female spayed

Persian cat

Presenting Complaints:

Proposed eye (eye popped out)

Step 2 – Gather Clues

Physical Examination:

Abdominal palpation: No significant findings (pliable on palpation, no distension or fluid wave noted, no obvious organomegally or masses noted).

Attitude: strangely calm and a little dull. If you had that eye you'd be completely freaking out. (Of course, if you had that face you'd be freaking out as well…even if your eye was fine.)

Cardiac: No murmur or arrhythmia noted. Palpable femoral pulse noted.

Ears: Canals appear clear of debris and no swelling noted.

Eyes: OS (left eye)- proptosis, with entrapment of the eyelids behind the globe. Episcleral injection with conjunctival edema noted. Dried appearance to the cornea noted with hyphema in the anterior chamber. Extraocular muscles are visible on three sides of the globe.[16]

Integument: Small laceration (~ 2 cm long) into the subcutaneous tissue noted on the back of the head, with some bruising around it. Otherwise no significant wounds noted.

Anterior chamber: the space between the cornea and the lens. The space behind the lens is called the posterior chamber.
Cornea: the clear front part of the eye, where the light first goes in.
Episcleral: connective tissue behind the sclera (white part of the eye). Scleral injection is redness to the sclera from inflammation.
Extraocular muscles: the little muscles controlling movement of the eye. They are smushed between the socket and attached along all four sides of the globe. In a cat there are seven of them.
Globe: the round bit of the eye, which we think of as the "eyeball."
Proptosis: a word for the eye being popped out of its socket.

[16] This is not a reference to Shakespeare's famous theater… At least, I don't think it is. Maybe hundreds of years ago an anatomist saw a play at the Globe, realized what a good use of his eyes it was, and named them globes? But it doesn't seem likely.

Lymph Nodes: No significant findings.

Musculoskeletal: No significant findings. The patient bears weight on all four limbs, and flexion and extension of joints is normal.

Neurologic: Dull but responsive. No visual tracking or menace response in the left eye (but both seem intact in the right eye). Pupillary light reflex (PLR) is absent in the left eye, but present in the right. Conscious proprioception is within normal limits in all four paws.

Oronasal: Slight epistaxis (bloody nose) front left nares. Narrowed nostrils (consistent with Persians). Teeth appear clean with no obvious trauma noted to jaw (no visible fractures, moves up and down fine).

Respiratory: No increased respiratory effort noted. A soft stertor is heard occasionally (consistent with the breed).

Urogenital: no significant findings.

Vitals: WNL

"Urp…" you repeat.

You reluctantly admit that, even though eye cases are gross, ophthalmologists have pretty much the coolest names for anything on the planet. You get to type lots of big, big words (some almost as big as Pueblo words) when you do notes on eye cases. Well, you've done the exam, now list your differentials. Take careful stock of all the things you've seen in this patient, and list the reasons his eye might look the way it does.

Before you turn the page that way, write each differential possibili-tay…

"If you were asked to prove that two and two made four, you might find some difficulty, and yet you are quite sure of the fact."

—Sherlock Holmes in *A Study in Scarlet*[xxv]

Stertor: a "snorty" congested sound when breathing.

Subcutaneous tissue: the fatty layer of tissue under the skin.

Did you feel a little silly making a differential list for a problem that was so obvious (bulging right out at you, so to speak)? Thinking through the possibilities can seem that way. Obviously this cat must have had some kind of trauma, right?

But one good reason for training yourself to stop and mentally list all the possibilities you can think of every time is that it will help you catch important problems you might miss otherwise.

Differential Diagnoses:

- Abscess
- Fungal granuloma
- Hematoma
- Neoplasia
- Trauma
    - Animal attack (dog, wild beast, etc.)
    - "High-rise syndrome" (i.e. falling off a house)
    - Hit by car
    - Kicked (or other form of deliberate trauma)

All the differentials outside of trauma are going to be "retrobulbar" problems. This is a fancy word for "something behind the eyeball." If this old cat had an infection or a tumor growing behind the eyeball, it could cause exophthalmos that predisposed him to proptosis. Of course, there is a more obvious problem in Náshdóitsoh that predisposes him to proptosis. Can you see what it is?

Why is this patient more prone to proptosis (eye popping out)?

____

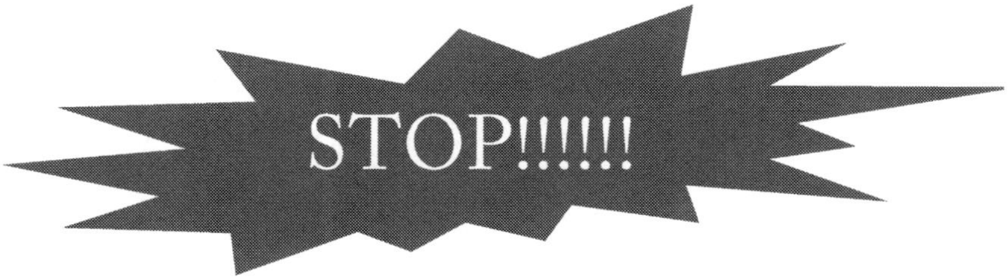

Exophthalmos: a big, ophthalmology word for "eyeball is bulging forward."
Retrobulbar: a fancy word for something behind the eyeball.

Some Animal Eye Emergencies

When you see these signs inside your pet, take them in to see the vet!

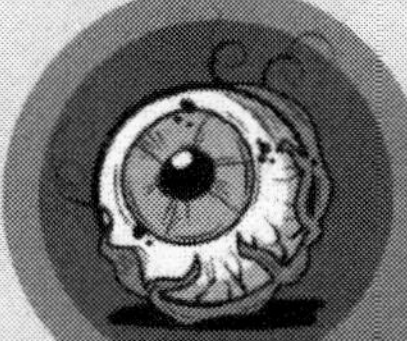

Globe (the round "eyeball" itself)

Traumatic proptosis ("popped" out of socket) is a true emergency. Sometimes the globe can be replaced, but it often needs to be removed (enucleated).

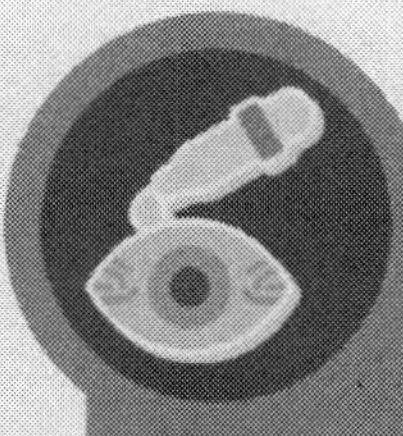

Cornea (the clear surface of the eye)

Lacerations or ulcers can be series emergencies (especially deep or penetrating ones, or those near the sclera). "Melting" ulcers, with infection deepening them can be very serious as well.

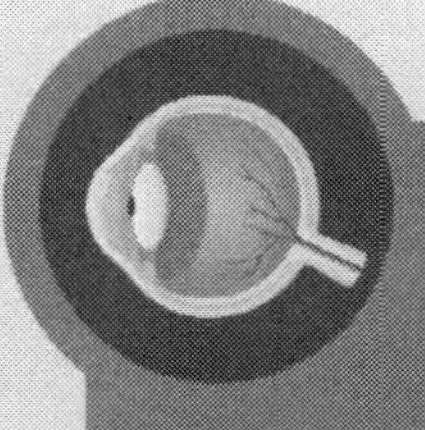

Glaucoma (increased pressure in the eye)

If the balance of fluid (aqueous humor) production and drainage is disrupted, pressure builds up in the eye. This can be primary or secondary and can be severe enough to need enucleation.

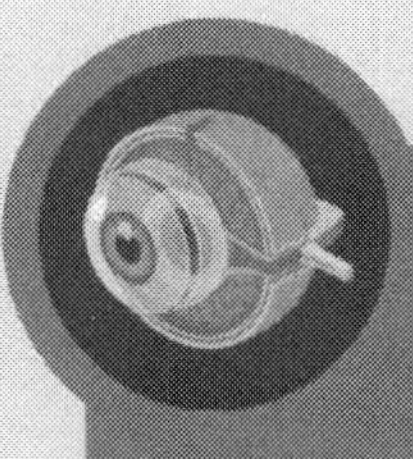

Anterior Chamber (space in the front of the eye)

Uveitis(anterior chamber inflammation) causes flare, visible floating material. It is can be a sign of serious systemic diseases. Hyphema (blood in this space) is a sign of severe inflammation or trauma.

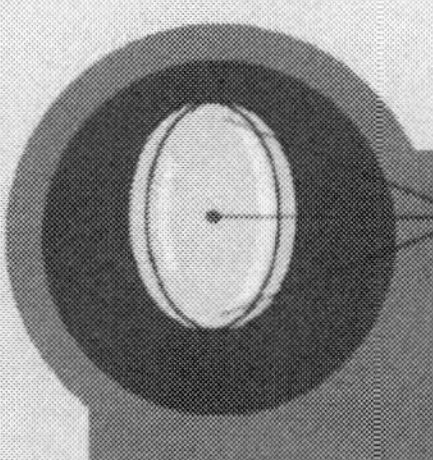

Others

Lens luxation is sometimes seen and can lead to problems like glaucoma or uveitis. Sudden blindness can result from genetic disease, systemic infections, toxins, or high blood pressure (which affects the vessels of the fungus, at the back of the eye).

This guy is a **brachycephalic cat breed (a Persian).**

Brachycephalic breeds have smashed-in faces and wide skulls. They also have orbits that cover less globe (a shallow eye socket), physiologic exophthalmos (bulgy, bulgy eye bulbs), macropalpebral fissures (gaps from wider than normal eyelids).

Told you ophthalmologists have good words! They're just fun to say. Set this book down and go tell your best friend "macropalpbral fissure" a few times. You'll be glad you did. Anyway, this constellation of eyeball mutation is something vets have turned BOS (brachycephalic ocular syndrome) in Persian and Himalayan cat breeds. And it's not really a good combination of problems to have for patients who like to keep their eyes inside their heads.

But, as you probably guessed, trauma is the most likely differential (or more immediate cause) of this cat's proptosis. What kind of trauma? He ain't tellin'. It's because of that very problem (your patients don't speak human) that veterinarians must channel their inner detective to think their way to the most likely solutions. So put on your Holmes hat and look over this cat's exam again.

There is an epistaxis (nosebleed) which can be a sign of blunt trauma. He also has a laceration on the back of his head. Some wild animals (like cats, ironically) like to pop their prey in the back of the head. It would need to be a larger animal to cause enough force to pop this guy's eye out. The cut looks suspicious of the sorts of tears you see from a canine tooth. Something you don't see is broken bones, extensive bruises, or seizures and neuro signs you'd relate to really severe trauma (like being hit by a car or purposefully kicked). The most likely trauma is from a dog attack. He was outside, after all. But it is a guess.

What is not a guess is that this guy has sustained some significant head trauma. You'll take that into consideration when recommending a plan.

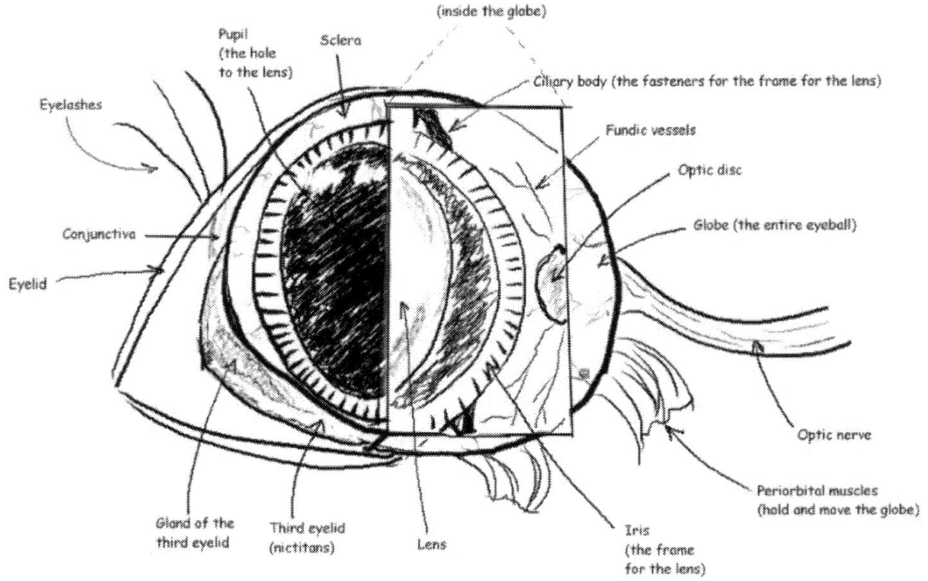

Decision time!

What tests do you want to run first?

Here's what you can do in your clinic:

- ✓ Basic bloodwork (a chemistry panel and CBC)
- ✓ Benchtop Ethylene glycol test
- ✓ Blood gas analysis
- ✓ Clotting times
- ✓ Cytology
- ✓ Fecal floatation and direct saline exam
- ✓ FeLV/FIV test
- ✓ Giardia test
- ✓ Heartworm test (with rickettsial diseases)
- ✓ Leptospirosis test
- ✓ Pancreatic lipase
- ✓ Parvo test
- ✓ Pregnancy test
- ✓ Radiographs (X-rays)
- ✓ Skin scraping
- ✓ Thyroid hormone level (T4)
- ✓ Ultrasound
- ✓ Urinalysis

What tests do you want to run?

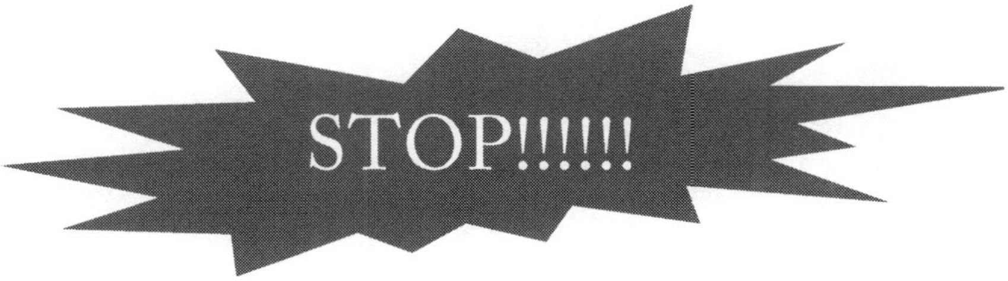

I'd probably pick **radiographs.** It would be helpful to know if there are skull (or other) fractures associated with this head trauma. You could also consider some **bloodwork** and an **ultrasound** (probably AFAST and TFAST) to assess internal trauma. Your client politely hears your diagnostic recommendations and then declines them all. You've learned to recommend the best, but work with less.

"My wife wanted this mountain lion. It cost a lot of money. Now I have to spend wisely. What will treatment cost?" Miguel Tafoya is a smart man.

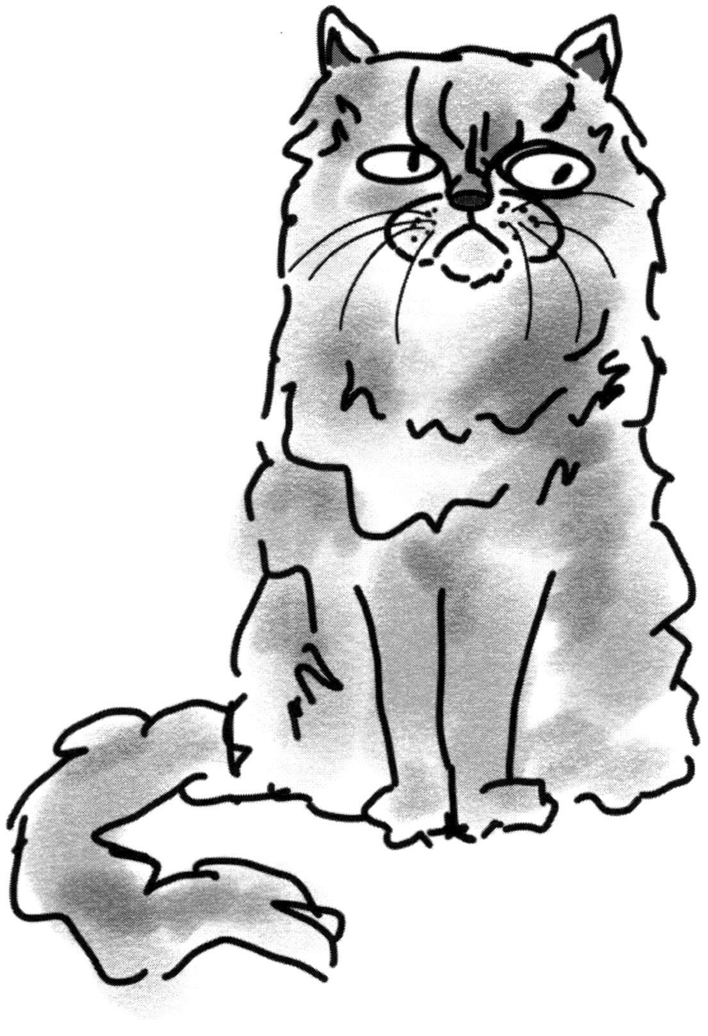

Choose some from this eye-popping list of treatment options.

What is your treatment plan? (pick several)

a) Antibiotics
b) Anti-inflammatory medications
c) Atropine eye ointment
d) Diphenhydramine
e) Have him tell you what letters he can see on a vision chart
f) Inject a steroid into the eye
g) IV fluids
h) Pain medications
i) Pop that eye back in
j) Subcutaneous fluids
k) Suction fluid out of the eye to relieve pressure
l) Take that eye right out
m) Wound repair

STOP!!!!!!

"It is hard to fail, but it is worse never to have tried to succeed."
— Theodore Roosevelt[xxvi]

C'mon, give it a try! Work those brain cells and pick some treatments!

You have two choices: **h and g, with either i or l.**

The most immediate treatment to perform at this point is **pain medications**. It's amazing how calm an animal acts when their eyeball is popped out, but you'd expect this to hurt like (and possibly a bit more than) the dickens! You plan to put him under general anesthesia with some **IV fluids** as you prep for surgery. There's an eyeball hanging out, and you're gonna need to **either put it back in or take it out the rest of the way**. Which is best? Well, that depends on a lot of factors.

Replacing the eye: Sadly, studies and expedience have shown that the chance of a cat healing from replacing the eye is very, very low. That may be because it takes more force to cause proptosis and more damage to the eye is sustained. Signs like exposure of more than two extraocular muscles, blindness, damage to the cornea (like severe drying or rupture) are clues that this eye is not going to be functional if you put it back. A big part of the challenge in replacing a proptosed eye into the globe is that the adnexa (all the tissue behind the eye) is swollen and damaged. If I am going to replace the globe, I will usually give an anti-inflammatory (steroid) as well to help reduce swelling. Then the patient has to go under anesthesia. You follow procedure to put the eye back in, then suture the eyelids over it. After two weeks, you remove the sutures and hope the eye stays in and functions. If not, it still needs to be removed with a second surgery.

Removing the eye: In the case of this cat, the eye is very far out of the socket, with three extraocular muscles showing. It's dried up (probably bad corneal damage) and not visual. You recommend enucleation (removal). It is better for Náshdóitsoh to get that broken eyeball out. The surgical procedure involves a full circle incision through the limbus (where the cornea and sclera meet), then dissection down through the conjunciva to sever the optic nerve and remove the eye. Then you'll cut of the edges of the eyelids and suture them together to make Náshdóitsoh a permanent pirate-lion.

Something likely hit this kitty in the head. And there is one organ that sits in a cat's head, and is pretty darn important for living, which you haven't considered yet. That's right! Mrs. Brain! You should consider the possibility of concussion, or traumatic brain injury (TBI). Náshdóitsoh is dull (meaning he's confused and lethargic) on your exam, which could be a sign of early or mild TBI. Bain trauma can be primary (i.e. damage to the tissue directly) or secondary (i.e. damage from the swelling, impaired blood flow, inflammation, and energy depletion associated with it).

There's not a lot we can do about primary damage to the brain, so we focus treatment of TBI on secondary effects of trauma by improving blood flow to the brain, treating low blood pressure, and trying to prevent high intracranial pressure (that can occur with things like inflammation and swelling). IV fluids are the most basic way to improve blood flow and treat low blood pressure.

You can consider drugs like mannitol or hypertonic saline, which are special fluids that reduce swelling in in tissue by attracting fluid to them. But that way lies danger! One study found intracranial bleeding in 96% of head trauma in dogs and cats. Bleeding involves blood leaking out of the vessels into the surrounding tissue in the brain. And if we give mannitol or hypertonic saline, where would some of it end up? That's right! Into the brain tissue with leaky blood. And fluid follows it. So, you could make swelling in the brain a lot worse with mannitol or hypertonic saline if there is significant bleeding. And if that's not enough, you can damage the lungs and the kidneys with those medications. Even so, most experts still say to risk mannitol if trauma is bad. In this specific case, it's probably not bad enough, and you'll stick to IV fluids, monitoring, and maybe some oxygen.

Mr. Tafoya approves enucleation and leaves for the night. You get busy and soon have his pet asleep on the surgery table. About 15 minutes later you hold a cat's eyeball in your hands. You resist the urge to say, "Congratulations, Fred, our patient has given birth to a healthy eyeball!" Instead, you clamp and ligate a bleeding vessel near the optic nerve.

"Er… We've got some gelfoam," Fred suggests, looking over your shoulder.

"Sure! Just a sec. Let me finish lighting this optic nerve and blood vessel," you say.

"OK, but I've heard that…"

"There we go! All done. Please pass the gelfoam."

Fred sighs and passes some sterile, dissolving foam that you pack into the socket before closing everything up. This will help control the bleeding inside while Náshdóitsoh heals. "Here, catch!"

You toss the eyeball to Lemon as she walks by. A normal young lady would be disgusted. But very few normal people work at the ER. She grins and says she's gonna get a formalin jar to keep it in. Very often the ER is a sanctuary for the world's most morbid comedians.

Fred takes the patient into Treatment. You hear footsteps behind you, and it suddenly dawns on you that there wasn't a fourth person in this clinic last you checked. Is this another visit from the clinic ghost? You turn in a panic, and let out a relieved gasp when you find Dr. Celia Short standing in the pharmacy.

"Hey," she half-smiles beneath heavy eyelids. "I came in to do some more admin work and heard surgery."

"Heya, Doctor Short! Burning that admin candle late, aren't you!"

"If anyone ever asks you to manage clinic, tell them to jump off a cliff."

"Oh, uh… Haha! Wise words," you fumble at her intensity.

She asks about surgery and you chat about Náshdóitsoh. "It's only my second enucleation, so I was a bit nervous. I forgot how much blood is in the socket. Had to ligate a big vessel along with the optic nerve."

She frowns. "You're not really supposed to do that, you know."

"Huh? Do what?"

"Ligating the optic nerve bundle… You can create traction across the optic chiasm and make the cat's other eye blind."

Your heart plummets into your shoes. "Uh, I…er… Ooooh…"

Dr. Short shrugs. "Too late now. You'll just have to wait and see if the cat goes blind or not." She rubs her shoulder and winces. "Arg. More cramps. I'm headed to the office. Have a good night."

You feel like the one with brain trauma as your mind insists on mulling over your surgical mistake again and again. You hang your head and drag yourself to the doctor's office feeling ashamed and worried. She's right. This is something you can't undo. You're just gonna have to wait it out. Which means you'll probably spend Christmas worrying.

"Told you so!" the little voice inside your head keeps singing (it's possible the fact he's singing is a sign you've been watching way too much Starship Beethoven).

"Been sayin' it since you started this gig.

ER med's for experts.

Your brain just ain't that big!"

Nobody else comes in, which means you have nothing but your own thoughts all night long as you sit alone in your back office. Well, maybe not alone. There is a clinic ghost back here too… You step out four or five times during the night and check on Náshdóitsoh. He seems able to see you but also seems really annoyed. Eventually you just sit and stare at the wall, wondering what other emergency might come in that you can mess up. And yet, despite beating yourself up, Náshdóitsoh can still see in the morning. His swelling from surgery is much better and he seems comfortable.

"Thank you, Doc!" Mr. Tafoya says when he picks his cat up. "You do good work here and Náshdóitsoh says he appreciates it."

Náshdóitsoh winks at you. You suspect he's still mad about you waking him up all night though.

Your client hands you a beautiful turquoise bracelet. "A gift for you. Merry Christmas and thanks again."

Tears glisten in your eyes, and you feel like wailing. Instead, you just say, "Thanks so much!"

Optic chiasm: a crisscross of the two optic nerves (one from each eye) inside the brain. Because they cross, tugging on one optic nerve can damage the other one.

Fitful sleep overtakes you after an hour or two of puttering around the house that morning. You wake up to the dazed feeling you're getting more used to. The phone woke you up this time, buzzing over your nightstand.

"Hey, it's Carley," says Carley, your friend fostering Samuel. "Sam's school called and he's feeling bad. Mac and I are unable to leave work. Is there any chance you could pick him up?"

You glance at the clock. There's still time before your shift and you tell her you'll help. Better be ready to go to work afterward though. You slip on your scrubs and pick up your pack (which you keep loaded up to bring on shift) and step outside. Snowflakes drift down from a gray sky, dancing in a chill breeze in a Christmas Eve greeting. You like snow and admire the thin blanket of white covering the desert cactus and sage under a thick layer of clouds. Everything seems so quiet.

Sam was feeling dizzy at school, and you take him right to his doctor. Everything checks out, and the doctor says it's probably just a side effect of his medication.

"Am I ever going to get better?" the little guy asks from the back seat.

You feel tired, and not ready to answer hard questions. But life doesn't wait for you to be ready. "Hey, Bud! Don't be sad. Your new medicine is really helping so far, and I'm sure you'll feel better soon. Carley is heading back from work, and she'll keep an eye on you this afternoon."

He sighs, feeling as bleak as the weather. "It's Christmas Eve. I wish you could hang out with us tonight. We're gonna put out the luminarias."

"Yeah. Me too. But I scheduled a shift tonight a while ago. ER doctors have to work a lot of holidays. At least I'll be there tomorrow!" You hope you'll be awake enough to be mentally there.

He sighs again. "Dad said he'd call on Christmas Eve, but he hasn't yet."

"Oh man, Sam. I'm sorry. There's still time…" But there's not a lot you can do. So you drop your little friend off with Carley and Mac and head to your next shift.

The bleak weather matches your mood as you try not to worry about Samuel. You also try not to worry about Náshdóitsoh and try not to worry about whatever cases might come in tonight. Maybe some music will help. You flip on the radio.

It's all Christmas songs. Songs filled with cheeriness and being-home-with-family that just make you feel sadder… You dangerously tap on your phone to open a playlist of Starship Beethoven music instead.[17]

"Ooooooh! Ooooooooh!

Our hearts are soft like goo.

[17] Tapping and driving is the new drinking and driving, by the way. Don't do this!!!!

From Quasar-3
aboard the B,
We wish good cheer to you!

"Warp factor 1! Warp factor 1!
This peaceful day has just begun.
A day without indifference,
We silence all the dissonance,
And look up to the Sun.

"Ooooh! Oooooh!
Before this song is through,
Peace and good cheer
Will meet us here,
We wish it all on you.

"Warp factor 1! Warp factor 1!
Today a better day's begun
A day without indifference,
We silence all the dissonance,
And look up to the sun."

You find yourself tearing up again and tap the skip button. It had to be "Warp factor 1…"

You glance down at the turquoise bracelet on your wrist, and a crack forms in the ice that seems so determined to coat your heart. The ER might bring you a string of cases from the mouth of hell itself tonight. You might feel so far out of your depth that you'll wish you'd brought scuba gear. But you are still going into that ER, and you're going to do your best to help people and their pets! Maybe you won't do as good a job as a TV emergency vet trained at Purdue who's got 30 years of experience. But you will do your best. And you'll be there when people and their pets need help. And that will be more than good enough. It's a new shift, a Christmas Eve shift with golden hope of being better than yesterday…

Case #12

Graham's grin and Lemon's look *and* Fred's felicitations (along with his goofy Santa hat) greet you when you walk into the lobby. "Hey, Doc! Happy Christmas Eve!" You'd forgotten that on special shifts like holidays, there's sometimes extra hands scheduled. Gearing up for a busy night…

You greet them back. They point out that a client left cookies, and you make a cup of coffee to go with one as you settle into your office.

Everything seems so still. Weirdly still.

Suddenly, nothing happens…

Then more nothing happens…

Nothing happens so much, in fact, that you fall asleep at your desk. You wake up sometime during the night, stuck to the desk in a glob of your own drool.

"Huh? Wha? Who? Why? When?" you eloquently utter.

SHHHHP! Thump! Thump! Thump!

That sounds familiar. A cold shiver runs down your spine. It's Christmas Eve… Traditional walk about time for ghosts.

"F-F-Fred? Lemon? Graham?!?!" You whisper, as you tiptoe across the room toward the door into Dr. Short's office. The sounds seem to be coming from inside.

SSSSSSSHP! Clunk!

You gulp down your fear and open the door. Suddenly, nothing happens all over again.

Everything seems dark and quiet and still. You flip on the light. Nothing moving… No more sounds. You notice a faint chill in the air, and find that the door to the backyard is cracked open.

"That's odd…" you mutter. "You been playing crochet outside, ghost?"

You open the door and step outside. The moon is out and casts a silver glow over the snow-dusted junk and scraggly bushes that fill the ugly back yard of Owlhoot Veterinary Emergency Clinic. Everything is still. No ghost in sight.

That bundle of clothes lying beside the cement slab near the door seems new. Or is it only clothes…?

You stoop down to look, then straighten up with a scream. A pale face stares lifelessly from the bundle. It's a face you recognize. Doctor Debbie Crimshaw lies dead on the cold ground.

A few minutes later all three of your technicians come running.

"What's up doc?" Fred asks in a funny voice, with highly inappropriate levity. To be fair, he has no idea you've just found a dead body at the back door.

"D-d-d-d-dead…G-ghost… Bluuuuh!" You can't get the words out.

"Oh man!" Lemon notices the body and stoops down to check for a pulse. Oh yeah. That would have been a good idea.

"I think we should call the police," Fred says, sensibly sobered now.

Not long later, the dark Christmas Eventide is lit up with police lights. Officer Fogarty from the Santa Fe PD sits you down in Dr. Short's office and asks about the body.

"She's a veterinarian named Debbie Crimshaw," you say, recovered some from your shock. "She used to own this building, before she got enough money to retire. I…I met her just last week, when she brought her dog here for an allergic reaction."

"Yeah? How did you find her body?"

"Well, I was following this ghost, see…"

Officer Fogarty raises an eyebrow, and you suddenly have a lot more talking to do. By the end of your explanation, Dr. Short has arrived, as have an EMS team and some firemen.

"Yep. She's dead," an EMS medic helpfully confirms.

"Detective Martinez and a CSI team are on the way," Fogarty announces. "You all need to stay here until Martinez gives the clear."

"Guess we should go on pause tonight," Graham says. "Not a night to see cases…"

"Ya think?" Dr. Short barks. She taps onto her phone a social media message to let the world know the ER is closed tonight.

The next 20 minutes is awkward as you all sit around munching Christmas cookies and trying to think of what to say. Finally a detective arrives, along with a bunch of other people. Detective Gabe Martinez isn't wearing a trench coat and a fedora. He's wearing an old rock band t-shirt with sweatpants.

"What's the deal, Fogarty?" he growls. "You wake me up in the middle of the night because some old lady dies of a heart attack at her clinic? Anyone have coffee here, by the way?"

You walk off to get the detective a cup of coffee. "Martinez is right," someone from the coroner's office behind you says. "Sure looks like a heart attack to me…"

You find your brain's gears suddenly whirring faster than the stone-gears of Ritardando that power the living planet Morgoth 16 (Starship Beethoven S2E10). Something's off here… By the time you return with the coffee, you feel sure of it.

"…needle marks in her left arm," the coroner guy was saying. "Maybe she was a druggie?"

"Would surprise me if she wasn't," Lemon comments. "But she was also diabetic. I heard her talk about her insulin when she was here the other day."

A light goes on across the investigator's faces as they make a note.

"But what was she doing here tonight?" Dr. Short asks.

"Wasn't this her clinic?" Martinez said.

"Not for years. She got a pile of cash through investments in Vetraxis, and lives outside town. There's absolutely no reason she should be in our backyard!"

"Dr. Crimshaw did a lot of things there were absolutely no reason for," Graham chuckles wryly.

"Oh wait, I think…" you hesitate just a little, thinking faster than your mouth can talk. "I think I may know."

Every eye turns to you, and you wish you'd not said anything.

"This wasn't a heart attack. This was murder!"

Detective Martinez sips the coffee you handed him. "Yeah? Murder, you say? Tell us all about it, Sherlock…"

You really need to stop talking.

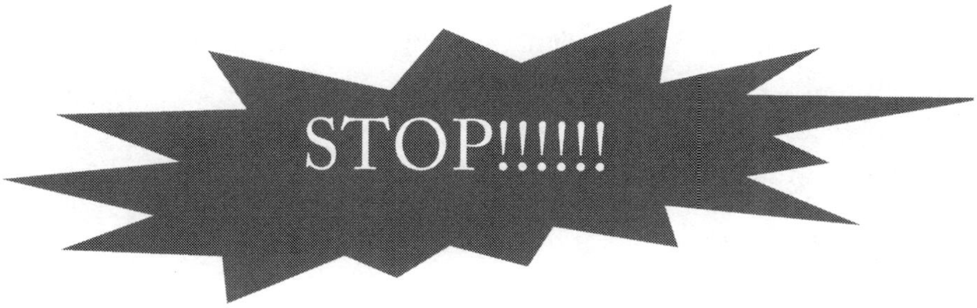

Do you know? What was Debbie Crimshaw doing in the clinic's yard?

You've trained your brain to think through mysteries. Sure, those mysteries have been medical cases so far, but the basic principles still apply. Take a step backward and use your brilliant, patented Fuzzy Logic differential thinking and case-organization to work this all out.

Just in case you forgot, these are the steps you follow with every case…

1. Organize the history and gather clues
2. Create a Differential List
3. Pick Some Tests
4. Make a Diagnosis
5. Make a Treatment Plan

Step 1 – Organize the History

Signalment:

Crazy old lady

Former owner of this clinic

Investor in a veterinary laboratory company

Diabetic

Presenting Complaint (what question needs answering?):

There is a dead person lying at your doorstep

Step 2 – Gather Clues

Physical Examination:

OK, so there's not even a little chance the police are going to let you examine the body, so you'll have to trust the coroner's office and CSI. Here's what you know…

Abdomen: Squishy? No significant findings.

Attitude: Dead.

Cardiac: asystole with no heartbeat on auscultation and no palpable pulses.

Ears: No significant findings

Eyes: OU– staring lifelessly up into the eerie moonglow

Integument: No lacerations or external signs of trauma noted, other than small bruises and punctures in her left arm.

Lymph Nodes: No significant findings.

Musculoskeletal: No significant findings.

Neurologic: Not responsive…even a little bit. She has, in fact, the reflexes one would expect of a very, very dead person.

Oronasal: Old person teeth, with some gum inflammation.

Respiratory: Apneic.

Vitals: None. Dead.

And that's what you have to work with.

Can you formulate a differential list to answer the question "Why was Dr. Crimshaw in the backyard tonight?" Make a list of possibilities before you turn the page…

Great job! I barely even noticed that look of utter confusion and hopelessness over your face. You're getting better at this!

Here's the list I came up with…

Crimshaw was meeting someone to buy drugs

Crmshaw was meeting someone who was secretly her child

Crimshaw was trying to break in and steal something

Crimshaw followed someone suspicious to the clinic yard

Crimshaw was looking for something she left the other day

Crimshaw was just confused and didn't know where she was

Crimshaw had secretly made a pact with the leader of a hippie-cult many years ago that she would die in the clinic yard, and came back tonight to fulfill her oath

Wow. Those are some pretty…um…interesting options there. Maybe my imagination is running a little too fast. Or maybe not!

Decision time!

What tests are you going to run to narrow down this beautiful list of detective differentials? Do you…

a) Go check the lock box where the drugs are kept? To do this, turn to page 224.
b) Look at Dr. Short's computer for any dubious receipts or suspiciously large bank account deposits? To do this, turn to page 226.
c) Go look over the pharmacy shelves? To do this, turn to page 228.
d) Wrestle Graham to the ground and take his wallet to see if his driver's license lists him as Graham Crimshaw? To do this, turn to page 227.
e) Look over the fence at the alley behind the backyard? To do this, turn to page 225.
f) Climb up to the roof and stare at the moon? To do this, turn to page 229.

"Though this be madness, yet there is method in 't."
—William Shakespeare, *Hamlet*[xxvi]

You trot through the treatment area, followed by your technicians, Dr. Short, and a cadre of law enforcement officials. The lock box is a small safe on the counter beside your CBC machine.

It's closed.

And locked.

There's a number combination lock that holds the keys that get into the safe. That's open.

"Where are the keys?" you gasp.

Graham holds up a small keyring with a few little keys. "Here they are. I'm the Keeper tonight."

Martinez stares questions at the younger man. Graham shrugs. "Clinic controlled drug policy is that the lead tech on the floor for a shift is the Keeper of the Keys. I get the drugs the doctor asks for and log them… At least I do tonight. Fred's Keeper tomorrow. Right, Doctor Short?"

Dr. Short seems a little red in the face, and rubs her tired eyes as she nods.

"Fine. Fine," Martinez says. "Now that you've randomly explained a bunch of stuff I didn't ask about, you mind opening the safe?"

Graham opens the safe. Dr. Short (officially in charge of stocking the controlled drugs) looks through it and declares that everything is there. "Nothing missing that I can see…"

"Well actually," Fred cuts in, holding open the logbook. "I've been meaning to talk to you about this, Dr. Short. There's been small discrepancies in the logs for methadone, ketamine, and pentobarbital lately."

The teams from CSI and Coroner's office all gasp in unison. Detective Martinez snags the logbook from Fred and flips through. "This is evidence now…"

You dash across the snow-dusted yard, followed by a gaggle of technicians, colleagues, and crime-scene investigators. All of you try not to look at the body still lying on the ground (all of you except the CSI guys: they *like* looking at dead bodies). You brush past an overgrown yucca plant to get to the gate, and find it cracked open.

"You enjoying tromping all over my crime scene, Doctor?" Martinez asks. "If you want, I can send Officer Fogarty here for your coat so's you can be more comfortable while you mess with all the evidence…"

You ignore his sarcasm, and shimmy through the gate to check the back alley.

A pickup truck reflects the silver moonglow. A pink sedan is parked behind it.

Then you become aware of the moaning. "Oooooh! Brrrrrr!"

Everyone's heart leaps to their throats, as you all turn toward the sound. A form is slumped against the fence in the shadows. It's Doug. He shivers in a thin windbreaker.

"Oh hey, Doc. Didn't see ya there!" he sighs. "Brrr it's cold tonight. Any chance I could come inside the clinic and warm up, just for a little… Oh, hi everyone!"

"Did you see anyone go into the yard tonight?"

He blinks at you. "Maybe. The ol' lady doctor that ran the place years ago walked past here."

"Do you know whose cars these are?"

He blinks at the cars, as if seeing them for the first time. "I saw that old lady get out of the pink car… I think it's got colder since you came out here. How about lettin' me inside for a while?"

Martinez grabs Doug roughly by the shirt collar. "Sure, pal! Sure! Come on in. You're a suspect now…"

You run into the room followed by a swarm of technicians, one doctor, and some spooks. You slide the mouse on Dr. Short's desktop.

"Hey, would you open your computer so I can look over your personal files and find all your bank account info?" You ask Dr. Short.

"No," she answers.

This wouldn't have surprised you if you'd thought it through a bit first.

The detective insists, his interest piqued. After some careful combing, you and (perhaps more importantly) the police, find exactly nothing. There's no bank accounts in the Cayman Islands, no suspicious deposits, no receipts for illicit drugs.

"But…but… Aren't you an opioid addict?" you ask your boss.

She glares at you.

"But…but you're always walking around like a zombie! You've got red bags under your eyes! You're always exhausted and cranky! You're always at the clinic! You've been complaining about headaches and stomach aches!

"Thanks for all that," she frowns. "I'm just overworked and ugly."

Perhaps if you'd have thought this over a little first, you might have a better chance of keeping your job.

[Turn back to pg 223 to try again.]

You leap on Graham and wrestle him to the ground. He shrieks as you flip him over and grab at the wallet in his blue jeans.

"You're her child! You must be her child!" you holler like a madman.

Then the police pull you off and arrest you for assault.

You probably should have thought this through a little more carefully…

Later, while you're waiting for your trial, you find out that Graham's driver's license reads "Graham Jones."

[Turn back to pg 223 to try again.]

You dash through the treatment area, and past surgery, followed by a herd of technicians, doctor, and dangerously irritated law-enforcement officers. Looking over the shelves you bob and weave while muttering to yourself, nearly exactly…no, exactly like a crazy person.

"Where was that…what did I think was…pretty sure it was right…here!"

You point at the top shelf, being careful not to move the bottle. An entire herd of eyeballs stare in the direction of your finger.

The bottle of tilmicosin is sitting on the shelf.

"The bottle of tilmicosin is sitting the shelf," you say, grinning wildly.

"Um… OK," says Detective Martinez. "And this is important, because?"

"Look beside it. Graham told me it doesn't get used. That's why there's dust around it. But look at this new, bottle-sized circle in the dust beside it! Someone has picked it up recently and put it back on the shelf!"

Graham and Lemon and Fred gasp.

"I think I'm missing something," Martinez growls.

"Tilmicosin is very toxic to humans. Accidental injections in people have been known to cause death within an hour."

"Yeah?"

"Yeah. And what, you may ask, are the symptoms it causes?"

"What are the symptoms it causes?" the detective takes the bait.

"Dizziness…" you say.

"Gasp!" says Graham, Lemon, and Fred

"Tackycardia…"

"Gasp!"

"Hypotension…"

"Gasp gasp!"

"Palpatations…"

"Oh gasp!"

"And cardiac collapse…"

"Gasp!" This last gasp came from Joe, one of the guys from the coroner's office. "Those are signs of a heart attack."

You do your very best Significant Look. "Exactly."

You jog across the clinic floor, down the fluorescent lit hallway, and out a side door: followed by a flock of technicians, an irritable doctor, and various police dudes. You pull a long ladder out of the storage room, and grunt as you drag it up to the wall outside.

Fred lends a helping hand, but with the qualification of a confused look. "What are we doing now?"

"You'll see?" you say, hopefully.

"Was that a question or an answer?" he frowns.

You sidle up the ladder and clamber onto the roof. Then three technicians, a doctor, four guys from the Coroner's Office, 3 CSI investigators, one detective and a policeman…and Doug all clamber up behind you. Years later you'll look back at this weird, moonlit scene and wonder how nobody fell off that ladder and broke their neck.

You plant your feet into the snow dusting the roof and feel the chilly wind in your face as you turn your gaze epically into the moonlight.

"Um… What are we doing?" Martinez asks.

You blink into the moonglow. Then you turn a puzzled look on him.

"I don't really know. Maybe I've been working too hard…"

[Turn back to pg 223 to try again.]

Solve Crimes like a Detective

Crime busting professionals often use these three tools to hunt and catch crooks...

1. Information

Facts and clues gathered through tools like crime scene investigation and research. You can organize these clues to help find which suspect had the best means, motive, and opportunity to commit the crime.

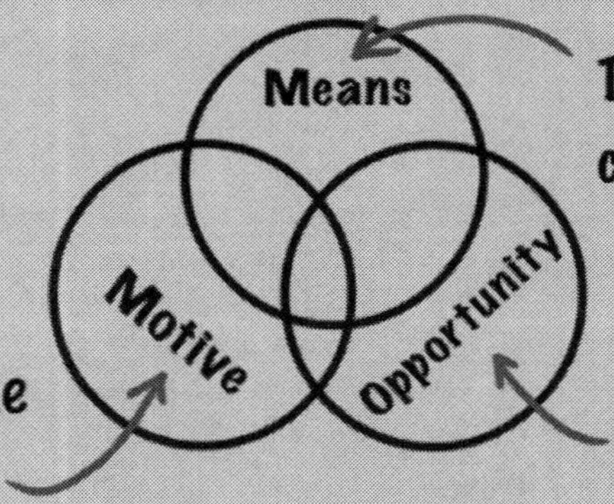

2. Interrogation

Talking to suspects and witnesses is a big part of the work of investigation. Skill at reading expressions, seeing through lies, and listening closely are vital!

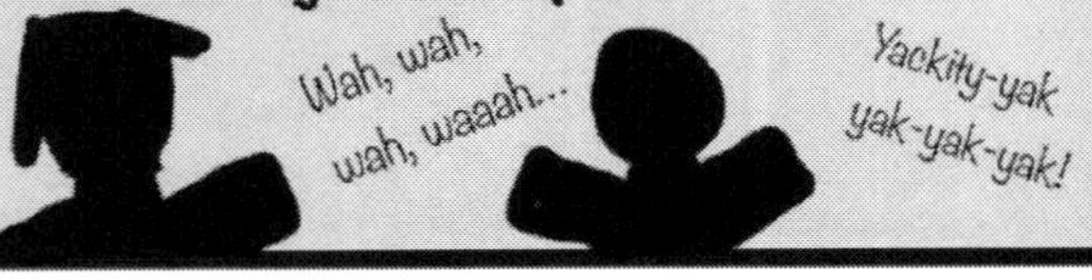

3. Implementation

When you've identified the most likely suspect, it's time to get busy gathering evidence, and planning to trap the culprit.

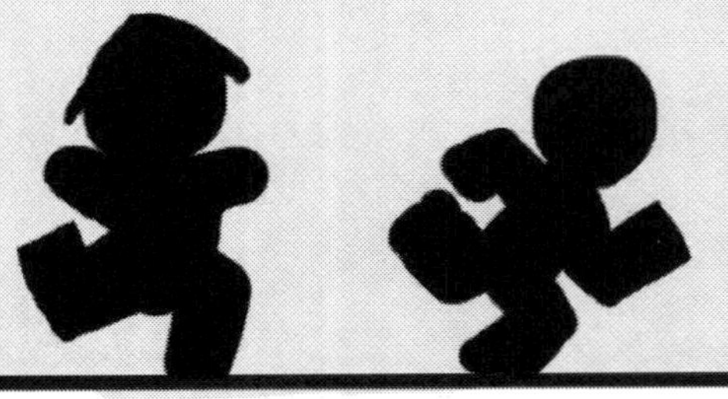

Alright! You've done your tests! You may be arrested, or possibly in an asylum somewhere trying to get some prescribed rest. But if not, you should have at least some idea of a diagnosis.

Take a moment to behold and wonder at the well-drawn infographic on the opposite page.

What is your answer? Why was Debbie Crimshaw in the clinic yard tonight?

And your diagnosis is?

____

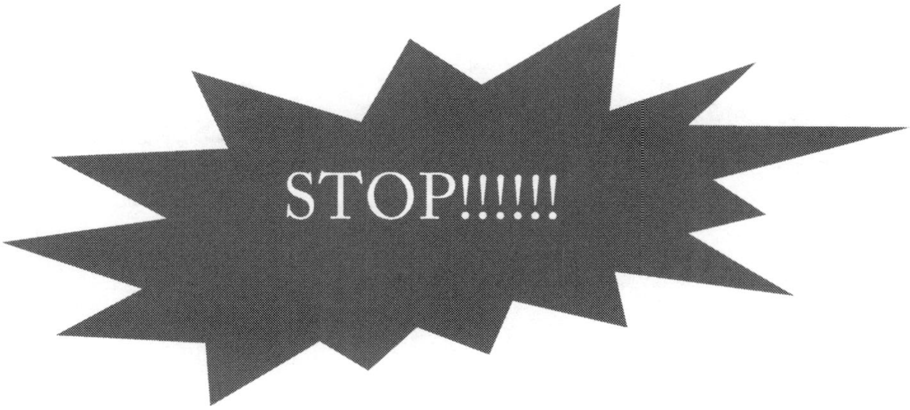

That's right! **Dr. Crimshaw followed someone suspicious to the clinic**!

You're pure, dead brilliant, you are.

- You couldn't find evidence that she was buying drugs. The box was locked and there was no evidence of weird sales on the computer.
- You didn't see anything important in the office, though perhaps there's something you don't know about.
- Graham is not her secret child. Of course, you could wrestle Lemon or Fred to the ground and check their wallets…
- Sure, she was a forgetful old lady and might have come to the clinic without knowing it. But it would be an awfully long drive in her little pink car…

Speaking of that little pink car, she parked it behind a truck. Did she park behind the truck because she was following somebody?

So, the new question is, *which somebody* was she following? Is it someone at the clinic tonight? Someone in this very room, perhaps?

It's time to compile a list of suspects. This, of course, already happened in your brain in a flash of brilliant inspiration, but we'll work through it more slowly. Before you turn the page, list out everyone you can think of who could have killed Debbie Crimshaw.

Form a differential list of suspects…

Check the next page for a hint…

Hint-

Use if you are stuck, or ready for more help.

Organize suspects in these three groups.

People you saw interact with Debbie Crimshaw (i.e., people at the clinic when she was here last):

-
-
-
-
-
-
-

People you know have interacted with Debbie Crimshaw (i.e., you've heard them talk about her):

-
-
-

Other people:

-

STOP!!!!!!

People you saw interact with Debbie Crimshaw (i.e., people at the clinic when she was here last):

- Doctor Short
- Graham
- Jane (whose last name you never actually heard)
- Senator Joe Dertoni
- Lemon
- The Clinic Ghost
- You

People you know have interacted with Debbie Crimshaw (i.e., you've heard them talk about her):

- Doug
- Fred
- Harlow

Other people:

- Anyone you don't know about who might have known Debbie Crimshaw

Maybe we should just ignore that last possibility. The category of "people you don't know" is far too big to work with.

Let's see where you get with people you do know.

What tests can you do to narrow down this differential list?

Well, where murder and mayhem are concerned, there are three time-honored questions that have been used to narrow down a list of suspects.

These are as follows:

1. Who had the means (the method used)?
2. Who had the opportunity to do the murderous murder?
3. Who had the motive for the killing?

First on the list of these all-important questions…

1. **Who had the means for this murder?**

First answer the question, “How was Debbie Crimshaw killed?”

Believe it or not, you have enough information to answer that already.

And so I say unto you…

Figure out how the murder was committed before you turn the page…

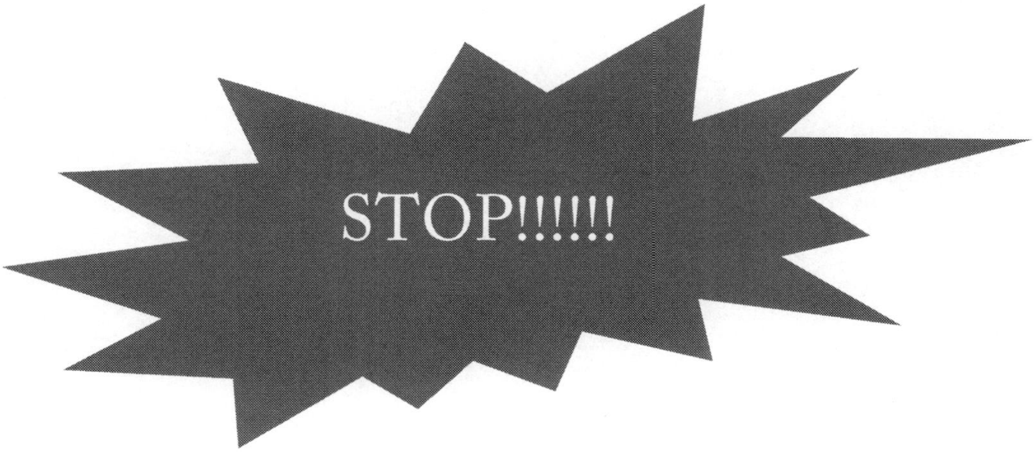

What?!?!? **Debbie Crimshaw was murdered by an injection of tilmocosin**?!?!? REALLY?!?!? HOW VERY CLEVER!

Oh yeah, I guess I knew that… I did write this story.

You got it right. Tilmicosin, an older type of antibiotic still used today (usually in large animal medicine), will cause a heart attack if injected into a human being. Signs start in about 60 minutes and can be rapidly fatal. In a frail old lady who's about 447, they would be very rapid.

But how the bloomin' onion did Debbie Crimshaw get injected with tilmicosin? Did the killer inject her, then hold her down in the backyard for an hour while waiting for her to die?

Seems unlikely.

"Or maybe…" you explain to the group of humans staring at you in the treatment area of the clinic. "Maybe the killer somehow switched something Debbie Crimshaw injected regularly with the tilmicosin. Twice every day, to be exact." You're doing your very best dramatic Detective-At-The-End-Of-The-Story-Explaining-The-Solution-Of-The-Murder bit.

"Oh! Oh!" Lemon jumps up and down in sudden understanding. "It was the insulin! She takes insulin injections for diabetes!"

"Gasp!" gasps everyone.

"Exactly!" you answer. "Someone put an insulin syringe filled with tilmicosin in her supplies. She must have used that syringe earlier and died just after she got here. She was probably feeling the effects as she parked in the alley and thus wound up dead at the back door."

"But how could whoever it was have made sure she took it?"

You put a finger into the air (hoping it's the proper one for dramatic effect), and pace up and down. "How indeed? How indeed? *That* is the salient question…"

Doug raises his hand.

"Salient means important, Doug."

Doug lowers his hand.

So who had access to the tilmicosin and Crimshaw's insulin?

Out loud you say, "That's the question that brings us to the test of opportunity…"

Graham raises his hand.

"The 'test of opportunity' means 'what chances came up to switch out the syringe.'"

Graham lowers his hand.

2. Who had the opportunity to commit this murder?

What were some points in the story (or outside of it) where someone could have put a poisoned syringe in Debbie Crimshaw's insulin supplies?

Do you have any guesses?

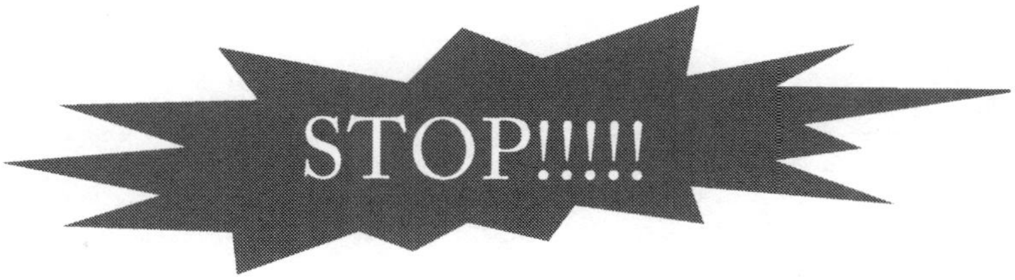

That's a tough one. Read on to work through some hints and whittle down the suspects list…

Debbie had been ready to take insulin at the clinic, which implies she brought syringes. Someone could have replaced one or more of them while she was at the clinic.

Reduce your 10 suspects to the 7 who were at the clinic when Debbie was there.

Can you logically rule any of them out?

-
-
-
-

Extra credit: Who can we add back onto the suspect list and why?

-
-

Extra extra credit: How's the updated list look after removing and adding suspects?

-
-
-
-
-

The suspects who had an opportunity to slip Debbie the murder weapon:

- Doctor Short
- Jane (whose last name you never actually heard)
- Graham
- Lemon
- Senator Joe Dertoni
- The Clinic Ghost
- You

Who of these suspects can we logically rule out?

- Jane. She came to the clinic in a flurry with her dead dog. She didn't really have a chance or brainpower to search for Crimshaw's medical supplies in between her sobs and wails.
- Senator Dertoni. The same can be said of Joe Dertoni. And neither he nor Jane seemed to know Crimshaw.
- You. You are very unlikely to have committed this murder, since you'd probably remember.
- Clinic ghost. It's very hard for a ghost to lift solid things like syringes (as far as you know).

One other suspect might have access to the victim's medical supplies.

- Harlow. She's Debbie's neighbor. She had access to her at home and potentially in the clinic parking lot, and could have snuck in to replace a syringe.
- Doug. Speaking of access, Doug practically lives in the clinic parking lot. While he had not been in the clinic, he could have accessed medical supplies Doc Crimshaw kept in her car.

This leaves us with:

- Doug
- Doctor Short
- Graham
- Harlow
- Lemon

The list is narrowing! The noose grows tight! The circle ever closeth! Verily yea!

You explain all this to your fans in the audience, and they gasp suitably.

"Gasp!" gasps everyone.

"Whew! Glad I'm off the list," says Fred. He starts to count off on his fingers (concentrating very hard). "That means and opportunity are starting to make sense. That leaves the motive…"

It does.

3. Who had motive to kill Dr. Crimshaw?

Can you think of any reasons why someone might have wanted Debbie Crimshaw killed?

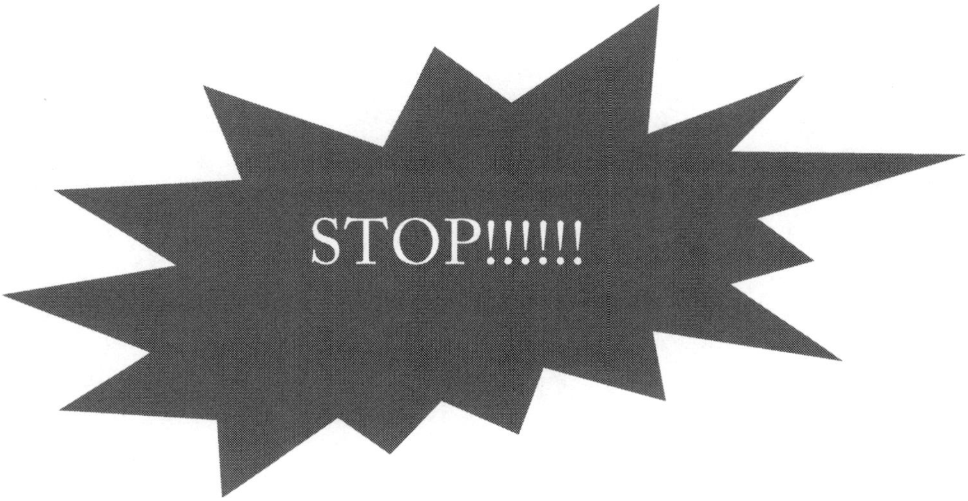

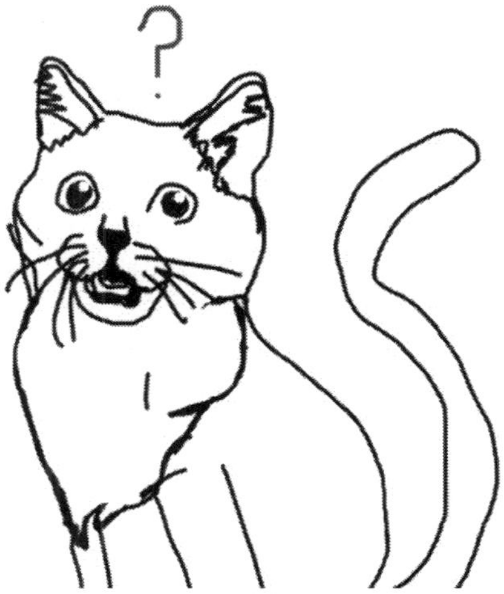

You hold your hands behind your back and pace back and forth in front of the increasingly interested audience. "Why? Why would someone want to kill Debbie Crenshaw? Was it because they wanted revenge for something she did in the past? Maybe it was someone who holds a grudge against her enough hard to talk about how cranky she used to be?"

You stare at Doug, and he sinks down in his chair.

"I may not have liked her, but I didn't kill her," he mutters.

"Or maybe it was a murder to cover up another crime! Could Doctor Crimshaw have followed someone to the clinic to blackmail, perhaps? Maybe someone stealing controlled drugs from the clinic?"

You glare at Celia Short. She glares back. "I'm not an addict."

"Aha!" you point at her so aggressively it makes even you jump. "I didn't say you were. You could have been siphoning off drugs to sell on the streets. You could have sold some to Doctor Crimshaw! She seemed awfully interested in controlled substances while she was in the building…" You scratch your chin, thinking through all the possibilities. "Or maybe this was a crime of greed. Could someone have gained financially from Doctor Crimshaw's death? Someone, perhaps, whose college studies left him desperate for money?"

You look at Graham, and he frowns. "Embarrassing…"

"Yes," Lemon cuts in, "but how would murdering Debbie Crimshaw get Graham money? Do you think she was carrying a bunch of cash, and he just happened to find her in the backyard?"

It's a good question. We know she was wealthy. But if the motive was her wealth, how could it be accessed? How could…

You look up at the back door of the clinic, and a sudden inspiration fwumps over you like a wet blanket on your head. "I think we may have struck someone off the list of suspects too soon!"

"What?" Martinez asks. He's chewing on a granola bar he pulled out of his pocket and seems to be thoroughly enjoying the show.

"Why?" Fred gasps.

"Who?" Dr. Short asks.

"The clinic ghost," you answer.

"Gasp!" gasps everyone.

"Wait… Are you being serious right now?" Lemon asks. "You're really saying our ghost is a suspect?"

"I just realized what some of the sounds we keep hearing are."

You go through the doctor's office into the manager's office, everyone following as quickly as they can.

You open the back door rapidly.

SHHHP! says the rubber insulation as it scrapes across the tile floor.

"Gasp!" everyone gasps again.

"Someone's been coming into the clinic on nights we hear 'the ghost.' That's the back door opening. And I'd bet the thumps we hear are footsteps, and maybe someone moving things on the desk and..." Something crazy clicks into place in your mind. "...knocking against the walls."

"What? Is this guy drunk and bumping into things?" Graham says. Everyone seems more confused than ever. You are about to lose your audience.

"Back it up a minute. Think of the times we've heard the ghost recently. It's always at the end of a shift, wasn't it?" Fred, Lemon, and Graham all nod. The rest of the room looks perplexed. "Someone without a set of keys, who knows we're only open at night, might sneak in just before the clinic closes. Then they could hide and wait for us to leave."

Lemon shivers. "Someone's been coming in here and hiding? But why?"

"They're looking for something. Something the forgetful (and probably drug-riddled) mind of Debbie Crimshaw forgot about when she sold this clinic years ago. The only shift I had this past two weeks that wasn't visited by the ghost was last night. Why was that?"

"Ghosts don't like Saturdays?" Officer Fogarty shrugs.

"Maybe!" you answer, realizing you don't know what days ghosts like best. "But I think the reason was that we had a different technician that night, a technician who'd not worked here recently before that."

"Wait..." says Fred.

"You're not talking about..." Dr. Short starts.

"Harlow???" Graham finishes the sentence.

"It makes sense! Harlow was here and could easily have filled an insulin syringe with tilmicosin. She's got a lot of experience in large animal medicine, and would have known what it could do. Harlow is Debbie Crimshaw's neighbor and had plenty of opportunities to replace her syringe. She had the means and the opportunity to do it. She didn't like Dr. Crimshaw, either."

"But (as Mr. Doug here so eloquently put it) not liking someone doesn't mean you'll kill them," Martinez points out.

"Yes. Yes indeed. But, you see, Harlow is the only one of us who worked with Dr. Crimshaw back when she owned this clinic. I think she found out about something Debbie Crimshaw left behind. And I think that's why she's been sneaking into the clinic in the early mornings. She didn't have to sneak in the other night when she was on a shift, and that's the night we didn't hear any ghost noises..."

"But I heard a ghost sound this morning," Lemon said.

Everyone quiets down. You nod. "I did too. I think it's what woke me up."

"Does that mean…?"

You nod. You cross the room to where the hot water heaters for the building are. You throw open the door with a sudden, dramatic fling.

Harlow glares up from where she's crouching inside, hiding like some grotesque goblin. "Miss Murderer, I presume," you say.

Then she attacks you.

"YAAAAAAAAAAAAAAAARG!" she screams, scratching at your face and pulling at your hair.

Fortunately, the room is full of police officers and detectives. A moment later, Harlow is in handcuffs and you're nursing a bruise on your face.

"I was so close, darn it!" Harlow fumes. "Was gonna find it today, I know I was! And you had to ruin it all. You with your stupid differential lists!"

"You were gonna find it today, because today you have old blueprints of this building, don't you? Probably stolen from Dr. Crimshaw when you swapped out her syringe…"

She smiles unpleasantly. "Left coat pocket."

You reach in and pull out a piece of printed paper. Everyone looks over your shoulder. It's a floor plan to the clinic.[18] You point at the doctor's office. "Look at what's on here, but not in this room…"

"A closet?" Celia Short mutters.

"It should be right here." You walk over to a blank wall and tap on it. It sounds hollow. Then you jump back as Fred rushes by with an office chair, which he slams through the wall.

WHUMP!

A cloud of white fiberglass and dry wall engulfs the room. You hack and cough, as you brush away the debris. Then you notice the door. It's an old closet door, walled in when the building was remodeled.

"Huh…" You open it and are hit with a very musty smell. Piles of papers and cardboard boxes are stacked inside.

"They're in there somewhere," Harlow sighs, with tears sparkling in her intense eyes. "I worked for that woman for years, and never got a break. I deserve those papers. They could have paid for my horses. I could have been rich."

"What's she talking about?" Martinez gapes at the hidden stash of what looks very much like junk.

---

[18] The blueprints of the clinic is in the first few pages of the book… See if you can find anything interesting on it.

"Shares. Original stock certificates for Vetraxis Labs…" you explain as Harlow nods sadly. "Dr. Crimshaw was one of the first investors. She mentioned, when she wandered back to Treatment the other night, that she'd left some papers in the office. We all assumed it was more senile rambling. But she was remembering something important! I'd bet my job (which I'm not going to have anyway after certain regrettable things said tonight)," you glance apologetically at Dr. Short, "that you'll find stock certs worth millions in those piles."

Everyone looks at you in astonishment. "What happened was this. Harlow knew about Doctor Crimshaw's Vetraxis certificates, but she didn't know until recently that not all of them had been cashed out and some were still hidden in the clinic. When she found out, she figured her ship had come in at last. She snuck into the clinic and searched for the last couple weeks, to no avail. But then a revelation struck her. The aging Debbie Crimshaw might never tell her where the treasure was, but she surely had clues in her home. Harlow also realized that she could never cash in on those certificates as long as Debbie Crimshaw was alive. So she booked a shift at the clinic and took some of the tilmicosin, putting it in an insulin syringe. Then she broke into Crimshaw's home, and found old clinic blueprints that showed a closet at the clinic she realized must have been walled up... Knowing Dr. Crimshaw might figure out she broke in and took things was added incentive to murder her. Harlow switched Crimshaw's insulin dose for tilmicosin while she was at the house. That ensured Crimshaw would die. My guess is that Dr. Crimshaw saw her leave the house and followed her, never realizing she was dying the moment she took her morning insulin dose."

Everyone was impressed. Martinez was impressed enough to slap some crime scene tape over the door. "Nobody goes in. This is evidence."

You shrug and walk out of the office. Case closed.

"Don't be so sure about losing your job," Dr. Short catches up to you. "You've got a good brain on you. And I can understand you thinking I'm a drug addict. Haven't been acting exactly normal lately…"

"I'm sorry, honest!" you say.

She extends a hand. "How about another try? Maybe with a raise?"

You take the hand with a grin of surprise. This might be a good Christmas after all. More police stomp through the building and carry off Harlow. You and your friends amble up to the front office.

"So, you thought I was a murderer?" Graham says.

You feel a blush of embarrassment. "Uh… Maybe for a sec. Sorry about that."

"I think it's pretty cool," he says. "Never been dope enough to be a murder suspect before."

"But what about the missing drugs in the logbook?" Fred asks.

"We'll look into it," Dr. Short answers. "But I'd be willing to bet those are normal hub losses."

"Wazzat?" you ask.

"Hub losses. When you inject a drug, a tiny bit gets lost in the hub of the needle. Over time it can cause a discrepancy in a logbook."

Doug walks up, cradling a cup of coffee in his hands. "So warm in here…" he mutters happily. Doctor Short frowns, obviously thinking she should kick him out. Then she shrugs, and nods instead.

"Yeah, Doug. The heating bill is paid. Stick around a while."

"Thanks! You're a good person, Doc. Not like that Doctor Crimshaw…"

"Poor Doctor Crimshaw," Lemon mutters.

Everyone mutters agreement.

"Heck of a thing. But you solved it!" Fred beams. "Your quick thinking brought her justice."

"And maybe a little peace," Graham shrugs. "We can hope, anyway?"

"At least we won't have any more visits from the ghost!" Lemon grins.

THUMP! THUMP!

Something sounds loudly from the other side of the wall near the reception desk. Maybe it's an echo from the policeman down the hallway?

Maybe…

EPILOGUE

Carols croon across the radio as you drive in the dim hours of the morning. These silent morning hours after a night shift always seem to have a sort of magical quiet. But today, Christmas Day, the silence feels sacred.

"It came upon a midnight clear,

that glorious song of old,

From angels bending near the earth,

To touch their harps of gold..."

You didn't know Debbie Crimshaw, but you hope she's singing with some angels somewhere. You wonder if she ever felt this confused mix of emotions that washes over your tired soul after a long week at the veterinary ER.

"'Peace on the earth, good will to men,

From Heaven's all-gracious King.'

The world in silent stillness lay,

To hear the angels sing."

It's hard to sing about peace on Earth, when you just saw hate and murder. But you also saw justice, and truth lighting up old, dark corners: and somehow you feel that's brought a peace of its own to the world.

"And ye, beneath life's crushing load,

Whose forms are bending low,

Who toil along the climbing way

With painful steps and slow."

Your first couple of weeks in emergency medicine had some painful steps and crushing loads. But there were also challenges that bettered you, and patients saved. Some days you feel inadequate, but you still seem to be doing some good and are improving your skills. They can be painful steps, but they're steps forward. And you hope the same for your life off the clinic floor.

"Look now! For glad and golden hours

Come swiftly on the wing.

Or rest beside the weary road,

And hear the angels sing!"

Someone's car is in your driveway when you pull up. Is that... It is! Carley and Mac have brought little

Sam over. All three of them greet you at your doorstep. It's not going to be a lonely Christmas after all.

"Happy Christmas, Doc!" they say. Sam gives you a hug and melts your heart. His smile seems genuine, and you're glad he's recovered from his gloom of yesterday.

"Dad called from jail," he beams. "He said he's proud of me."

"Well, of course he is, Sam. We all are."

"He says things are getting better for him."

Mac explains. "Friend of yours named Robert McCutchen called and told us he's taken an interest in Arturo's case. I think he works for the government somehow?"

"Yeah. CIA." You feel a glimmer of hope for the future.

"I got this for you," Sam holds up a hideously wrapped package. "Merry Christmas!" You open his gift to find a small model of the Starship Beethoven for you to hang on your stethoscope.

"He bought it with his own allowance money," Carley smiles.

"It's perfect!" You run to the closet and pull out a package (which you quickly remember to put into a gift bag). "I got you something too, buddy…"

His little eyes light up when he looks inside, and it seems to you they light up this dark old world just a little bit (maybe a bit like another Kid on the first Christmas Day). "A squishwidget!"

"A what?" Carley and Mac ask.

You shrug your shoulders. "*He* likes it."

"I'm gonna squish it, and twist it, and draw on it with crayons too!"

"You do that. Have fun."

Snow drifts down outside the living room window, from where you curl up on the sofa and gratefully accept a cup of hot cocoa from your friends. Feelings of gratitude wash over you as your mind, fuzzy with exhaustion, takes in the warm conversation of your friends and family. It's a happy fuzziness, a warm Christmas haze: a fuzziness like the fur on the patients you get the privilege of treating every week.

This is a good life, with good work. Though it has its highs and its lows, you'll go on fighting through them using your fuzzy logic to make this world just a little brighter: one patient at a time.

"The world is indeed full of peril, and in it there are many dark places; but still there is much that is fair, and though in all lands love is now mingled with grief, it grows perhaps the greater."
-J. R. R. Tolkien, *The Fellowship of the Ring*[xxvii]

DISCLAIMER:

If and when you become a veterinarian, please do not attribute nefarious and criminal reasons to the odd behavior of your clients. Clients behave oddly all the time, and most of the time the reasons for it are perfectly innocent. I added a mystery to this book within the framework of the clients' histories just to make it more interesting (and to underscore the point that veterinarians and detectives both use inductive and deductive reasoning to solve cases). However, should you happen to solve a case or catch a criminal through these methods, I expect part of the reward money.

More Veterinary Adventures

Check out the other books in the Fuzzy Logic series!

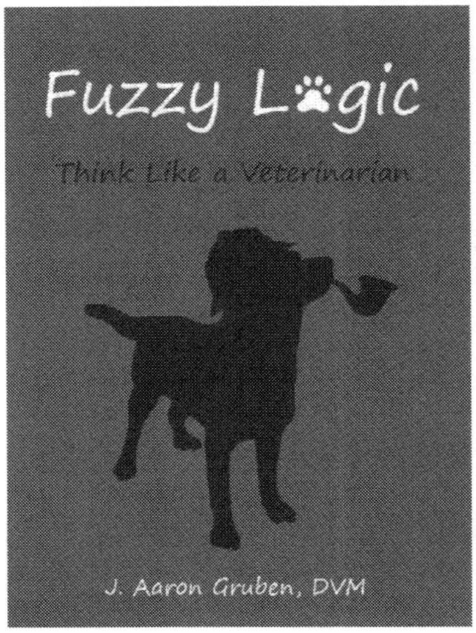

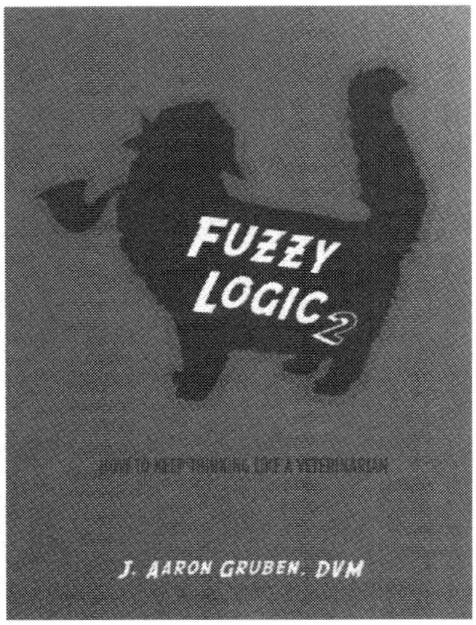

(scan for more Fuzzy Logics and vet books)

If you enjoyed characters like Fred Kawalkovitch, Sam, and the mysterious CIA agent Robert McCutchen, you'll want to check out J. Aaron Gruben's time-bending fictional series **TANGLED EONS** to find them in adventures with veterinarians through time and more!

(scan to discover the Tangled Eons!)

Already read 'em? Please consider leaving a review on Amazon or other book sites, it helps a lot. Thanks!!

GLOSSARY

Abdominocentesis: inserting a needle into the abdomen to check and/or remove fluid.

AFS: abdominal fluid score

Anterior chamber: the space between the cornea and the lens. The space behind the lens is called the posterior chamber.

Antihistamine: a drug to treat allergic reactions.

Apnea: cessation of breathing. Sleep apnea is not very bad. Death apnea is very, very bad.

Arrythmia: abnormal heart rhythm (like beating too fast or slow, or skipping beats)

AU: both ears.

Auscultation: an "old-school" trick to listen for gas distention with your stethoscope. A "ping" is an airy high-pitched echo when thumping on the abdomen just behind the ribs, while listening with your stethoscope, *if* the stomach is filled with too much gas.

BAR: Bright, alert, and responsive.

Bilaterally: including two sides.

Blood gas analysis: a blood panel specifically designed to check chemistry related to respiration and blood pH (like oxygen and bicarbonate levels).

Bolus: a single large dose.

Capillary refill time (CRT): capillary refill time. A simple way to check blood flow (perfusion) by pushing down on the gums and counting how long it takes to pink up again in that spot. It should be less than 2 seconds in a healthy beast.

Caudal vena cava: big, important vein that drains blood back in the right side of the heart from organs in the abdomen.

Ceruminous: waxy; this refers to ear wax in particular.

CC: Cysto-Colic view (bottom part of abdomen when patient is on the back) on AFAST ultrasound.

Chemistry panel: a blood panel that usually has basic information on the function of the liver, the kidneys, electrolyte levels, protein levels, and blood glucose.

Circulatory system: the heart and blood vessels.

Clotting times: a test of the ability of blood to clot properly.

Coagulation: blood clotting.

Concave pinna: inside of part of the ear flap.

Congestive heart failure: right sided heart failure in particular can fill an abdomen up with fluid (which is called ascites).

Conjunctival: a transparent membrane lining the inside of the eyelids and stretching across the sclera to the globe.

Cornea: the clear front part of the eye, where the light first goes in.

Corneal reflex: poking the eyeball with a finger doesn't make him blink. You usually don't want clients to see you do this.

Cyanosis: a blue or purple color to the mucous membranes (usually seen in the gums and/or tongue best) from lack of oxygen circulating.

Cytology: looking at cells under a microscope. If you pick this, you have to pick where to get the cells from. Will it be scrapings from the skin? Or cells from a tumor with a needle (fine needle aspirate)? Or cells from a swab of ear gunk or snot?

Debris: a fancier way to say "gunk."

Decompensate: deterioration of organs.

DDx: shorthand for differential diagnoses.

DH: Diaphragmatico-Hepatic view (the top of the abdomen when patient is on the back) on AFAST ultrasound.

Differential list: the list of possible causes ("differentials") for a patient's problems. List of diseases that might make the patient sick.

Distention: gastric distention means the stomach is dilated and bloated.

Dyspneic: breathing abnormally.

Edema: fluid building up in tissue, causing severe swelling.

Endotracheal tube: a flexible plastic tube that goes down into the windpipe through the mouth, and has a balloon on the tip you blow up with a syringe to make a seal.

Episcleral: connective tissue behind the sclera (white part of the eye). Scleral injection is redness to the sclera from inflammation.

Episcleral injection: redness to the white bit of the eyes.

Eupneic: a fancy way to say "breathing normally" in a single word.

Exophthalmos: a big, ophthalmology word for "eyeball is bulging forward."

Extraocular muscles: the little muscles controlling movement of the eye. They are smushed between the socket and attached along all four sides of the globe. In a cat there are seven of them.

Exudative: "goopy," a process that leaks fluid of some kind.

Feline Idiopathic Cystitis (FIC): a condition causing inflammation in the bladder (and often urethra) without an infection. It's related to stress in cats, neurologic and hormonal abnormalities, and has genetic predispositions.

FeLV/FIV: feline leukemia virus and feline immunodeficiency virus. These contagious diseases suppress the immune system in cats.

Gastric antrum: lower, funnel-shaped portion of the stomach.

Gastric dilatation: a stomach filled up and distended with gas.

Gastric dilatation-volvulus (GDV): a stomach filled up and distended with gas AND twisted out of its normal, happy position.

Gastric overdistension: This means a stomach "all swollen up" with food. It's often called "food bloat" and is exactly what it sounds like: a dog that ate way more than could fit in his stomach comfortably.

Gastropexy: a surgery to attach the stomach to the body wall so it can't flip and cause GDV.

Gastrosplenic ligament: a band that connects the spleen to the stomach.

Giardia: a microscopic parasite that looks like a flying saucer with googly eyes. It causes a nasty infection in the intestines that produces diarrhea and vomiting.

Globe: the round bit of the eye, which we think of as the "eyeball."

Greater curvature: the big part of the stomach.

Heart arrhythmia: irregular heartbeat, either too slow or too fast.

Hemoabdomen: This is a belly full of blood, from internal bleeding.

Hepatocytes: liver cells.

HR: Hepato-Renal view (left side of abdomen when patient is on the back) on AFAST ultrasound.

Hyphema: blood inside the eyeball.

Hypovolemic shock: a whole-body drop in blood pressure in response to a disease, starving the tissues of oxygen.

Hypoxia: not enough oxygen.

Integument: a fancy word for skin.

Lateral: on the side.

Leptospirosis: a bacterial disease that causes kidney and liver failure, often contracted through contaminated water (much like giardia). This bug looks like a coiled, swimming pigtail.

Ligate: to bind/tie off, usually using a suture.

Lymph node: important structures for the immune system. "Hubs" of white blood cells and lymphatic drainage, to fight infection in specific places of the body. Small and bean-shaped, like the author of this book.

MAP: mean arterial blood pressure—average blood pressure.

Menace response: a reflex that makes a patient close his eye when your hand is coming toward it.

Mucous membranes: the wet bits of a critter at the junction of skin and mucosa (like the gums in the mouth).

Necrosis: death of body tissue.

Neoplasia: cancer.

NSF: no significant findings (it's all normal looking).

Obstipation: really bad constipation.

Obtund: "out of it." Superfly is spacey, dude, like totally psychedelic.

Odiferous: bad smelling.

Optic chiasm: a crisscross of the two optic nerves (one from each eye) inside the brain. Because they cross, tugging on one optic nerve can damage the other one.

Organomegaly: fun way to say "organs that are too big."

Oronasal: the mouth and nose.

OU: "oculus uterque," a fancy Latin phrase that means "both eyes."

Palpebral reflex: closing an eye when you touch the inside edge of the eyelid.

Pancreatic Lipase: a test for pancreatitis. There's an fPL (feline pancreatic lipase) and a cPL (canine pancreatic lipase).

Pancreatitis: inflammation in the pancreas, which is an organ that makes hormones and helps digestion.

Parvo test: a test for canine parvovirus, which is a virus that attacks the GI tract in puppies.

PE: Physical Examination.

Perfusion: flow of blood to organs.

Petechiation: tiny spots covering the mucous membranes, usually a sign of blood clotting problems.

Plasmalyte: a fluid solution similar to plasma.

Portal vein: a big vein that carries blood from the other organs in the abdomen to the liver, for filtering out bad juju.

Proprioception: a big neurology term (woo hoo!) for a reflex that causes an animal's paw to flip "right side up" when you turn it over. This is a postural reflex a related to the brain and the spinal cord useful to check in emergency cases.

Proptosis: a word for the eye being popped out of its socket.

Pylorus: the narrowed part of the stomach that flows out to the intestines.

Radiographs: X-rays. A way to use radiation to take pictures of an animal's insides.

Retrobulbar: a fancy word for something behind the eyeball.

Respiratory: all the bits for breathing; the body system that takes in oxygen and breathes out carbon dioxide.

Rickettsial diseases: some infectious diseases carried by ticks (lyme is one of them).

Right lateral: lying on the right side.

Rodenticide: rat poison.

Serosanguinous: "kind of bloody;" thin and blood colored, usually because it has serum and blood in it.

Serous: clear; a serous discharge is a watery secretion.

Signalment: the descriptive characteristics of the patient.

Skin turgor: the tension or "stretchiness" of the skin, how well it falls back down when you tent (pull) it upward. This is a way we check the hydration status of a patient.

Splenic torsion: a twisted spleen; rare but life-threatening, often occurs with a GDV. NOT morally twisted like an evil supervillain spleen, though a villainous spleen might be kinda cool.

Splinting: tensing or tightening of the abdomen (often a specific region) because of pain or sometimes anxiety.

SR: Spleno-Renal view (right side of abdomen when patient is on the back) on AFAST ultrasound.

Stertor: a "snorty" congested sound when breathing.

Subcutaneous tissue: the fatty layer of tissue under the skin.

Suppurative: "nasty and goopy," a process that creates pus leaking from infection.

Synchronous: coordinated with the heartbeat.

Systemically: everywhere in the body.

Tachycardia: a faster than normal heart rate.

Tachypnea: breathing fast.

Transect: cutting, often after ligation.

Turgid: a fancy word for "hard and tense."

Ultrasound: a way to use sound in ultrasonic frequencies to view pictures of an animal's insides.

Urinalysis: a test on urine, generally looking for infection or crystals from bladder stones.

Urogenital: urinary and genital organs.

Urolithiasis: a fancy word for urinary stones. Often, in cats, this manifests as sandy, crystalline substance, but can be actual little rocks.

Ventral: lower body surface; situated close to the abdomen.

WNL: Within Normal Limits.

Xiphoid: pokey bit at the front of the breastbone.

Appendix A: Bloodwork Panel Details

Client:	Species:	Sex:
Patient:	Breed:	
Patient ID:		

When you look at bloodwork, run your eyes over this "flag" column first: this cues you into which results were high (above the reference range) and which were low (below the reference range). Sometimes lab results are right on the border of the reference range. This might just as important as a number outside the range.

Chemistry Panel

Test	Result	Flag	Reference Range	
ALT			5-60	IU/L
ALP			10-150	IU/L
GGT			0-10	IU/L
tBili			0-0.4	mg/dl
Glucose			60-125	mg/dL
Cholesterol			112-328	mg/dL
Total Protein			5.1-7.8	g/dL
Albumin			2.6-4.3	g/dL
Globulin			2.1-3.7	g/dL
Calcium			7.5-11.3	mg/dL
BUN			7-27	mg/dL
Creatinine			0.4-1.8	mg/dL
Phosphorus			2.1-6.3	mg/dL
Sodium			141-156	mEq/L
Potassium			4.0-5.6	mEq/L
Chloride			105-115	mEq/L

These are normal ranges for a patient. The specific numbers will be different based on species.

ALT, ALP, GGT, tBili: These values will go up with liver disease or dysfunction (and a few other diseases).

Glucose: Glucose is blood sugar.

Cholesterol: A fat derivative, useful for cell walls and other stuff.

Total Protein: All the proteins: albumin is one type of protein.

Albumin: A protein made in the liver.

Globulin: A type of protein produced by the immune system to fight infection.

Calcium: An important mineral stored in bones

BUN, Creatinine, Phosphorus: Kidney values: they go up when the kidneys are failing (or from a few other things).

Sodium, Potassium, Chloride: These are electrolytes.

Client:	Species:	Sex:
Patient:	Breed:	
Patient ID:		

CBC

TEST	RESULT	FLAG	REFERENCE RANGE	
WBC			6.0-17.0	$10^3/\mu L$
Neutrophils			3-11.5	$10^3/\mu L$
Monocytes			0.18-1.35	$10^3/\mu L$
Lymphocytes			1-4.8	$10^3/\mu L$
Eosinophils			1-1.25	$10^3/\mu L$
Hematocrit			37-55	%
MCV			60-77	fL
Platelet Count			200-500	$10^3/\mu L$

This is the count of white blood cells which defend the body from disease.

Different types of white blood cells.

The hematocrit (similar to PCV) is the concentration of red cells in the blood.

Mean Corpuscular Volume is a measure of the size of red blood cells: in general it will go up when the body is making new red cells.

Platelets help blood clot.

Client:	Species:	Sex:
Patient:	Breed:	
Patient ID:		

Blood Gas

On a real-life blood gas panel, CO2 is often listed as PCO2 (P = partial pressure) and O2 listed as PO2.

TEST	RESULT	FLAG	REFERENCE RANGE[xxix]	
pH				
CO2				
O2			85-95	mmHg
HCO3-			17-24	mEq/L

pH: The measure of the body's acidity, reflecting the amount of hydrogen ions.

CO2: Carbon dioxide is dissolved in the blood, then exhaled. It is a good estimate of breathing efficiency.

O2: The oxygen dissolved in the blood. It is low in the blood when you can't get enough oxygen.

HCO3-: Bicarbonate is a base in solution, produced by the tissues.

Client:	Species:	Sex:
Patient:	Breed:	
Patient ID:		

Clotting Times

These time how long it takes blood to clot. A high number means the blood is not clotting normally and clotting factors are missing.

TEST	RESULT	FLAG	REFERENCE RANGE
APTT	214	H	84-72 seconds
PT	21	H	11-17 seconds

Activated partial prothrombin time (aPTT) measures the effectiveness of clotting factors:

- IX, XI, XII (in a set of reactions called the intrinsic pathway).
- I, II, V, X (in a set of reactions called the common pathway).

The **prothrombin time (PT)** measures the effectiveness of clotting factor VII (which controls the chemical reactions called the extrinsic pathway).

ENDNOTES-WORKS CITED

[i] A. Conan Doyle. "The Sign of Four." *Wikisource*. Web. 7 May. 2026.

[ii] "Ludwig Wittgenstein Quotes." Goodreads.com. 6 May 2026. www.goodreads.com/author/quotes/7672.Ludwig_Wittgenstein

[iii] A. Conan Doyle. *The Boscombe Valley Mystery.* Fullreads.com. www.fullreads.com/literature/the-boscombe-valley-mystery/9/

[iv] All Chemistry Panel Reference Ranges in the book are taken from *The Merck Veterinary Manual*. Khan, Cynthia M., Editor. *The Merck Veterinary Manual, 9th Edition*. Merck & Co. Inc, Whitehouse Station, NJ. 2005. P. 2586

[v] All CBC Reference Ranges in the book are taken from *The Merck Veterinary Manual*. Khan, Cynthia M., Editor. *The Merck Veterinary Manual, 9th Edition*. Merck & Co. Inc, Whitehouse Station, NJ. 2005. P. 2584

[vi] Albert Einstein. *Evolution of Physics.* Today in Science History. Web. www.todayinsci.com/E/Einstein_Albert/EinsteinAlbert-ProblemQuote800px.htm

[vii] Dickens, Charles. *Great Expectations.* Project Gutenberg. Web. www.gutenberg.org/files/8608/8608-readme.txt

[viii] Dewey, John. *Logic: The Theory of Inquiry.* Internet Archive. www.archive.org/details/JohnDeweyLogicTheTheoryOfInquiry

[ix] Khan, Cynthia M., Editor. *The Merck Veterinary Manual, 9th Edition*. Merck & Co. Inc, Whitehouse Station, NJ. 2005. P. 2586

[x] Khan, Cynthia M., Editor. *The Merck Veterinary Manual, 9th Edition*. Merck & Co. Inc, Whitehouse Station, NJ. 2005. P. 2586

[xi] Khan, Cynthia M., Editor. *The Merck Veterinary Manual, 9th Edition*. Merck & Co. *Inc, Whitehouse Station, NJ.* 2005. P. 2584

[xii] Grotheer M, Hirschberger J, Hartmann K, et al: Comparison of signalment, clinical, laboratory and radiographic parameters in cats with feline asthma and chronic bronchitis. Journal of Feline Medicine and Surgery 2020 Vol (7) pp 649-55

[xiii] Wodehouse, P. G. *Jeeves and the Unbidden Guest.* Fullreads. www.fullreads.com/literature/jeeves-and-the-unbidden-guest

[xiv] Star Trek: The Next Generation (S2E21). Goodreads.com. 6 May 2026. www.goodreads.com/quotes/8660482

[xv] Landy, Derek. *Skulduggery Pleasant*. Goodreads.com. www.goodreads.com/work/quotes/909082

[xvi] Adams, John. "Adams' Argument for the Defense: 3–4 December 1770." Founders Online. 6 May 2026. https://founders.archives.gov/documents/Adams/05-03-02-0001-0004-0016

[xvii] Lewis, C. S. *The Magician's Nephew*. Goodreads. 6 May 2026. www.goodreads.com/quotes/78195

[xviii] A. Conan Doyle. *The Sign of Four.* Project Gutenberg. www.gutenberg.org/cache/epub/2097/pg2097-images.html

[xix] Khan, Cynthia M., Editor. *The Merck Veterinary Manual, 9th Edition*. Merck & Co. Inc, Whitehouse Station, NJ. 2005. P. 2586

[xx] Wodehouse, P. G. *The Inimitable Jeeves.* Project Gutenberg. www.gutenberg.org/cache/epub/59254/pg59254-images.html

[xxi] "J. R. R. Tolkien Quotes." Goodreads. Web. 6 May 2026. www.goodreads.com/quotes/207055

[xxii] Christie, Agatha. *The Murder of Roger Ackroyd.* Project Gutenberg. www.gutenberg.org/cache/epub/69087/pg69087-images.html

[xxiii] Allingham, Margery. *The Crime at Black Dudley.* Project Gutenberg. www.gutenberg.org/cache/epub/75359/pg75359-images.html

[xxiv] Tolkien, J. R. R. *The Return of the King.* AZ Quotes. Web. 6 May 2026. www.azquotes.com/quote/433907

[xxv] A. Conan Doyle. *A Study in Scarlet.* Project Gutenberg. www.gutenberg.org/cache/epub/244/pg244-images.html

[xxvi] Roosevelt, Theodore. "The Strenuous Life." Theodore Roosevelt Association. Web. www.theodoreroosevelt.org/content.aspx?page_id=22&club_id=991271&module_id=339361

[xxvii] Shakespeare, William. *Hamlet.* Project Gutenberg. www.gutenberg.org/cache/epub/2265/pg2265-images.html

[xxviii] "J. R. R. Tolkien Quotes." Goodreads. Web. 6 May 2026. www.goodreads.com/quotes/207055

[xxix] Fielder, Susan E. From *Merck Veterinary Manual* online. 2025. www.merckvetmanual.com/reference-values-and-conversion-tables/reference-guides/hematology-reference-ranges. Accessed 11/1825

ABOUT THE AUTHOR

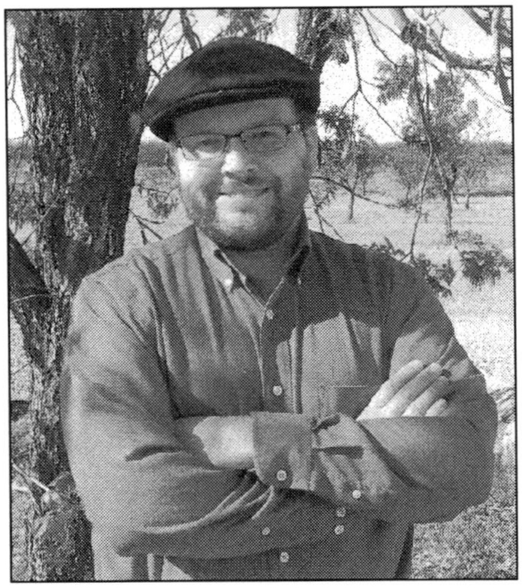

J. Aaron Gruben grew up in the Southwest and currently lives in Texas with his wife and six children. His interest in animals and science began when he was young, leading to a veterinary medicine career choice that never changed. Today, he works full time as an emergency veterinarian in northern Texas and would have loved to have had this book when he was younger.

A veritable Renaissance man, he is the author of works in multiple genres, including historical fiction, humorous fantasy, alternate history, Christian living, and chivalry and Viking school studies. When he is not repairing sick animals or writing, Aaron enjoys reading, hiking, acting goofy with his kids, playing board games, drinking a plethora of coffee, and making music on a variety of instruments. Christ brought Aaron into his camp at the age of 9, and his relationship with his beloved Savior has been the center of his life ever since.

Follow him on Facebook (*facebook.com/authoraarongruben*) and Instagram (*instagram.com/authoraarongruben*) to keep up with new projects and random thoughts.

If you enjoyed the book, please consider taking a moment to leave a review on Amazon, Goodreads, or other book sites. Thanks!

Made in the USA
Monee, IL
05 November 2026

67811483R00146